Prentice Hall's *Nursing Notes*
NURSING LEADERSHIP
AND MANAGEMENT

Organizing Nursing Care Shift Responsibilities and Activities

1. Arrange nursing care environment with easy access to supplies, equipment, and client designated areas.
2. Use previous intershift report to determine tasks and priorities.
3. Develop a shift action plan that includes optimal and reasonable expected outcomes as well as identification of times by which specific care activities will be completed.
4. Assign who will perform nursing interventions or other care activities.
5. Implement the shift action plan beginning with initial client care rounds:
   - Make client care rounds—rapid assessment of information gathered.
   - Schedule treatments and monitoring—firm time commitment for treatments and monitoring.
   - Plan for appropriate equipment and supplies to be available for care.
6. Evaluate outcomes and re-examine shift action plan:
   - Were optimal outcomes achieved? If not, why?
   - Determine if there were staffing problems or client care crises.
   - Were realistic outcomes set? If not, why?
   - Identify what was learned from this shift action plan and determine what can be applied in the future.

Calculating Nursing Care Hours

After a health organization determines the client classification system, the number of nursing care hours can be determined for each classification. Nursing care hours (NCH) per client (patient) day (PPD) is the number of nursing care hours worked in 24 hours divided by the client census, where NCH is the nursing hours worked in 24 hours and PPD is the client census.

Step 1: Identify the number of nursing care hours needed for each acuity level and determine the number of clients in each category.

Example with a client census of 20:
   Category 1 = 2.3 hours, 8 clients
   Category 2 = 3.0 hours, 4 clients
   Category 3 = 4.2 hours, 4 clients
   Category 4 = 5.1 hours, 4 clients

Step 2: Calculate the number of nursing care hours per client: multiply each category (acuity level) by the number of clients in that category.

Example continued:
   Category 1 = 2.3 hours × 8 clients = 18.4
   Category 2 = 3.0 hours × 4 clients = 12
   Category 3 = 4.2 hours × 4 clients = 16.8
   Category 4 = 5.1 hours × 4 clients = 20.4

Step 3: Add all hours from the four categories together.

Example continued:
   18.4 + 12 + 16.8 + 20.4 = 67.6

Step 4: Divide the total number of nursing care hours by the number of clients receiving care;

Example continued:

$$\frac{67.6 \ (\text{nursing care hours})}{20 \ (\text{client census})} = 3.38 \text{ hours per client day}$$

The nurse leader is responsible for knowing budgeted hours per client per day; calculating the number of NCH required for any given day assists the nurse leader to determine unit staffing needs and avoid either understaffing or overstaffing the unit.

Delegation and Assignment-Making

Process of delegating duties and activities of client care to individual personnel
1. Give clear, concise directions.
2. Delegate responsibility.
3. Delegate authority for the performance of the care.
4. Retain accountability for the assignment as the RN.

Delegation of Nursing Assignments
1. Delegate nursing care assignments based on knowledge of the competency of the delegate, including:
   - Education level
   - Knowledge level
   - Skill level
2. Three tasks that cannot be delegated to nonprofessional staff:
   - Initial nursing assessment, subsequent assessments, and those requiring professional judgment
   - Nursing diagnosis, nursing care goals, and progress plans
   - Interventions requiring professional knowledge and skill

Five Rights of Delegation
1. **Right Task:** Nurses determine those activities team members may perform. For each situation, the nurse must consider the client's condition, the complexity of the activity, the unlicensed assistive person's (UAP's) capabilities, and the amount of supervision the nurse will be able to provide.
2. **Right Circumstances:** The nurse evaluates the individual clients and the individual UAPs and matches the two. The nurse assesses the client's needs, looks at the care plan, and considers the setting, ensuring that UAPs have the proper resources, equipment, and supervision to work safely.
3. **Right Person:** The nurse follows organizational policies, which are congruent with state law, in determining the appropriate staff to which to delegate a nursing activity.
4. **Right Direction and Communication:** The nurse communicates the acceptable tasks and activities. The nurse must clearly understand the organization's policies and procedures to carry out effective delegation. In turn, staff nurses need to direct UAPs' actions and communicate clearly about each delegated task. Nurses must be specific about how and when UAPs should report back to them. Nurses should feel comfortable asking: *Do you know how to do this? Where did you learn? How many times have you done it in the past? Where is your experience documented?*
5. **Right Supervision and Evaluation:** Nurse managers ensure that each unit has adequate staffing and time, identify tasks inherent to each staff role, and evaluate the impact of the organization's nursing service on the community. The delegating nurse then must supervise, guide, and evaluate the UAPs' task implementation. The nurse must ensure that UAPs meet expectations and intervene if they aren't performing well.

Delegation Process
1. Determine and identify the task and level of responsibility of each task.
2. Evaluate delegate's fit with assigned task.
3. Decide what level of supervision is needed and describe expectations.
4. Reach agreement on performance and outcome.
5. Provide continuous feedback—monitor performance and adjust accordingly.

ISBN-13: 978-0-13-119601-8
ISBN-10: 0-13-119601-4

Clients as a Safety Check

Clients themselves can be major safety check; nurses have a critical role ensuring that clients:

- Know which medications they are taking.
- Know appearance of their medications.
- Know side effects of medications.
- Are responsible for notifying their healthcare providers of medication discrepancies.

Ethical Principles Important to Nursing Practice

- *Autonomy:* ability of an individual to determine his or her own course of action or self-determination
- *Beneficence:* when an individual helps others to further their important and legitimate interests by promoting good consequences
- *Justice:* obligation to treat all people fairly; *distributive justice* is fair and equitable distribution of limited resources and material benefits among all citizens of society
- *Nonmaleficence:* obligation to do no harm
- *Veracity:* truthfulness or power of perceiving and conveying truth
- *Fidelity:* respecting, maintaining, and carrying out promises one makes; nurse leaders are expected to be:
  - Respectful toward clients, staff, and other health professionals
  - Competent in clinical supervision and clinical skills
  - Able to implement quality standards
  - Able to protect clients from incompetent, illegal, or unethical practice
  - Able to honor agreements made as part of the nurse-client relationship

Calculating Average Daily Census

The average daily census (ADC) is the average number of clients cared for in budgeted beds on a nursing unit over a period of time. It provides a key measure of the unit's activity or productivity and provides a measure to project the workload of the unit.

Formula for calculating average daily census:

Client days for given period of time
Number of days in time period

Example:

1050 client days in January = 1050 ÷ 31 = ADC of 33.9

- Use a problem-solving approach to work toward joint agreement or solution, rather than focusing on winning or losing
- Keep the client as your chief concern
- Be mindful of agency policies, procedures, standards, and systems, and use this knowledge during the resolution process
- Distinguish between people and their positions in the organization
- Work to establish mutual trust and respect
- Actively listen to understand the other side and ask questions or seek clarification if uncertain of what is being said
- State own position in a concrete manner, using data or evidence to strengthen it, but without pressure or being defensive
- Avoid emotional outbursts, overreacting, and premature judgments or blame

Adapted from Finkelman, A.W. (2006). Leadership and management in nursing. *Upper Saddle River, NJ: Pearson Education, Inc.*

Quality Improvement Methods

- *Standards of care:* descriptions of minimum acceptable performance during client care from a healthcare provider who has specific knowledge and skills; developed by professional organizations, legal sources, regulatory agencies, and healthcare agencies
- *Credentialing and licensure:* review process used by an insurance carrier or healthcare organization to guarantee that a healthcare professional may practice or provide care to clients
- *Utilization review/management:* process of evaluating healthcare services to specific client populations for necessity, appropriateness, and efficiency
- *Clinical guidelines:* produced most notably by the Agency for Healthcare Research and Quality (AHRQ) and also by professional organizations; improve care by identifying outcomes and supporting best practices
- *Clinical pathways:* tools for use with specific client diagnoses to focus on client outcomes and appropriate use of resources in a timely manner; promote cost effectiveness as an added benefit
- *Benchmarking:* tool that identifies best practices and allows the healthcare organization to compare its performance with other units or areas within the organization and also with other organizations

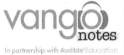
Hear it. Get It.

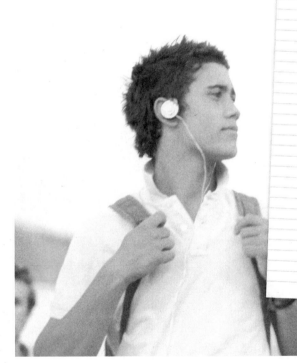

Prentice Hall Nursing Reviews & Rationales

Nursing Leadership and Management

Mary Ann Hogan, MSN, RN

Clinical Assistant Professor
University of Massachusetts–Amherst
Amherst, Massachusetts

Donna M. Nickitas, RN, PhD, CNAA, BC

Professor of Nursing
Hunter College
New York, New York

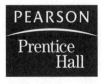

PEARSON

Prentice Hall

Upper Saddle River, New Jersey 07458

Library of Congress Cataloging-in-Publication Data
Hogan, Mary Ann.
    Nursing leadership and management / Mary Ann Hogan, Donna M. Nickitas.
        p. ; cm. — (Prentice Hall nursing reviews & rationales)
    Includes bibliographical references and index.
    ISBN-13: 978-0-13-119601-8
    ISBN-10: 0-13-119601-4
    1. Nursing services—Administration—Examinations, questions, etc.   2. Leadership—Examinations, questions, etc.
    [DNLM: 1. Nursing, Supervisory—organization & administration—Examination Questions.   2. Leadership—Examination Questions.   WY 18.2 H714n 2009]
    I. Costello-Nickitas, Donna M.   II. Title.   III. Series.
    RT89.3.H64 2009
    362.17′3068076—dc22
                                                    2008019159

Notice: Care has been taken to confirm the accuracy of the information presented in this book. The authors, editors, and the publisher, however, cannot accept any responsibility for errors or omissions or for the consequences for application of the information in this book and make no warranty, express or implied, with respect to its contents.

The authors and the publisher have exerted every effort to ensure that drug selections and dosages set forth in this text are in accord with current recommendations and practice at time of publication. However, in view of ongoing research, changes in government regulations, and the constant flow of information relating to drug therapy and drug reactions, the reader is urged to check the package inserts of all drugs for any change in indications of dosage and for added warnings and precautions. This is particularly important when the recommended agent is a new and/or infrequently employed drug.

The authors and publisher disclaim all responsibility for any liability, loss, injury, or damage incurred as a consequence, directly or indirectly, of the use and application of any of the contents of this volume.

Publisher: Julie Levin Alexander
Assistant to Publisher: Regina Bruno
Editor-in-Chief: Maura Connor
Editorial Assistant: Marion Gottlieb
Developmental Editor: Danielle Doller
Managing Editor, Production: Patrick Walsh
Production Liaison: Anne Garcia
Production Editor: Karen Berry, Pine Tree Composition
Manufacturing Manager: Ilene Sanford

Design Coordinator/Cover Designer: Maria Guglielmo
Director of Marketing: Karen Allman
Senior Marketing Manager: Francisco Del Castillo
Marketing Specialist: Michael Sirinides
Media Product Manager: John Jordan
New Media Project Manager: Stephen Hartner
Composition: Pine Tree Composition, Inc.
Printer/Binder: Edwards Brothers
Cover Printer: Phoenix Color Corp.

Pearson Prentice Hall™ is a trademark of Pearson Education, Inc.
Pearson® is a registered trademark of Pearson plc.
Prentice Hall® is a registered trademark of Pearson Education, Inc.

Pearson Education Ltd., *London*
Pearson Education Australia PTY, Limited, *Sydney*
Pearson Education Singapore, Pte. Ltd
Pearson Education North Asia, Ltd., *Hong Kong*
Pearson Education Canada, Inc., *Toronto*

Pearson Educación de Mexico, S.A. de C.V.
Pearson Education—Japan, *Tokyo*
Pearson Education Malaysia, Pte. Ltd.
Pearson Education, *Upper Saddle River, New Jersey*

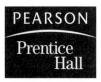

10 9 8 7 6 5 4 3 2 1
ISBN-13: 978-0-13-119601-8
ISBN-10:   0-13-119601-4

Contents

This series has been specifically designed to provide a clear and concentrated review of important nursing knowledge in the following content areas:

- Anatomy & Physiology
- Nursing Fundamentals
- Nutrition & Diet Therapy
- Fluids, Electrolytes, & Acid-Base Balance
- Medical-Surgical Nursing
- Pathophysiology
- Pharmacology
- Maternal-Newborn Nursing
- Child Health Nursing
- Mental Health Nursing
- Physical Assessment
- Community Health Nursing
- Nursing Leadership & Management

The books in this series are designed for use either by current nursing students as a study aid for nursing course work, for NCLEX-RN® licensing exam preparation, or by practicing nurses seeking a comprehensive yet concise review of a nursing specialty or subject area.

This series is truly unique. One of its most special features is that it has been developed and reviewed by a large team of nurse educators from across the United States and Canada to ensure that each chapter is edited by a nurse expert in the content area under study. The series editor, Mary Ann Hogan, designed the overall series in collaboration with a core Prentice Hall team to take full advantage of Prentice Hall's cutting edge technology. The consulting editors for each book, also experts in that specialty area, then reviewed all chapters and test questions submitted for comprehensiveness and accuracy. Finally, Mary Ann Hogan reviewed the chapters in each book for consistency, accuracy, and applicability to the NCLEX-RN® Test Plan.

All books in the series are identical in their overall design for your convenience. As an added value, each book comes with a comprehensive support package, including a bonus *NCLEX-RN® Test Prep* CD-ROM and a tear-out *NursingNotes* card for clinical reference and quick review.

Study Tips

Use of this book should help simplify your review. To make the most of your valuable study time, also follow these simple but important suggestions:

1. Use a weekly calendar to schedule study sessions.
   - Outline the timeframes for all of your activities (home, school, appointments, etc.) on a weekly calendar.
   - Find the "holes" in your calendar, which are the times in which you can plan to study. Add study sessions to the calendar at times when you can expect to be mentally alert and follow it!
2. Create the optimal study environment.
   - Eliminate external sources of distraction, such as television, telephone, etc.
   - Eliminate internal sources of distraction, such as hunger, thirst, or dwelling on items or problems that cannot be worked on at the moment.
   - Take a break for 10 minutes or so after each hour of concentrated study both as a reward and an incentive to keep studying.
3. Use pre-reading strategies to increase comprehension of chapter material.
   - Skim read the headings in the chapter (because they identify chapter content).
   - Read the definitions of key terms, which will help you learn new words to comprehend chapter information.

- Review all graphic aids (figures, tables, boxes) because they are often used to explain important points in the chapter.
4. Read the chapter thoroughly but at a reasonable speed.
   - Comprehension and retention are actually enhanced by not reading too slowly.
   - Do take the time to reread any section that is unclear to you.
5. Summarize what you have learned.
   - Use questions supplied with this book and the *NCLEX-RN® Test Prep* CD-ROM to test your application of chapter content.
   - Review again any sections that correspond to questions you answered incorrectly or incompletely.

Test-Taking Strategies

We provide test-taking strategies along with the rationales for every question in the series. These strategies will enable you to select the correct answer by breaking down the question, even if you don't know the correct response. Use the following strategies to increase your success on nursing tests or examinations:

- Get sufficient sleep and have something to eat before taking a test. Take deep breaths during the test as needed. Remember, the brain requires oxygen and glucose as fuel. Avoid concentrated sweets before a test, however, to avoid rapid upward and then downward surges in blood glucose levels.
- Read the question carefully, identifying the stem, the 4 options, and any key words or phrases in either the stem or options.
   - Key words in the stem such as "most important" indicate the need to set priorities, since more than 1 option is likely to contain a statement that is technically correct.
   - Remember that the presence of absolute words such as "never" or "only" in an answer option is more likely to make that option incorrect.
- Determine who is the client in the question; often this is the person with the health problem, but it may also be a significant other, relative, friend, or another nurse.
- Decide whether the stem is a true response stem or a false response stem. With a true response stem, the correct answer will be a true statement, and vice-versa.

- Determine what the question is really asking, sometimes referred to as the issue of the question. Evaluate all answer options in relation to this issue, and not strictly to the "correctness" of the statement in each individual option.
- Eliminate options that are obviously incorrect, then go back and reread the stem. Evaluate the remaining options against the stem once more.
- If two answers seem similar and correct, try to decide whether one of them is more global or comprehensive. If the global option includes the alternative option within it, it is likely that the more global response is the correct answer.

The NCLEX-RN® Licensing Examination

The NCLEX-RN® licensing examination is a Computer Adaptive Test (CAT) that ranges in length from 75 to 265 individual (stand-alone) test items, depending on individual performance during the examination. Upon graduation from a nursing program, successful completion of this exam is the gateway to your professional nursing practice. The blueprint for the exam is reviewed and revised every three years by the National Council of State Boards of Nursing according to the results of a job analysis study of new graduate nurses practicing within the first six months after graduation. Each question on the exam is coded to a *Client Need Category* and an *Integrated Process*.

Client Need Categories. There are 4 categories of client needs, and each exam will contain a minimum and maximum percent of questions from each category. Each major category has subcategories within it. The *Client Needs* categories according to the NCLEX-RN® Test Plan effective April 2007 are as follows:

- Safe, Effective Care Environment
   - Management of Care (13–19%)
   - Safety and Infection Control (8–14%)
- Health Promotion and Maintenance (6–12%)
- Psychosocial Integrity (6–12%)
- Physiological Integrity
   - Basic Care and Comfort (6–12%)
   - Pharmacological and Parenteral Therapies (13–19%)
   - Reduction of Risk Potential (13–19%)
   - Physiological Adaptation (11–17%)

Integrated Processes. The integrated processes identified on the NCLEX-RN® Test Plan effective April 2007, with condensed definitions, are as follows:

- Nursing Process: a scientific problem-solving approach used in nursing practice; consisting of assessment, analysis, planning, implementation, and evaluation.
- Caring: client-nurse interaction(s) characterized by mutual respect and trust and that are directed toward achieving desired client outcomes.
- Communication and Documentation: verbal and/or nonverbal interactions between nurse and others (client, family, health care team); a written or electronic recording of activities or events that occur during client care.

- Teaching and Learning: facilitating client's acquisition of knowledge, skills, and attitudes that lead to behavior change

More detailed information about this examination may be obtained by visiting the National Council of State Boards of Nursing website at http://www.ncsbn.org and viewing the *NCLEX-RN® Examination Test Plan for the National Council Licensure Examination for Registered Nurses.*[1]

---

[1]Reference: National Council of State Boards of Nursing, Inc. *NCLEX Examination Test Plan for National Council Licensure Examination for Registered Nurses.* Effective April, 2007. Retrieved from the World Wide Web at http://www.ncsbn.org/RN_Test_Plan_2007_Web.pdf.

HOW TO GET THE MOST OUT OF THIS BOOK

Each chapter has the following elements to guide you during review and study:

Chapter Objectives describe what you will be able to know or do after learning the material covered in the chapter.

Objectives

➤ Discuss legal considerations related to maternity nursing.

➤ Delineate ethical issues that influence maternal-newborn nursing practice.

➤ Identify culturally diverse health beliefs that impact the maternity cycle.

➤ Describe a philosophy of care that maintains maternal–newborn safety and fosters family unity.

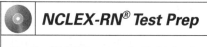

NCLEX-RN® Test Prep

Use the CD-ROM enclosed with this book to access additional practice opportunities.

Review at a Glance contains a glossary of key terms used in the chapter, with definitions provided up-front and available at your fingertips, to help you stay focused and make the best use of your study time.

Review at a Glance

belief something accepted as true, especially as a tenet or a body of tenets accepted by an ethnocultural group

cultural competency the awareness, knowledge and skills necessary to appreciate, understand and communicate with people of diverse cultural backgrounds

family a group of individuals related by blood, marriage, or mutual goals

family-centered maternity care maternity care that is family oriented and views childbirth as a vital, natural life event rather than an illness

scope of practice legally refers to permissible boundaries of practice for nurses and is defined by statute (written law), rules and regulations, or a combination of the two

Pretest provides a 10-question quiz as a sample overview of the material covered in the chapter and helps you decide in what areas you need the most—or the least—review.

PRETEST

1 The nurse performs a vaginal examination and determines that the fetus is in a sacrum anterior position. The nurse draws which conclusion from this assessment data?

1. The fetal sacrum is toward the maternal symphysis pubis.
2. The fetal sacrum is toward the maternal sacrum.
3. The fetal face is toward the maternal sacrum.
4. The fetal face is toward the maternal symphysis pubis.

Practice to Pass questions are open-ended, stimulate critical thinking, and reinforce mastery of the chapter information.

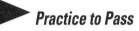

Practice to Pass

The client scheduled for a hysterosalpingogram reports an allergy to shellfish. What should the nurse do?

NCLEX Alert identifies concepts that are likely to be tested on the NCLEX-RN® examination. Be sure to learn the information highlighted wherever you see this icon.

Case Study, found at the end of the chapter, provides an opportunity for you to use your critical thinking and clinical reasoning skills to "put it all together." It describes a true-to-life client case situation and asks you open-ended questions about how you would provide care for that client and/or family.

Case Study

A 14-year-old primigravida is admitted in early labor with severe preeclampsia at 42 weeks gestation. The client's blood pressure is 168/102.

1. What other assessment data would you obtain?
2. Describe the complications this client is at risk for.
3. Discuss the medications you expect to administer to this client.
4. What concerns do you have for this fetus? Why?
5. What would you teach this client and her family about her condition?

For suggested responses, see page 343.

Posttest provides an additional 10-question quiz at the end of the chapter. It provides you with feedback about mastery of the chapter material following review and study. All pretest and posttest questions contain comprehensive rationales for the correct and incorrect answers, and are coded according to cognitive level of difficulty, NCLEX-RN® Test Plan category of client need and integrated process.

POSTTEST

1 A client who is a brittle diabetic is seeking to get pregnant. The nursing working in a primary care provider's office suggests that which of the following healthcare providers would be an optimal choice?

1. A certified nurse-midwife
2. A family nurse practitioner
3. An obstetrician
4. A maternal-fetal medicine specialist

NCLEX-RN® Test Prep CD-ROM

For those who want to practice taking tests on a computer, the CD-ROM that accompanies the book contains the pretest and posttest questions found in all chapters of the book. In addition, it contains 30 NEW questions for each chapter to help you further evaluate your knowledge base and hone your test-taking skills. We included some of the newly developed alternate NCLEX Test Items, so these items will give you valuable practice with different types of questions.

Prentice Hall NursingNotes Card

This tear-out card provides a reference for frequently used facts and information related to the subject matter of the book. These are designed to be useful in the clinical setting, when quick and easy access to information is so important!

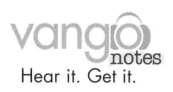

VangoNotes

Study on the go with VangoNotes. Just download chapter reviews from your text and listen to them on any mp3 player. Now wherever you are—whatever you're doing—you can study by listening to the following for each chapter of your textbook:

- **Big Ideas**: Your "need to know" for each chapter
- **Practice Test**: A gut check for the Big Ideas—tells you if you need to keep studying
- **Key Terms**: Audio "flashcards" to help you review key concepts and terms

VangoNotes are **flexible**; download all the material directly to your player, or only the chapters you need. And they're **efficient**. Use them in your car, at the gym, walking to class, wherever. So get yours today. And get studying.

About the Leadership & Management Book

Chapters in this book cover "need-to-know" information about nursing leadership and management. Chapters focus on important content such as creating a culture of care, leadership and management theories, ethics, legal rights and responsibilities, delegation, performance improvement, building an effective care team, assuring competence in care givers, resource management, and creating a caring future for nursing. Mastery of the information in this book and effective use of the test-taking strategies described will help you be confident and successful in testing situations, including the NCLEX-RN®, and in actual clinical practice.

Acknowledgements

This book is a monumental effort of collaboration. Without the contributions of several individuals, *Nursing Leadership & Management: Reviews and Rationales* would not have been possible. A grateful acknowledgement goes to Sharon F. Beasley, MSN, RN of Technical College of the Lowcountry, Beaufort, South Carolina who contributed to the NCLEX items. Their work will surely assist both students and practicing nurses alike to extend their knowledge in the areas of leadership and management.

We owe a special debt of gratitude to the wonderful team at Prentice Hall Nursing for their enthusiasm for this project, as well as their good humor, expertise, and encouragement as the series developed. Maura Connor, Editor-in-Chief for Nursing, was unending in her creativity, support, encouragement, and belief in the need for this series. Danielle Doller, Developmental Editor, devoted many long hours to coordinating different facets of this project, and tirelessly and cheerfully encouraged our efforts as well. Her high standards and attention to detail contributed greatly to the final "look" of this series. Editorial Assistant, Marion Gottlieb, helped to keep the project moving forward on a day-to-day basis, and we are grateful for her efforts as well. A very special thank you goes to the designers of the book and the production team, led by Anne Garcia, Production Editor, and Mary Siener, Designer, who brought the ideas and manuscript into final form.

Thank you to the team at Pine Tree Composition, led by Project Coordinator Karen Berry, for the detail-oriented work of creating this book. We greatly appreciate their hard work, attention to detail, and spirit of collaboration.

Finally, Mary Ann would like to acknowledge and gratefully thank her children, who sacrificed hours of time that would have been spent with them, to bring this book to publication. Their love and support kept me energized, motivated, and at times, even sane.

Donna would like to thank her husband Michael, whose support and encouragement allowed her to pursue this important endeavor, and her children, Nick, Katie, and Jon-Philip, for their wisdom and insight on mastering the lessons of leadership and management from all spheres of influence including home, work, and community. "Leaders are not leaders unless they have followers." Thank you for reminding me when to lead, when to follow, and when to get out of the way.

MaryAnn Hogan
Donna M. Nickitas

Piri Barger, RN, MSN, CCRN
Humboldt State University
Arcata, California

Dr. Mary Lou Bost, DrPH, RN
Carlow University
Pittsburgh, Pennsylvania

Mary T. Boylston, RN, MSN, EdD
Eastern University
St. Davids, Pennsylvania

Cathy Dyches, RN, PhD
Clemson University
Clemson, South Carolina

Lori A. Escallier, PhD, RN, CPNP
State University of New York
    at Stony Brook
Stony Brook, New York

Linda Johanson, RN, EdD
Lenoir-Rhyne College
Hickory, North Carolina

Ruby Shaw Morrison, DSN, RN, CMAC
The University of Alabama
Tuscaloosa, Alabama

Linda Wagner, EdD, MSN, RN
Southern Connecticut State University
New Haven, Connecticut

P.J. Woods, PhD, MBA, RN
University of New Mexico
Albuquerque, New Mexico

Creating a Culture of Care

1

Chapter Outline

Healthcare Settings

Healthcare Management

Establishing Priorities and Supervising

Skills for Nurse Leaders and the Emerging Workforce

Empowerment

Strategies to Ensure Safety for Clients and Nurses

Focusing Practice to Provide Effective Evidenced-based Care

Objectives

➤ Describe current models of healthcare management and current settings in which healthcare is delivered.

➤ Describe the leadership expectations and desires of the emerging nurse workforce.

➤ Explain how nurse leaders determine priorities and manage supervision responsibilities.

➤ Discuss why empowerment is essential to clinical nursing leadership.

➤ Describe how nurses can effectively prevent work-related illnesses or injuries.

➤ Identify two reasons why evidenced-based care is important to nursing practice.

NCLEX-RN® Test Prep

Use the CD-ROM enclosed with this book to access additional practice opportunities.

Review at a Glance

charisma possession of individual traits or skills such as articulate speech, flair, self-confidence, and strong convictions that promote a vision that strongly connects with followers

client outcome measures indicators of effectiveness of healthcare; examples include improved health status, improved quality of life, and meeting client preferences

compassionate leadership a style characterized by openness and respect toward others with receptivity toward their ideas and values; encourages a sense of "ownership" and loyalty; sets staffing levels based on nurse competency and skill mix relative to client mix and acuity; and acknowledges and rewards nursing staff according to their excellence in client care and safety

culture an organization's transmitted beliefs and assumptions about the organizational environment and the employees within it; these shared beliefs provide role expectations to guide employee behavior and assist employees in responding to the work environment

emergent workforce the next generation of nurses between the ages of 18 and 35 years and members of a group labeled Generation X

empowerment a concept whereby individuals recognize and feel their strengths, abilities, and personal power; a way to transform the work environment of nurses and enhance client safety

empowerment process promotes professional accountability and development, thereby placing the ownership of ongoing clinical knowledge, information, and competencies on the frontline professional nurse

evidenced-based care clinically competent care supported by the best scientific evidence available

mentoring power relationship of equal support between two persons of unequal rank

mission statement a written statement that describes the purpose of an organization and outlines the types of activities to be performed for clients

nurse safety health and well-being of nurses that results from the use of practices that protect them against illness or injury in the workplace environment

outcomes research scientific study that seeks to understand the end results of specific health practices and interventions

shared governance an organizational culture that supports supervision with a sense of "ownership" for clinical practice and fosters a partnership between and among employees and the employer

supervisor an individual having the authority in the interest of the employer to hire, transfer, suspend, lay off, recall, promote, discharge, assign, reward, or discipline other employees

supervising the provision of guidance or direction, evaluation, and follow-up of assistive personnel for accomplishment of one or more delegated nursing tasks

vision articulation of the mission of an organization in an appealing and intuitive picture that conveys what the organization can be in the future and instills a common purpose, self-esteem, and a sense of membership within the organization

PRETEST

1 A staff nurse plans to interview for the position of Pediatric Nurse Manager. In self-reflection, the nurse concludes that which emergent workforce attributes are pertinent for this position? Select all that apply.

1. Democratic orientation
2. Type A personality
3. Commitment
4. Stoicism
5. Charisma

2 After a nurse manager notes leadership characteristics in one of the charge nurses, the nurse manager provides the charge nurse with guidance and leadership development courses. This nurse manager is using which concepts to improve the workforce? Select all that apply.

1. Charisma
2. Development
3. Mentorship
4. Improvement
5. Fairness

3 The vision statement of a healthcare system is: "Provide quality, cost-effective care to clients in our region." The nurse manager best demonstrates this vision statement by:

1. Instituting a cost-center checklist containing the unit's direct care costs to assist charge nurses.
2. Instituting care maps for clients with diabetes mellitus.
3. Purchasing fewer personal items and eliminating office supplies.
4. Providing a series of in-services dedicated to cost containment.

4 A nurse leader has the authority to assign beds on all the units, transfer clients, and respond to "codes." This nurse leader functions in which role?

1. Unit manager
2. Supervisor
3. Chief operating officer
4. Charge nurse

5 A nurse manager plans quarterly in-services to enhance clinical competence of the staff. The nurse would report the outcomes of these in-services to which of the four councils that set policies for shared governance?

1. Nursing practice
2. Quality improvement
3. Education
4. Management

6 The culture of a healthcare organization is changing. Nurses are now allowed to self-schedule, and administrators seek input from the staff on major decisions. A nurse who has been interviewed for a nursing position in this organization concludes that there has been a shift to which type of managerial model?

1. Shared governance.
2. Empowerment.
3. Compassionate leadership.
4. Workforce support.

7 A nurse leader observes a staff nurse as an articulate public speaker. The nurse leader asks the nurse to prepare in-services on a new program and present the information to the staff. By this action the nurse leader demonstrates:

1. Shared governance.
2. Compassionate leadership.
3. Empowerment.
4. Charismatic leadership.

8 A nurse leader evaluates a certified nursing assistant (CNA) and notes positive qualities in the CNA. The nurse leader encourages the CNA to pursue a nursing degree. A registered nurse on the unit who observes this interaction concludes that the leader is using which behavior to empower the CNA?

1. Motivation
2. Communication
3. Charisma
4. Partnership

9 A nurse manager rewards a staff nurse for creating teaching boards for parents. The nurse considers that this manager's actions demonstrate which type of leadership?

1. Compassionate
2. Empathetic
3. Charismatic
4. Influential

10 A nurse has difficulty scanning the client's identification bracelet prior to administering medications. Frustrated, the nurse scans a sticker with the client's account number, name, and date of birth obtained from the face sheet of the client's chart. A nurse coworker notes that which element of medication safety has been compromised by the nurse?

1. Right time
2. Right dose
3. Right person
4. Right documentation

➤ *See pages 19–20 for Answers and Rationales.*

PRETEST

I. HEALTHCARE SETTINGS

A. Hospitals

1. Deliver acute care health services (necessary treatment of disease for short period of time in which client is treated for brief, severe episode of illness)

2. Hospitals are acute care facilities that have the goal of discharging clients with appropriate discharge instructions when they are deemed healthy and stable

3. The term *acute* often means care is rendered in an emergency department, ambulatory care clinic, or other short-term stay facility

B. Extended-care facilities

1. Include skilled nursing (intermediate care) and extended (long-term) care facilities

2. May be located inside or outside the hospital complex

C. Sub-acute facilities: provide extensive care to clients newly released from hospitals who require continued intensive nursing care and may need high-tech equipment

D. Ambulatory care

1. Provides healthcare on an outpatient basis including diagnostic and/or one-day surgery

2. Clinics provide care inside or outside the hospital setting with a variety of specialized care services including immunizations, primary care, and ambulatory care centers

E. Home healthcare agencies

1. Provide healthcare in the client's home by healthcare professionals

2. Home care is nonmedical or custodial care (provided by persons who are not nurses, doctors, or other licensed medical personnel), whereas home healthcare refers to care provided by such licensed personnel

F. Retirement and assisted-living facilities

1. Refer to noninstitutionalized facilities used by people not able to live on their own, but who are not yet in need of a level of continuous nursing care offered by skilled nursing facilities (nursing homes)

2. Usually they offer no special medical monitoring equipment, nor 24-hour nursing staff as in a nursing home; however, trained staff are usually on-site around the clock to provide other needed services

3. Private apartments generally are self-contained (i.e., having their own small kitchen, bathroom, living area, and bedroom)

4. Individual living spaces may resemble dormitory or hotel rooms consisting of a private or semi-private sleeping area and a shared bathroom; they usually include common areas for socializing, as well as a central kitchen and dining room for preparing and eating meals

G. Hospice services

1. Provide care to clients with life-limiting illness and take place in various settings (client's home, nursing home, or inpatient unit or hospital)

2. Regardless of setting, hospice services always provide care to ensure the best quality of life; care encompasses provision of physical, spiritual, and emotional support by interdisciplinary teams including nurses, home health aides, social workers, chaplains, therapists, volunteers, and physicians

3. The client and family are integral in the plan of care, and decisions are based on their wishes

4. Each team member has a part in the client's care

H. Psychiatric hospitals

1. Inpatient hospitals specialize in the treatment of persons with mental illness needing emergency and urgent treatment

2. Community mental health care agencies are outpatient facilities that provide healthcare to clients who have mental health problems requiring ongoing, long-term treatment; these agencies allow clients to receive their treatment and care in their own community, not in a hospital

I. Substance abuse treatment centers

1. Offer effective treatment and recovery services for clients with alcohol and drug problems

2. They support a variety of activities aimed at improving the lives of individuals and families affected by alcohol and drug abuse by ensuring access to clinically sound, cost-effective addiction treatment that reduces healthcare and social costs to communities

II. HEALTHCARE MANAGEMENT

A. Health Maintenance Organizations (HMOs)

1. Term developed by pediatric neurologist Paul Ellwood that reflects principles of a prepayment system

2. Formally established through federal legislation to reorganize healthcare services to reduce rate of healthcare cost increases and control utilization of services

3. Is a geographically organized system providing enrollees with an agreed-on package of health maintenance and treatment services

4. Offers healthcare services to groups of individuals who voluntarily enroll in the program

   a. They are designed to provide care directed toward health promotion and disease prevention

   b. Each is an integrated delivery system that offers health services at fixed, prepaid premiums for enrollees

   c. Types of HMOs

      1) Staff model: primary healthcare providers such as physicians and nurse practitioners are HMO employees and are paid a salary

      2) Independent Practice Associations (IPAs): primary healthcare providers maintain individual or group practices, but contract with the HMO to serve enrollees for a negotiated fee

      3) Group model: HMO contracts with a multi-specialty group to provide enrollees' services for negotiated fee

      4) Network model: HMO contracts with two or more independent or group practices to provide enrollee services at fixed monthly fee per enrollee, called capitation

B. Preferred Provider Organizations (PPOs) contract with established medical care providers, referred to as preferred providers

   1. Incentives are given to participants for selecting preferred providers
   2. PPOs offer participants greater flexibility in provider and hospital selection

C. Point of Service (POS) combines selection choice of PPO with lower cost of HMO

   1. POS is like an HMO in that participants are required to choose a primary care provider from within the healthcare network; however, participants are not limited to only providers in their network
   2. Clients may be referred to other healthcare providers outside the network by the primary care provider but there is a deductible for out-of-network care even if the participant's deductible is met

D. Managed care

   1. Refers to a variety of strategies, systems, and mechanisms for monitoring and controlling utilization of health services
   2. Is the newest form of healthcare delivery system; objective is to restructure healthcare services to:
      a. Enhance cost containment
      b. Maintain quality
      c. Facilitate management of client care needs
   3. Providers must submit written justification to request prior approval for diagnostic tests and interventions or to extend client's length of stay (LOS)
   4. See Box 1-1 for objectives of a managed care system

E. Nursing care delivery systems

   1. Are in constant flux and are impacted by healthcare economics, staffing shortages, and organizational philosophy and goals
   2. They are designed as models of the mix of nurses and ancillary caregivers who provide nursing care and completion of various nursing activities and tasks
   3. Common nursing care delivery systems
      a. Functional nursing
         1) Began in mid-1940s
         2) Client needs are defined by tasks to be allocated to Registered Nurses (RNs), Licensed Practical/Vocational Nurses (LPNs/LVNs), and Unlicensed Assistive Personnel (UAPs); the focus is on the job to be accomplished, and is a task-oriented approach to nursing care

---

Box 1-1

Key Objectives of Managed Care

1. Reduce unnecessary healthcare costs through a variety of mechanisms, including economic incentives for healthcare providers and clients.
2. Select less costly forms of care.
3. Review medical necessity of specific services; increase beneficiary cost sharing between healthcare provider, client and payor.
4. Place controls on in-patient admissions and lengths of stay.
5. Establish cost-sharing incentives for outpatient surgery.
6. Engage in selective contracting with healthcare providers.
7. Use intensive management strategies for high-cost healthcare cases.

      3) Advantage: efficient and effective at regularly performed tasks

      4) Disadvantage: uneven continuity of care, absence of holistic view of client, time-consuming communications, problems with follow-up

   b. Primary nursing

      1) The primary nurse designs, implements, and is accountable for nursing care of clients

      2) Is a model in which care is given by Primary Nurse/Associates; the primary nurse plans and designs care, sets goals, and evaluates goal achievement over 24 hours of care

      3) Advantage: is a knowledge-based practice model, with decentralization of nursing care decisions, authority, and responsibility to the staff nurse

      4) Disadvantage: requires excellent communication between nurses; continuity of care and accountability may be challenged

   c. Team nursing

      1) Most common nursing care delivery system in United States

      2) A team of nursing personnel provides total client care to a group of clients

      3) Advantage: allows use of non-RN staff, coordination of activities requires more than one person

      4) Disadvantage: is time-consuming with respect to communication; continuity of care may be diminished; role confusion and resentment may occur

F. Case management

  1. Organizes client care by major diagnoses and focuses on attaining predetermined client outcomes within specific time frames

  2. Advantage: all professionals are equal members of the team; emphasis is on managing interdisciplinary outcomes

  3. Disadvantage: requires that essential baseline data is available to team members

III. ESTABLISHING PRIORITIES AND SUPERVISING

A. Establishing leadership priorities

  1. Contemporary nurse leaders address challenges and opportunities presented within the healthcare organization of their employment

  2. To meet demands successfully, nurse leaders possess and must be willing to instill a deep-seated sense of ownership in the organization's work; a culture of ownership becomes the major driver for providing client services

  3. Workforce behaviors include having the right to act and a belief in the obligation to act on behalf of the organization's mission and vision

  4. Information is fully shared and communicated to all within the organization

    a. Monthly statements of organization's financial status and activity level

    b. Alerts and analyses of pending regulatory and legislative updates

    c. Industry trends, local competitive market conditions, and organization's strategic priorities

B. Creating a common vision

  1. Critical job-related responsibility of a nurse leader is to create a common vision for nursing, develop a big picture mentality and a sense of urgency.

2. In fulfilling responsibility toward a common vision, the nurse leader influences workplace priorities and outcomes by:

   a. Connecting work objectives to the strategic plan

   b. Ensuring unit-based or clinical objectives support the common vision and ensure safe, high-quality care

   c. Delegating authority to prioritize and deploy resources in order to manage all on-going critical client care situations

C. Supervising and supervision

1. **Supervising** is a process consisting of a set of actions by a nurse leader to offer guidance or direction, evaluation, and follow-up of nursing personnel for accomplishment of delegated nursing tasks

2. **Supervisor** is defined as any individual having authority in the interest of the employer to hire, transfer, suspend, lay off, recall, promote, discharge, assign, reward, or discipline other employees

3. Supervisors are responsible for:

   a. Competent and disciplined staff

   b. Clear directions and communication

   c. Timely follow-up to ensure prompt execution of delegated activities and orders

   d. Consistent use of active listening skills

   e. Having a thorough scope of knowledge necessary to supervise work

   f. Demonstrating fairness and respect toward all and providing feedback for work well done as well as resolving problems and conflicts

D. *Shared governance*

1. A **culture** that supports supervision with a sense of ownership and that fosters partnership

2. Has decentralized power sharing and decision making

3. Priorities of the organization are accomplished through a series of councils

   a. One council for each nursing unit

   b. Four councils set policies and address organizational issues:

      1) Nursing practice

      2) Quality improvement

      3) Education (ensures continuing education requirements and staff competency)

      4) Management of organization's service specific areas, such as general medical-surgical, mother-baby, critical care, intermediate care, and ancillary

   c. An overall coordinating council is composed of a chairperson elected by nursing staff, clinical specialist(s), and four chairs of house-wide councils

IV. SKILLS FOR NURSE LEADERS AND THE EMERGING WORKFORCE

A. Generational challenges

1. Today's nursing workplace provides unique leadership and management challenges for the nurse leader

2. First time nurse leaders are faced with an emerging workforce with two generations (baby boomers and gen-Xers) with major differences in regard to professional goals, motivational needs, and communication styles

3. Baby boomers:

   a. Generation born after end of World War II

   b. Largest generation in today's workforce

   c. Known as "sandwich generation" because they care simultaneously for children and aging parents

   d. Value group participation and consensus

   e. Recognition is highly valued, and they care about what others think

   f. Have heavy family obligations and require time to meet them

4. Gen-Xers are the **emergent workforce**

   a. Between 18 and 35 years old

   b. Have a distinctive set of values and expectations concerning work (see Table 1-1)

   c. Desire effective and intelligent leaders who are approachable, supportive, receptive, and motivating

   d. Require frequent feedback from leadership

   e. Want to be trusted and respected for work contributions and performance

B. Nurse leaders have responsibility to create a work environment that:

1. Facilitates and encourages nursing staff to demonstrate accountability for their own practice

2. Empowers nurses at all levels of the organization to critically think and participate in decision making that affects nursing practice

3. Expects emergent workforce as employees to include behaviors that promote and induce:

   a. Ongoing feedback

   b. Trust

   c. Respect

   d. Flexibility

   e. Ongoing training and professional development

   f. Coaching and mentoring

   g. Merit-induced monetary rewards for excellence in client care delivery

C. Emerging skills for the nurse leader

1. Has high personal integrity

2. Empowers and encourages others to act

3. Promotes group participation in problem solving and moves toward consensus when possible

Table 1-1	Desire for Work by Gen-Xers	Perceptions of Hospitals
Generation X Desires for Work versus Hospital Expectations for Employees	1. Demand flexibility and are fiercely independent	1. Highly structured and controlled environments
	2. Disdain authority for the sake of authority and focus on results	2. Hierarchical systems
	3. Tend to side-step rules with no connection to mission	3. Mission driven
	4. Seek a healthy work–life balance	4. Professional career
	5. Anchor themselves to relationships with individuals, instead of institution	5. Institution goals and objectives come first
	6. Internalize rules that make sense and don't always follow compliance requirements	6. Compliance is a core requirement
	7. Focus on results	7. Focus on the bottom line
	8. Monitor feedback constantly and adjust rapidly to changing circumstances	8. Change takes time; slow to adjust to circumstances
	9. Easily learn new technologies	9. Technologies are slow to develop
	10. Take charge of their own skill building	10. Institutions impose training programs
	11. Set personal goals and deadlines for tasks and responsibilities	11. Goals are determined by board of governance/directors
	12. Solve problems more independently	12. Problems are solved by committee. Emphasis is on solutions that work for "all," not "some"
	13. Acclimate quickly to new environments	13. Imposed orientation programs
	14. Seize emerging opportunities	14. Slow to evaluate and embrace new "best practices"
	15. Build long-term relationships with individuals who can help them	15. Mentor and peer support are short-term and difficult to cultivate

   4. Brings people of different backgrounds together
   5. Honors and respects those differences of all
   6. Sets high standards and holds people to them
   7. Sets directions and persuades others to follow them
   8. Exhibits **charisma**

D. Nurturing and supportive workplace environment promotes and encourages nurse leaders whose work ethic and competencies have demonstrated:

   1. Honesty
   2. Self-motivation
   3. Excellent communication

E. Key aspects for improving work environment for emergent nurse workforce in the 21st century

   1. Renewed attention to **mission statement** of organization (describes purpose of organization and outlines types of activities to be performed for clients)
   2. Greater managerial engagement with nurse clinicians
   3. Recognition of vital role nurses play in inpatient and outpatient outcomes
   4. Priority placed on creating organizations that enable clinicians to deliver high-quality care

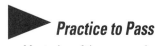

Practice to Pass

Mentoring of the new graduate by experienced professional nurses can be a key component in producing beneficial outcomes for both the mentor and mentoree. Identify the key components of leadership that would be beneficial to a new nurse leader. Discuss how to identify a potential nurse leader mentor.

5. Encouraging, coaching, and **mentoring** (guiding, and supporting) new nurse leaders as they learn their role

   a. Mentoring is a career development tool to develop critical nursing leadership skills

   b. Involves sharing knowledge and expertise (teaching), providing psychological support and providing access to resources for self-development

   c. When effective, mentoring fosters independence, job satisfaction, self-confidence, improved decision-making and problem-solving skills, and further upward mobility in the workplace

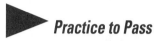

Practice to Pass

As the nurse manager, you witness a staff nurse delegating to an unlicensed assistive personnel (UAP) an assigned task for which the UAP is not prepared and that is beyond the UAP's scope of practice. What should be your response?

F. **Astute supervision allows for effective management of day-to-day priorities and clinical care needs of assigned clients; supervisors are responsible for:**

   1. Ensuring a competent and disciplined staff

   2. Clear directions and communication

   3. Timely follow-up to ensure prompt execution of delegated activities and orders

   4. Active listening skills

   5. Thorough scope of technical knowledge of supervised work

   6. Demonstrated fairness and respect toward all

   7. Feedback for work well done and resolution of problems and conflicts

V. EMPOWERMENT

A. *Empowerment* **involves enabling individuals to recognize and feel their strengths, abilities, and personal power; is an effective method or strategy to maintain client safety and transform the work environment of nurses**

B. **Empowered nurses have freedom and autonomy to practice professional nursing through:**

   1. Collaboration rather than competition

   2. Connectedness rather than isolation

   3. Sharing information and power openly and freely

   4. Encouraging development of sense of community rather than individualism

   5. Establishing equitable partnerships with other healthcare providers

C. **An empowerment model acts as a compass to nurse leaders, allowing them to create a philosophy where nursing workforce principles and practices are consistent with the values of empowerment:**

   1. Letting go of command-and-control leadership

   2. Promoting self-efficacy and sense of self-control

   3. Encouraging self-mastery

   4. Enabling others to recognize their talents and contributions in the workplace while experiencing a sense of personal power

D. **Encourages frontline nurses to be engaged in any decisions that affect their work life and client care; by promoting use of empowerment nurse leader encourage nurses to have clear and profound voice and opportunity to participate in clinical decision making**

E. **The** *empowerment process* **promotes professional accountability and development, thereby putting ownership of ongoing clinical knowledge, information, and competencies on frontline professional nurse to ensure a culture where a standard of excellent client care can be created and maintained**

F. **Nurse leaders foster an empowered workplace environment by modeling key behaviors of empowerment**

1. Human motivation is a multidimensional experience with multiple levels of responsibility:

   a. Each individual is responsible for envisioning the future and all possibilities life has to offer

   b. The nurse leader is responsible for recognizing each team member's learning style and helping each one to reach full potential

   c. The organization is responsible for designing and implementing policies that energize, motivate, and demonstrate commitment to empowerment

2. The human condition is to grow and excel; leaders challenge team members to create career plans, and help them reach their full potential and meet their professional development needs by suggesting evidence-based practice readings, research, and educational training programs

3. **Compassionate leadership** is a style of leadership in which the nurse leader acts as a driver to engage team members to become empowered, strengthened, and determined to make difference in the lives of clients and other team members; it is characterized by:

   a. Openness and respect toward others

   b. Receptivity to ideas and values

   c. Encouraging a sense of ownership and loyalty

   d. Setting staffing levels based on nurse competency and skill mix relative to client mix and acuity

   e. Acknowledging and rewarding nursing staff according to excellence in client care and safety

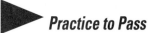

Practice to Pass

Empowering new nurse leaders with the self-confidence they need to be leaders is critical to future leadership. Describe the knowledge and skills needed to enhance self-confidence and the ability to lead others.

VI. STRATEGIES TO ENSURE SAFETY FOR CLIENTS AND NURSES

A. **Strategies to ensure client safety are designed to prevent, detect, and minimize hazards and the likelihood of error**

1. The first report by Institute of Medicine (IOM), *To Err Is Human,* suggests that the first principle for designing safe systems for clients within healthcare organizations is to provide leadership from the uppermost level of the organization

2. Clients should not be harmed by a healthcare system that promises "First, do no harm"; more annual deaths occur from medication errors than from HIV/AIDS, breast cancer, or highway accidents

3. Errors are most often caused by:

   a. Faulty systems and processes

   b. Conditions that lead people to make mistakes and fail to prevent them

   c. In 1999, IOM report estimated that medical errors might kill as many as 98,000 Americans each year

4. Setting and enforcing explicit performance standards for error prevention and client safety can improve the reliability and safety of care for clients through processes such as:

   a. Licensing

   b. Certification

Practice to Pass

The nurse leader has just completed listening to the end of shift report by the night unit charge nurse. The charge nurse has reported that a client died six hours post-op after receiving two units of the wrong blood during surgery and two more in the post-anesthesia care unit (PACU). Explain how these tragic errors, for which the hospital is responsible, can be prevented.

Box 1-2	
Simple Rules for the 21st-Century Healthcare System	1. Initiatives in client safety: Near-miss reporting of medication or transfusion reactions, communication or consent issues, wrong client or procedures, communication breakdown, or technology malfunctions. 2. Technology in healthcare settings: Electronic medical record (EMR) reduces several types of errors, including those related to prescription drugs, preventive care, and tests and procedures. 3. Evidence-based nursing practice. 4. Mandatory reporting: Hospitals voluntarily report serious client harm collected by client safety organizations under contract to analyze errors and recommend improvements. Reports remain confidential and cannot be used in liability cases. Federal government serves to coordinate data collection and maintain the national database. 5. Quality and safety initiatives in community pharmacy practice: Use of automated drug dispensing devices, computerized drug utilization review tools, and electronic prescriptions from prescribers may decrease the risk for error and increase the likelihood of delivering high quality of care. 6. Health literacy: An individual's ability to read, understand, and use healthcare information to make decisions and follow instructions for treatment. Clients should be encouraged to ask three questions each time they talk to a doctor, nurse, or pharmacist: What is my main problem? What do I need to do? Why is it important for me to do this? 7. Pay for performance: Compensation according to measures of work quality or goals. 8. Liability protection for disclosing errors: Disclosure of the most serious adverse events.

   c. Accreditation

   d. Health professional training in client safety

   e. Collaboration across health disciplines

   5. Implement strategies to reduce errors in today's healthcare systems (Box 1-2)

B. Client safety is protected by effective surveillance systems and staffing adequacy; nurses are accountable for keeping clients safe

   1. Nurses constitute a surveillance system for early detection of complications and errors in client care and are in best position to initiate actions that minimize negative outcomes for clients

   2. The higher the number of RNs in the overall staffing mix, the better client outcomes, with a 3 to 12% reduction in certain adverse outcomes, including urinary tract infection, pneumonia, shock, and upper gastrointestinal bleeding

   3. Client safety priorities:

   a. Medication administration safety includes using technology that identifies the client and medication prior to administration; improved naming, labeling, packaging, and distribution of medications; physician order entry and automated medication administration records; education of client and families about medication safety; use of written computerized protocols; reporting of errors, near misses, and adverse drug reactions

   b. Blame-free cultures (that eliminate blame and punishment) hold systems rather than individuals accountable; root cause analysis is a process conducted to identify systems and processes that contribute to error

   c. Adverse occurrences sensitive to or amenable to prevention by nursing, including assessment and interventions to prevent falls or skin breakdown, utilization of aseptic techniques to reduce infections and use of restraints

   4. Suggestions from the IOM for redesigning and improving client care are outlined in Box 1-3

Box 1-3

**New Rules
to Redesign
and Improve Care**

1. **Care based on continuous healing relationships.** Clients receive care whenever they need it and in many forms, not just face-to-face visits. Healthcare system should be responsive at all times (24 hours a day, every day) and access to such care should be provided over the Internet, by telephone, and by other means in addition to face-to-face visits.

2. **Customization based on client needs and values.** The system of care is designed to meet the most common types of needs, but has the capability to respond to individual client choices and preferences.

3. **Client as source of control.** Clients are given the necessary information and the opportunity to exercise the degree of control they choose over healthcare decisions that affect them. The health system accommodates differences in client preferences and encourages shared decision making.

4. **Shared knowledge and the free flow of information.** Clients have unfettered access to their own medical information and to clinical knowledge. Clinicians and clients communicate effectively and share information.

5. **Evidence-based decision making.** Clients receive care based on the best available scientific knowledge. Care does not vary illogically from clinician to clinician or from place to place.

6. **Safety as a system property.** Clients are safe from injury caused by the care system. Reducing risk and ensuring safety require greater attention to systems that help prevent and mitigate errors.

7. **Need for transparency.** The healthcare system makes information readily available to clients.

8. **Needs are anticipated.** The system anticipates client needs, rather than simply react to events.

9. **Waste is continuously decreased.** The system does not waste resources or client time.

10. **Cooperation among all clinicians is a priority.** Clinicians and institutions actively collaborate and communicate to ensure an appropriate exchange of information and coordination of care.

Source: Institute of Medicine. (2001). *Crossing the quality chasm: A health system for the 21st century.* Washington, DC: National Academy Press. Reprinted with permission from the National Academies Press, Copyright 2001, National Academy of Sciences.

C. Nursing leadership has the obligation to create a safe and effective nursing environment for clients and staff through organizational support for nursing care

1. Financial and other adequate resources must be dedicated to supporting nursing staff in acquisition of new knowledge and skills to maintain clinical competence

2. Nurse autonomy empowers staff to set criteria for closing the unit to new admissions as necessitated by workload levels

3. Nurse control involves direct-care staff in identifying staffing levels, causes of nursing staff turnover, and methods to improve retention and safety

4. Collegial health discipline relationships promote interdisciplinary collaboration through interdisciplinary rounds, formal education and training programs, and staff satisfaction surveys

D. *Nurse safety* ensures health and well-being of nurses and protects them against illness or injury in the workplace

1. Major workplace health and safety issues confronting nurses are:
   a. Back injuries
   b. Needle sticks

    c. Respiratory diseases

    d. Workplace violence

  2. The American Nurses Association recommends that nurses take the following precautions against workplace violence:

    a. Make sure healthcare facilities track all assaults on clients, employees, and visitors

    b. Insist that the Occupational Safety and Health Administration (OSHA) *Guidelines for Preventing Workplace Violence for Health Care and Social Service Workers* are being implemented at all healthcare facilities

    c. Encourage employees to report threats (both verbal and physical), as well as injuries

    d. Insist that full medical treatment and post-assault counseling be provided in the event of an assault

  3. Hazardous exposure is minimized through appropriate policies and procedures

E. Nurses can protect themselves against work-related illness if they have active role in uncovering, assessing, and addressing these illnesses proactively by:

  1. Assessing the workplace for hazards and harmful conditions

  2. Using available resources to reduce work-related risks, such as following work redesign practices by regulators and oversight organizations such as the Joint Commission on Accreditation of Healthcare Organizations (JCAHO) and state licensing agencies

  3. Identifying potential equipment or activities that can reduce risks and injuries, such as using proper handwashing technique to reduce infection, following five rights to medication administration to reduce errors, and providing employee training in error detection, analysis, and reduction

  4. Inquiring about task force or committee formation to explore and focus attention on workplace ergonomics, such as voluntary adoption and use of lifting devices as an alternative to manual client lifting by nurses and UAPs

  5. Being informed about policies and regulations in occupational safety and health issues such as caring for clients with tuberculosis (TB) or severe acute respiratory syndrome (SARS); fitting of an N-95 particulate filter mask; or training in use of needleless parenteral medication administration systems

  6. Knowing how to use client lifting and transfer devices to prevent back and other physical injuries

  7. Knowing resources to use to address health and safety issues (see Box 1-4)

VII. FOCUSING PRACTICE TO PROVIDE EFFECTIVE EVIDENCED-BASED CARE

A. Evidence needed to inform practice

  1. Evidence-based practice allows nurse leaders to identify and assess high-quality, relevant research that can be applied to clinical practice

  2. **Evidenced-based care** is defined as the process of providing clinically competent care supported by the best scientific evidence available, such as outcomes research and expert advisers

  3. Data is analyzed and determined to be credible as evidence

  4. Data accompanied by its usefulness guides clinical practice

Box 1-4	The ANA's Health and Safety Web Page
Resources for Nurse Protection and Safety	*http://nursingworld.org/osh*

The ANA's Health and Safety Web Page
  http://nursingworld.org/osh
OSHA Website for Information on Healthcare Facilities
  http://www.osha.gov/SLTC/healthcarefacilities/index.html
Centers for Disease Control Website for SARS
  http://www.cdc.gov/ncido&sars/workplace.htm
National Institute for Occupational Safety and Health
  http://www.cdc.gov/niosh/
Joint Commission on Accreditation of Healthcare Organizations
  http://www.jcaho.org
Agency for Healthcare Research and Quality
  http://www.ahrq.gov

B. *Outcomes research*

1. Is defined as seeking to understand results of particular healthcare practices and interventions that are analyzed and used to improve client care through ongoing systematic reviews

2. Provides evidence about benefits, risks, and results of treatment so that both nurses and clients can make more informed decisions

   a. Estimates effect of healthcare interventions

   b. Provides general answers, based on the number of studies in different settings and includes a variety of participants

   c. Identifies individual, clinical, and contextual factors that influence effectiveness

   d. Identifies any gaps and uncertainties found in research

C. Role of nurse leaders related to evidence-based practice

1. Nurse leaders are responsible for establishing and supporting a culture for evidence-based care; creating culture for evidence-based care involves:

   a. Integrating clinically observed and research-directed evidence

   b. Applying knowledge and evidence to clinical practice

   c. Evaluating and measuring clinical care outcomes

2. Examples of outcome indicators that measure impact of care include mortality, complications, and cost as well as quality of life and client satisfaction

3. Nurse leaders can ensure that staff use evidence-based practice by demonstrating how to implement best practices into daily nursing practice using a seven-step evidence-based process:

   a. Precisely define the client problem

   b. Identify information necessary to solve the problem

   c. Conduct an efficient and thorough search of the literature

   d. Critically appraise the evidence

   e. Find a clinical answer as it applies to the client problem

   f. Use clinical guidelines or evidence-based protocols when available

   g. Monitor and evaluate evidence-based practice

      1) Monitor for errors

      2) Monitor occurrence/incident reports

      3) Monitor interventions and outcomes

      4) Monitor system performance and response

   D. Healthcare organizations have an obligation to engage clinical providers to apply evidence-based care processes to all levels within the institution

      1. Customization of care occurs based on client needs

      2. Practice guidelines are developed and utilized

      3. There is a continuous focus on promoting excellence in nursing practice to improve client care outcomes

      4. Client outcome measures include improved health status and quality of life, and respecting client preferences whenever possible

Case Study

Managed care has attempted to change the healthcare delivery system because total expenditures on healthcare have drastically increased, consuming greater portions of the nation's resources. The impetus for this change was continually increasing hospitalization costs and prescription drug expenses to treat chronic diseases, primarily incurred by increasing numbers of older adults who have a lengthening lifespan.

1. Discuss how managed care attempts to control healthcare costs.

2. Explain how managed care demonstrates that health promotion is a primary goal.

3. Define the following types of managed care organizations: (a) Health Maintenance Organization (HMO), (b) Preferred Provider Organization (PPO), (c) Point-of-Service Organization (POS), and (d) Physician Hospital Organization (PHO).

4. Describe the impact of managed care on cost containment and healthcare consumers.

5. Explain the responsibilities of nurses who function as case managers.

For suggested responses, see page 234.

POSTTEST

1 A hospital uses a scan system to identify clients prior to administering medications. Nurses are frustrated because the new system is adding time to medication administration. Instead of scanning the client's identification bracelet, the nurses scan the client's identification sticker, which is found on the client's chart. Subsequently, a nurse administers the wrong medication to the client. The nurse manager concludes this error was possibly caused by which of the following? Select all that apply.

  1. Inefficient systems
  2. Inadequate processes
  3. Inept conditions
  4. Improperly labeled medications
  5. Transcriber oversight

2 A nurse is a unit representative to a hospital committee that reviews medication errors. One error under current review occurred on a medical unit that is poorly staffed, requiring each nurse to be assigned to 8 clients. The nurse anticipates that this medication error most likely occurred because of which of the following?

  1. Faulty systems
  2. Unit-specific conditions
  3. Failure in processes
  4. Pharmacy errors

POSTTEST

POSTTEST

3 During an investigation of a medication error made by a nurse using a new medication administration system, the nurse states, "I wasn't comfortable using this new system." The nurse manager should plan to prevent this type of medication error by doing which of the following?

1. Verifying all nurses are licensed
2. Encouraging all nurses to become certified
3. Providing professional training for new equipment
4. Collaborating across health disciplines

4 A nurse working in a nursing home on the 7 PM–7 AM shift observes a person outside lurking behind the trees. Which action should the nurse take to prevent workplace violence?

1. Take shifts guarding the doors.
2. Call the local police immediately.
3. Report the suspicious behavior to the on-call administrator.
4. Keep all doors locked at all times.

5 Which strategies should the chief nursing officer (CNO) utilize to create a culture of evidence-based practice? Select all that apply.

1. Provide in-services defining evidence-based practice.
2. Delegate this task to the unit managers.
3. Seek changes in policies to reflect clinical research.
4. Include evidence-based practice in the strategic plan.
5. Seek buy-in from unit managers and coordinators.

6 A nurse leader notes that the average length of hospital stay for clients with diabetes mellitus is higher than for non-diabetic clients. In investigating the reasons for this discrepancy, the nurse leader should first plan to review which of the following?

1. Current policies and procedures
2. Specific outcome indicators
3. Evidence-based research
4. Current clinical practice

7 A nurse is preparing to lift a client who has right hemiplegia. Which measures should the nurse take to prevent injuries? Select all that apply.

1. Apply a back support.
2. Use a lifting device such as a Hoyer lift.
3. Keep knees straight.
4. Use a partner.
5. Keep feet together.

8 The nurse has been chosen to be the nursing unit representative to a hospital committee focusing on quality and effectiveness of care. The nurse plans to gather data about which client care outcome indicators as part of the work of the committee? Select all that apply.

1. Infection rates
2. Medication administration
3. Support systems
4. Diagnosis
5. Length of hospital stay

9 The nurse manager reviews the unit's policy and procedure for central line dressing changes. In determining the need for revisions, the manager should consider which of the following priority areas?

1. The development of practice guidelines
2. Joint Commission on Accreditation of Healthcare Organizations (JCAHO) guidelines
3. The most current clinical research
4. Clinical indicators of care

10 When interviewing for a position on a hospital nursing unit, the nurse learns that members of the nursing staff are allowed to develop and deliver in-services and participate on hospital committees. The nurse concludes that this nursing unit utilizes which of the following models?

1. Nurse manager decision-making model
2. Decision-making model
3. Client accountability model
4. Shared governance model

➤ *See pages 20–22 for Answers and Rationales.*

ANSWERS & RATIONALES

Pretest

1 **Answer: 1, 3, 5** For a position of leadership, a nurse manager needs to have a predominately democratic approach in working with and supervising others. Nurse managers need commitment and a bit of charisma for influential power. Type A personality and stoicism are not emergent workforce attributes needed for the role of a nurse manager.
Cognitive Level: Application **Client Need:** Safe Effective Care Environment: Management of Care **Integrated Process:** Nursing Process: Evaluation **Content Area:** Leadership/Management **Strategy:** The critical words in the question are *emergent workforce attributes*. First, recall that democracy, charisma, and commitment are all necessary for positions of leadership to choose them as correct options. Recalling that type A personality and stoicism both stand out as rigid characteristics that may not be effective traits for leadership, these two options would not be selected. **Reference:** Finkelman, A. W. (2006). *Leadership and management in nursing.* Upper Saddle River, NJ: Pearson Education, pp. 5–7.

2 **Answer: 2, 3** The nurse manager uses mentorship to prepare the nurse for leadership roles. The manager identifies strengths and supports the nurse by providing educational opportunities to develop leadership skills. Charisma is a personal trait or skill that attracts followers. Improvement is a not a concept utilized in the question. Fairness is another name for the ethical principle of justice, but this term does not apply to the situation in the question.
Cognitive Level: Comprehension **Client Need:** Safe Effective Care Environment: Management of Care **Integrated Process:** Nursing Process: Implementation **Content Area:** Leadership/Management **Strategy:** Identify the best answers that fit the scenario. Note that charisma and the ability to make fair decisions are leadership traits, but are not specific concepts used to improve the workforce. Next, recall that improvement is not a workforce concept. This leaves development and mentorship as correct options. **Reference:** Finkelman, A. W. (2006). *Leadership and management in nursing.* Upper Saddle River, NJ: Pearson Education, pp. 22–23.

3 **Answer: 2** Care maps are guides to provide nationally accepted, standardized care. The care provided is scheduled, aggressive care to prevent increased length of hospital stay while maintaining satisfactory client outcomes. Options 1, 3, and 4 focus on cost containment but do not include any effect on quality of care to clients.

Cognitive Level: Application **Client Need:** Safe Effective Care Environment: Management of Care **Integrated Process:** Nursing Process: Implementation **Content Area:** Leadership/Management **Strategy:** Eliminate option 1 first because it focuses only on supply checks, not quality. Next, eliminate option 3 because it precludes quality by reducing items that are needed in the process of care delivery. Note that a series of in-services (option 4) does not address the issue of quality. Finally, choose option 2 because it addresses both quality care and cost containment through the use of care maps. **Reference:** Finkelman, A. W. (2006). *Leadership and management in nursing.* Upper Saddle River, NJ: Pearson Education, pp. 134–135.

4 **Answer: 2** A supervisor monitors the influx of clients admitted and discharged. In addition, the supervisor oversees changing conditions on the various units. The supervisor in most facilities must respond to codes. The unit manager supervises the day-to-day operations of the unit. The chief operating officer (COO) supervises the functions of the entire facility, and the charge nurse supervises the activities on the unit during a specific shift.
Cognitive Level: Comprehension **Client Need:** Safe Effective Care Environment: Management of Care **Integrated Process:** Nursing Process: Analysis **Content Area:** Leadership/Management **Strategy:** This question specifically asks for a leader who makes assignments on *all* units. Unit managers and charge nurses make assignments on their specific units. The COO has the authority to make assignments on all units, but this is not the role of the COO. The best choice is option 2. **Reference:** Finkelman, A. W. (2006). *Leadership and management in nursing.* Upper Saddle River, NJ: Pearson Education, pp. 227–228.

5 **Answer: 3** In-services fall under the auspices of education because they provide staff with information about policies, procedures, and products that are used in the course of delivering client care. The other options do not apply. A nursing practice council addresses standards of client care (option 1). A quality improvement council seeks to monitor the effectiveness of nursing care that has been delivered (option 2). A management council determines policy and addresses workforce issues (option 4).
Cognitive Level: Application **Client Need:** Safe Effective Care Environment: Management of Care **Integrated Process:** Nursing Process: Implementation **Content Area:** Leadership/Management **Strategy:** Identify the critical

words *in-services* and *clinical competence*, which are cues indicating that education is the correct option. The question does not describe nursing practice, quality improvement, or management. **Reference:** Finkelman, A. W. (2006). *Leadership and management in nursing*. Upper Saddle River, NJ: Pearson Education, pp. 148–150.

6 **Answer: 1** A shared governance model is characterized by input from all employees of the facility and a culture of "this is the workplace of the employees." Employees are treated as associates. Empowerment is a feature of a shared governance model but is not the name of a model. Compassionate leadership and workforce support are desirable traits or behaviors in nurse leaders but, again, they are not models of organizational behavior.
Cognitive Level: Analysis **Client Need:** Safe Effective Care Environment: Management of Care **Integrated Process:** Nursing Process: Assessment **Content Area:** Leadership/Management **Strategy:** The core issue of this question is knowledge of models of organizational behavior. Identify the critical words *self-scheduling* and *input from staff*, and note that they imply shared governance. Empowerment, compassionate leadership, and workforce support are concepts that not directly addressed in this question. **Reference:** Finkelman, A. W. (2006). *Leadership and management in nursing*. Upper Saddle River, NJ: Pearson Education, pp. 148–150.

7 **Answer: 3** The nurse leader has empowered the nurse to function in a role in which the nurse is obviously comfortable. This action also gives the nurse a challenging job with interesting facets. Shared governance refers to a structure of management within a healthcare organization. The nurse manager's action does not represent either compassionate or charismatic leadership because the manager is not relying on social relationships or personal charm, respectively.
Cognitive Level: Comprehension **Client Need:** Safe Effective Care Environment: Management of Care **Integrated Process:** Nursing Process: Analysis **Content Area:** Leadership/Management **Strategy:** First, consider that shared governance obviously does not fit this situation. Compassionate leaders focus on social relationships in the workplace. This leader does not use charm in this question; however, the leader does empower the staff nurse to use personal attributes to help serve the needs of the staff. **Reference:** Finkelman, A. W. (2006). *Leadership and management in nursing*. Upper Saddle River, NJ: Pearson Education, pp. 86–87.

8 **Answer: 1** Motivation is implied by the critical word, *encourage*, making option 1 the best option. Partnership does not fit the description because the manager and CNA have not formed an alliance to meet a particular goal. Communication seems plausible, but it is not the

best choice because there is an intention for action, not merely an exchange of words. Charisma, a personal attribute, is not used in this question.
Cognitive Level: Application **Client Need:** Safe Effective Care Environment: Management of Care **Integrated Process:** Nursing Process: Assessment **Content Area:** Leadership/Management **Strategy:** The core issue of the question is the use of best practices in staff development. Identify best practices in staff development and use the process of elimination to select the correct option. **Reference:** Finkelman, A. W. (2006). *Leadership and management in nursing*. Upper Saddle River, NJ: Pearson Education, pp. 86–87.

9 **Answer: 1** Compassionate leadership is characterized by the use of rewards to motivate staff for excellence in practice. Empathetic and influential leadership are not formalized leadership models. Charismatic leaders utilize personal traits to draw their staff to them.
Cognitive Level: Application **Client Need:** Safe Effective Care Environment: Management of Care **Integrated Process:** Nursing Process: Evaluation **Content Area:** Leadership/Management **Strategy:** A critical word in the question is *rewards*. Recall that compassionate leaders reward individuals for excellence in practice to help you choose correctly. **Reference:** Yoder-Wise, P., & Kowalski, K. (2006). *Beyond leading and managing: Nursing administration for the future*. St. Louis, MO: Elsevier Mosby, pp. 120–121.

10 **Answer: 3** The nurse has not verified the right person. As with many systems, nurses and other staff occasionally find and utilize loopholes that compromise safety, although they save time. Retrieving the information from the chart sticker instead of the client's identification bracelet does not properly identify the client. There is no specific reference in the question to time, dose, or documentation.
Cognitive Level: Application **Client Need:** Safe Effective Care Environment: Management of Care **Integrated Process:** Nursing Process: Assessment **Content Area:** Leadership/Management **Strategy:** The question does not indicate a problem with time or dose, and documentation is completed after the medication has been administered. The only option remaining is "right person." **Reference:** Finkelman, A. W. (2006). *Leadership and management in nursing*. Upper Saddle River, NJ: Pearson Education, pp. 471, 498–499.

Posttest

1 **Answer: 1, 2** A system failure or process failure appears to be the etiology of the error. The scenario does not describe inept conditions. There are no indications that medications are improperly labeled or there is a transcriber oversight.

Cognitive Level: Application **Client Need:** Safe Effective Care Environment: Management of Care **Integrated Process:** Nursing Process: Analysis **Content Area:** Leadership/Management **Strategy:** Eliminate options 4 and 5 first, since transcription and medication labeling are clearly not addressed in the question. Next, eliminate option 3 because the term inept implies an inability to do something, but this usually refers to a person or action, not a "condition." Identify best practice options to select the remaining correct responses. **Reference:** Finkelman, A. W. (2006). *Leadership and management in nursing.* Upper Saddle River, NJ: Pearson Education, pp. 498–500.

2 **Answer: 2** The nurse was probably rushed to administer medications, which can lead to an increase in medication errors. Pharmacy errors and faulty systems errors are not addressed in this scenario. There could be a failure in processes, but this information isn't revealed in the scenario. Thus, the best option is 2.
Cognitive Level: Application **Client Need:** Safe Effective Care Environment: Management of Care **Integrated Process:** Nursing Process: Analysis **Content Area:** Leadership/Management **Strategy:** In this case, a specific answer is best. The unit is poorly staffed, making it more likely that errors are due to conditions that potentiate unsafe practice. The question does not provide information to support faulty systems, failure in processes, or pharmacy errors. **Reference:** Finkelman, A. W. (2006). *Leadership and management in nursing.* Upper Saddle River, NJ: Pearson Education, pp. 498–500.

3 **Answer: 3** Before using new equipment, nurse leaders should provide staff with education about the new equipment to prevent any client or nurse incidents. All practicing nurses must be licensed, but do not require certification to prevent medication errors. Collaboration across health disciplines is not necessary in this case.
Cognitive Level: Application **Client Need:** Safe Effective Care Environment: Management of Care **Integrated Process:** Nursing Process: Planning **Content Area:** Leadership/Management **Strategy:** Identify the root problem—the nurse isn't comfortable using the new equipment. Look at the options to determine which choice fits this question. Options 1, 2, and 4 do not fit because the question does not include any information to support these choices. However, option 3 is the closest answer that addresses the root of the problem—lack of understanding of new equipment. **Reference:** Finkelman, A. W. (2006). *Leadership and management in nursing.* Upper Saddle River, NJ: Pearson Education, pp. 498–500.

4 **Answer: 2** Employees of healthcare organizations are encouraged to report any suspicious behavior. Violence in the workplace is a real phenomenon that could have detrimental outcomes. It may not be feasible to keep all doors locked at all times. It is not reasonable to post staff at facility entrances. However, the administration should research security options to keep employees and residents safe at all times.
Cognitive Level: Application **Client Need:** Safe Effective Care Environment: Management of Care **Integrated Process:** Nursing Process: Implementation **Content Area:** Leadership/Management **Strategy:** The first response by the nurse is to keep all staff and residents safe. The only option that may prevent workplace violence in this case is notifying the police immediately. Prioritizing based on Maslow's hierarchy of needs may help in choosing the correct answer. In this case, there is someone suspicious on the premises, and the nurse should call the police immediately in an effort to get prompt help. Option 1 may not be feasible. Staff, residents, and visitors should all report suspicious behavior; however, in this case, a possible intruder is on the premises and help is needed immediately. Locking the doors may help, but the nurse needs help on the grounds from the authorities. **Reference:** Finkelman, A. W. (2006). *Leadership and management in nursing.* Upper Saddle River, NJ: Pearson Education, pp. 498–499.

5 **Answer: 1, 3, 4, 5** All options are recommended with the exception of option 2. Enhancing utilization of evidence-based practice should not be delegated. The CNO should lead the nurse managers and staff in creating the culture.
Cognitive Level: Application **Client Need:** Safe Effective Care Environment: Management of Care **Integrated Process:** Nursing Process: Implementation **Content Area:** Leadership/Management **Strategy:** First, consider that options 1 and 3 are within the role of the CNO. Next, recognize that the CNO identifies pertinent elements that should be added to the strategic plan. In creating a culture of evidence-based practice, the CNO should get buy-in from the unit managers and coordinators to assist in moving the plan along. Eliminate option 2 because delegating this task to lower-level management could prove to be disastrous for the CNO and hospital. Change should come from the source. **Reference:** Finkelman, A. W. (2006). *Leadership and management in nursing.* Upper Saddle River, NJ: Pearson Education, pp. 496–498.

6 **Answer: 4** The manager should review the current clinical practice. This data will alert the leader of the safe or unsafe practices that occur on the unit that may be contributing to the problem. Once the current practice is examined, the leader should review evidence-based research to determine congruence of the current practice with the standards of care for clients with diabetes. Policies and procedures should reflect the standardized practice of care.

Cognitive Level: Application **Client Need:** Safe Effective Care Environment: Management of Care **Integrated Process:** Nursing Process: Assessment **Content Area:** Leadership/Management **Strategy:** Note the word *investigating* in the question and associate this with assessment. The leader should first review the current practice on the unit in regard to clients with diabetes. This option is a priority. Policies and procedures could then be reviewed to determine if practice is in concert with these. Finally, evidence-based practice guidelines can be reviewed to determine whether agency policies and procedures are up to date. **Reference:** Finkelman, A. W. (2006). *Leadership and management in nursing.* Upper Saddle River, NJ: Pearson Education, pp. 264–268.

7 **Answer: 1, 2, 4** The correct interventions to prevent injury are the application of back support, use of the lifting device, and a partner. The other options will increase the risk of sustaining a back injury.
Cognitive Level: Application **Client Need:** Safe Effective Care Environment: Management of Care **Integrated Process:** Nursing Process: Evaluation **Content Area:** Leadership/Management **Strategy:** Recall these basic safety principles. When lifting, one should wear back support, use a lifting device, and get help to assist in lifting. In addition, knees should be bent and feet should be apart when lifting, which make options 3 and 5 incorrect choices. **Reference:** Finkelman, A. W. (2006). *Leadership and management in nursing.* Upper Saddle River, NJ: Pearson Education, pp. 510–511.

8 **Answer: 1, 5** Outcome indicators determine the effectiveness of care. The number of infections is an indicator of quality of care as is length of hospital stay. Better care should be associated with reduced infection rates and length of stay. Medication administration, support systems, and diagnosis are not pertinent to the question as written.
Cognitive Level: Application **Client Need:** Safe Effective Care Environment: Management of Care **Integrated Process:** Nursing Process: Evaluation **Content Area:** Leadership/Management **Strategy:** Recall that outcome indicators determine the effectiveness of care. Medication administration is a process (not an outcome), which makes it incorrect in this case. Medication errors would be a better indicator. Support systems do not fit the description of an outcome indicator. Diagnosis, although used by utilization review, is not used as an outcome indicator. Hospital-acquired infection rates are monitored because they increase length of stay. Length of stay is

impacted by effectiveness of treatment, exacerbation of co-morbid conditions, and other complications. **Reference:** Finkelman, A. W. (2006). *Leadership and management in nursing.* Upper Saddle River, NJ: Pearson Education, pp. 501–502.

9 **Answer: 3** To provide evidence-based nursing care, revisions to policies and procedures should be guided by the results of current clinical research. Practice guidelines (option 1) provide direction about care that is needed by a client with a specific health problem. JCAHO (option 2) is an accrediting organization that does not recommend specific clinical care guidelines. Clinical indicators of care (option 4) would not provide information about what needs to be changed in the current policies and procedures.
Cognitive Level: Application **Client Need:** Safe Effective Care Environment: Management of Care **Integrated Process:** Nursing Process: Planning **Content Area:** Leadership/Management **Strategy:** Recall first that revisions should not be based on the development of practice guidelines. The word *development* is the word that makes option 1 incorrect. Option 2 is incorrect because JCAHO determines which policies agencies should have in place. Recall that JCAHO allows agencies to develop its own policies. While policy revisions may be modified based on data retrieved from clinical indicators of care, policy revisions are based on evidence-based research. **Reference:** Finkelman, A. W. (2006). *Leadership and management in nursing.* Upper Saddle River, NJ: Pearson Education, pp. 506–509.

10 **Answer: 4** Shared governance is a leadership model that involves employees in decision making and fosters open communication with staff. Nurse manager decision making (option 1) is not a formal decision-making model. Decision-making model (option 2) is too broad and is not a formal model. Client accountability (option 3) is not a formal model and does not apply to the scenario.
Cognitive Level: Application **Client Need:** Safe Effective Care Environment: Management of Care **Integrated Process:** Nursing Process: Analysis **Content Area:** Leadership/Management **Strategy:** Recall that shared governance supports a sense of ownership and fosters partnerships among the nurse leader and the nursing staff. Use this knowledge to systematically eliminate each of the incorrect options. **Reference:** Finkelman, A. W. (2006). *Leadership and management in nursing.* Upper Saddle River, NJ: Pearson Education, pp. 148–150.

References

Aiken, L. H. (2002). Superior outcomes for magnet hospitals: The evidence base. In M. L. McClure & A. S. Hinshaw (Eds.), *Magnet hospitals revisited: Attraction and retention of professional nurses.* Washington, DC: American Nurses Publishing.

Aiken, L. H., Clarke, S. P., & Sloane, D. M. (2002). Hospital staffing, organization, and quality of care: Cross-national findings. *Nursing Outlook, 50,* 187–194.

Aiken, L. H., Clarke, S. P., Cheung, S. P., Sloane, O. M., & Silber, J. (2003). Educational levels of hospital nurses and surgical patient mortality. *Journal of the American Medical Association, 290*(12), 1617–1623.

Cordeniz, J. A. (2002). Recruitment, retention, and management of generation X: A focus on nursing professionals. *Journal of Healthcare Management, 47*(4), 237–245.

Coupland, D. (1992). *Generation X: Tales for an accelerated culture.* New York, NY: St. Martin's Press.

Finkelman, A. W. (2001). *Managed care: A nursing perspective.* Upper Saddle River, New Jersey: Prentice Hall, pp. 246–247.

Finkelman, A. W. (2006). *Leadership and management in nursing.* Upper Saddle River, NJ: Pearson Education.

Hubbard, H., Walker, P., Clancy, C., & Stryer, D. (2002). Outcomes and effectiveness research: Capacity building for nurse researchers at the Agency for Healthcare Research and Quality. *Outcomes Management, 6*(4), 146–151.

Institute of Medicine. (1998). *To err is human: Building a safer health system.* Washington, DC: National Academy Press.

Institute of Medicine. (2001). *Crossing the quality chasm. A new health system for the 21st century.* Washington, DC: National Academy Press.

Institute of Medicine. (2002). *Unequal treatment: Confronting racial and ethnic disparities in health care.* Washington, DC: National Academies Press.

Joint Commission on Accreditation of Healthcare Organizations (JCAHO). (2002). *Health care at the crossroads: Strategies for addressing the evolving nursing crisis.* Chicago: Author.

Kimball, B., & O'Neill, E. (2002). *Health care's human crisis: The American nursing shortage.* Princeton, NJ: The Robert Wood Johnson Foundation.

Kowalski, K. (2001). Nursing work force of the future: The administrative perspective. *Journal of Perinatal and Neonatal Nursing, 15*(1), 8–15.

Norrish, B., & Rundall, T. (2001). Hospital restructuring and the work of registered nurses. *The Milbank Quarterly, 79*(1), 55–79.

Chen, K. (2002, April 19). Nursing-home industry to get 14 of voluntary ergonomics rules. *Wall Street Journal.*

Needleman, J., & Buerhaus, P. (2001, February 28). *Nurse staffing and patient outcomes in hospitals, Final Report.* Washington, DC: U.S. Dept. of Health and Human Services, Health Resources and Services Administration.

Nicklin, W. (2002). Canadian nurses' perceptions of patient safety in hospitals. *Canadian Journal of Nursing Leadership, 15*(3), 11–21.

Sullivan, E. J., & Decker, P. (2005). *Effective leadership and management in nursing* (6th ed.). Upper Saddle River, NJ: Pearson Education.

Wieck, K. L., Prydun, M., & Walsh, T. (2002). What the emerging workforce wants in its leaders. *Journal of Nursing Scholarship, 34*(3), 283–288.

2 Leading and Managing for a Safe and Effective Care Environment

NCLEX-RN® Test Prep

Use the CD-ROM enclosed with this book to access additional practice opportunities.

Objectives

➤ Differentiate between leadership and management.

➤ Describe the characteristics of an effective leader.

➤ Describe the management process.

➤ Differentiate among various theories of leadership and management.

➤ Explain reflective thinking and problem solving.

Review at a Glance

autocratic leadership a leadership style motivated by external forces; the leader makes all decisions and directs the followers' behavior

bureaucratic leadership a leadership style motivated by external forces; the leader trusts neither followers nor self to make decisions and instead relies on organizational policies and rules

clinical practice all direct and indirect client care activities undertaken to provide nursing care to individuals, families, or groups

controlling a process of establishing standards of performance, determining means to be used in measuring performance, evaluating performance, and providing feedback

democratic leadership a leadership style motivated by internal forces; the leader uses participation and majority rule to achieve work goals and activities

followers those who offer their personal commitment to a cause and acknowledge a central leader as source for guidance, motivation, and authority

formal leadership a leadership style used by an individual with legitimate authority conferred by position within an organization

informal leadership a leadership style used by an individual who does not have a specified management role

laissez-faire leadership a leadership style motivated by internal forces that leaves individuals alone to complete their work; the leader provides no direction or facilitation

leader an individual who uses interpersonal skills to influence followers to accomplish specific goals

leadership an ability to articulate a vision, embrace the values of that vision, and nurture an environment where followers can reach both the organization's goals and their own personal goals

manager an individual employed by an organization who is responsible for efficiently accomplishing the goals of the organization

organizing the process of coordinating work to be done within an organization

planning a process that includes decision making and problem solving in order to achieve specific goals

servant leadership a practical philosophy and model, which supports people who choose to serve first and then lead as a way of expanding services to individuals and institutions; encourages collaboration, trust, foresight, listening, and ethical use of power and empowerment

transactional leadership a leadership style that influences followers by using contingent rewards and punishment to achieve desired work levels or performance

transformational leadership a leadership style that is influential in motivating and transforming followers to be more aware of task outcomes, activate their highest order needs and go beyond their own self-interest for the benefit of the organization

PRETEST

1 A nurse leader persuades other staff nurses to buy into the agency's vision, mission, and special projects and to embrace change. The nurse working with this leader concludes that these characteristics are consistent with those expected of a

1. Case manager.
2. Chief operating officer.
3. Nurse manager.
4. Chief financial officer.

2 Which of the following strategies would the nurse leader select as having the greatest likelihood of being effective when empowering staff nurses' participation in clinical decision making? Select all that apply.

1. Implement decentralized unit-based programs or team organizational structures for decision making.
2. Allow organizational or system-wide committees and communication structures that include staff nurse representation.
3. Utilize review systems for nursing analysis and correction of clinical care errors and client safety concerns.
4. Create additional team leaders among nurses and nursing assistants to report to the nurse manager weekly.
5. Create staff forums that allow members to vent their frustrations about the facility.

3 The nurse striving to be a leader would focus on continued development of which of the following characteristics? Select all that apply.

1. Compassion
2. Loyalty
3. Employee-driven
4. Mission-driven
5. Process-oriented

4 A nurse who is self-analyzing personal leadership characteristics would correctly conclude that the presence of which characteristics are consistent with those of an effective nurse leader? Select all that apply.

1. Power and influence on others
2. Reluctance to change without substantial evidence of need
3. Ability to motivate others
4. Avoidance of changing the behavior of others
5. Consistent actions and beliefs

5 A nurse leader openly shares clinical expertise with staff nurses and provides learning opportunities for these nurses. The staff nurse concludes that this nurse leader is using which strategy to improve staff members?

1. Personal attention
2. Role modeling
3. Precepting
4. Mentoring

6 An interim nurse manager has been given authority to schedule the work of employees and reprimand staff as needed. The nurse manager is aware that the type of leadership that results from this situation is which of the following?

1. Formal
2. Informal
3. Compassionate
4. Shared

7 A nurse leader seeks to gain respect of the staff by providing rewards and supporting each staff member's personal goals. Which of the following rationales is the nurse leader likely using to support these actions?

1. A good leader must gain the respect of others.
2. A leader should use the "country club" approach of leadership.
3. A leader should be able to identify with the simple individual.
4. Socialization will boost support from the staff.

8 A nurse leader would draw on which management skill set to identify goals that must be accomplished and encourage staff to apply for positions suited to their work ability?

1. Planning and setting direction
2. Organizing and aligning people
3. Getting others to believe in the message
4. Controlling

9 A nurse leader has been appointed as the manager of the Quality Improvement Department by the chief operating officer (COO). In thinking about the skills needed to fulfill the responsibilities of this position, the nurse leader first considers that the type of leadership associated with this position is

1. Informal.
2. Formal.
3. Charismatic.
4. Compassion.

10 A nurse leader needs to restructure the units of an acute care medical center as determined by executive level management. In considering how to design the restructuring, the nurse leader should base the restructure on which of the following primary goals?

1. Focusing on nurse safety
2. Rewarding success
3. Improving client care outcomes
4. Revising inadequate policies and procedures

➤ *See pages 42–44 for Answers and Rationales.*

I. LEADERSHIP VERSUS MANAGEMENT

A. These are important but different concepts

1. **Leadership** is based on relationships and assisting people and organizations to achieve their visions

2. Management focuses on achieving order, planning, organizing, coordinating resources, and following rules and procedures (see Table 2-1)

B. Contemporary nursing leadership

1. Is about engaging people, building relationships, and influencing change; not only about formal titles, job duties, and functions

2. The terms *leader*, *administrator*, *supervisor*, and *manager* are sometimes used interchangeably, yet they are different but complementary

3. A **leader** uses his or her skills to influence others to perform to best of their ability toward goal achievement

4. Leadership is an attempt to change the behavior of another

5. Leadership is the art of getting others to want to do what one deems important

6. Leadership includes coping with change

7. Leadership requires action; a leader's actions and beliefs must be congruent and compatible

8. Leadership is the exercise of power and influence

C. To be a leader one must earn the trust of another

1. Leadership is about learning to earn the respect and trust of others; otherwise there be no followers; gaining respect and trust results in **followers** who exhibit extraordinary commitment and loyalty to their leader; leaders must have followers who are willing to trust and follow their lead

   a. Followers must share a sense of stewardship and accountability toward their leader

   b. Leaders must have a keen ability to know what type of followers they have and know how to intervene accordingly; followers have all types of behaviors related to nurse leadership styles, including but not limited to:

      1) Effective follower: thinks critically and functions independently

      2) Alienated follower: thinks critically but is passive rather than active; may appear angry, unhappy, or uninvolved

      3) Yes follower: complies with requests eagerly; enjoys structure and tends not to offer new ideas; does not enjoy being in a position of decision-making

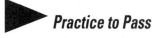

Practice to Pass

Describe at least three important terms that best describe leadership potential and leadership style.

Table 2-1	Leaders	Managers
Differences Between Leaders and Managers	Facilitator	Director
	Coordinator	Controller
	Inspiring and integrating	Telling and selling
	Macro management	Micro management
	Peer or followers	Subordinates
	Coaching and challenging	Blaming
	Problem solving and quality improvement	Problem identifying

▶ *Practice to Pass*

Describe your followership style. Explain why you assume this type of behavior. How can you become more effective in your follower style so that you can improve your potential leadership?

4) Partner follower: has a positive and interactive relationship with leader; may become a leader later

5) Contributer follower: is active in work processes and works well with others, but does not align as closely with leader as a partner follower

6) Politician follower: focuses on communication and interpersonal skills, but may not demonstrate high level performance of work role

7) Subordinate follower: focuses on job performance but may not have strong commitment to improvement

D. **Leaders must know and understand themselves before they can adequately lead and direct others; they must possess self-knowledge and self-awareness, including:**

1. Being aware and knowledgeable about their own core values and principles

2. Incorporating values and principles into their leadership style

3. Keeping abreast and monitoring their ability and impact on human and fiscal resources

4. Articulating their values and actions with trust, integrity, honesty, and commitment

E. **Leaders can be formal and informal**

1. **Formal leadership** is bestowed upon nurse by organization and described in job description; provides for influence through:

   a. Legitimate authority

   b. Power of position

   c. Ability to reward and punish

2. **Informal leadership** does not hold official title in organization but can substantially influence others through:

   a. Thoughtful and convincing ideas

   b. Knowledge

   c. Status

   d. Personal skills

II. FOUNDATIONS OF EFFECTIVE LEADERSHIP AND MANAGEMENT

A. **Effective leadership is a responsibility rather than rank or privilege; effective leaders:**

1. Desire strong associates and encourage them, push them, and glory in their success

2. Articulate the organization's vision in manner that stresses the values of followers

3. Involve followers in deciding how to achieve the organization's vision

4. Support followers' efforts to realize the vision through coaching, feedback, and role modeling

5. Recognize and reward success

6. Do not blame others when things go wrong

B. **A nurse leader's first objective is to assist and support frontline staff in the workplace by learning to:**

1. Put clients first

2. Focus on client safety

3. Enhance care quality and improve client care outcomes (see Box 2-1)

Box 2-1 **Principles and Elements of a Healthful Practice/Work Environment**	The Nursing Organizations Alliance believes that a healthful practice/work environment is supported by the presence of the following elements:

1. Collaborative Practice Culture

Respectful collegial communication and behavior

Team orientation

Presence of trust

Respect for diversity

2. Communication-Rich Culture

Clear and respectful

Open and trusting

3. A Culture of Accountability

Role expectations clearly defined

Everyone accountable

4. The Presence of Adequate Numbers of Qualified Nurses

Ability to provide quality care to meet client/client's needs

Work/home life balance

5. The Presence of Expert, Competent, Credible, Visible Leadership

Serve as an advocate for nursing practice

Support shared decision making

Allocate resources to support nursing

6. Shared Decision Making at All Levels

Nurses participate in system, organizational, and process decisions

Formal structure exists to support shared decision making

Nurses have control over their practice

7. The Encouragement of Professional Practice and Continued Growth/Development

Continuing education/certification is supported/encouraged

Participation in professional association is encouraged

An information-rich environment is supported

8. Recognition of the Value of Nursing's Contribution

Reward and pay for performance

Career mobility and expansion

9. Recognition by Nurses for Their Meaningful Contribution to Practice

Source: American Organization of Nurse Executives, *Principles and Elements of a Healthful Practice/Work Environment.* http://www.aone.org/aone/pdf/PrinciplesandElementsHealthfulWorkPractice.pdf. Reprinted by permission.

C. **Effective nurse leadership empowers nurse participation in clinical decision making and organization of clinical care systems by:**

1. Using decentralized, unit-based programs or team organizational structures for decision making

2. Providing for organization or system-wide committee and communication structures that include staff nurse representation

3. Involving nurses in performance improvement of clinical care and organization of clinical care systems

4. Having a utilization review system for nursing analysis and correction of clinical care errors and client safety concerns

5. Providing professional nurses with authority to develop and execute nursing care orders and actions and to control their practice

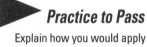

D. **Leadership development and performance require learning a body of knowledge and using effective management strategies including core leadership skills:**

1. Communication
2. Team building
3. Knowledge of healthcare economics
4. Financial accounting
5. Organizational management
6. Human resource management
7. Evidence-based outcomes

E. **Nurse leaders have an obligation to invest and build upon the human capital of their nursing staff; which includes:**

1. Utilizing models of care that promote collaboration and participation by nursing staff
2. Promoting shared decision making, ownership, initiative, and follow-through
3. Establishing clear responsibilities, accountabilities, and education for all nursing and support services
4. Focusing nursing resources on clinical care functions
5. Providing for ongoing professional development and training for frontline staff
6. Removing gaps and barriers created by professional, cultural, and generational differences
7. Promoting sincere, authentic relationships that cultivate trust and respect
8. Rewarding and acknowledging team members for their impact on client care
9. Creating a work environment that meets the physical and emotional needs of nursing staff
10. Communicating in ways that are culturally and linguistically appropriate

Practice to Pass

Explain how you would apply the core leadership skill of communication to effectively manage client care assignments, lunch, and break times for unlicensed assisted personnel.

III. MANAGEMENT PROCESS

A. **A *manager* is an individual employed by an organization who is responsible and accountable for efficiently accomplishing the goals of the organization; responsibilities include:**

1. Coordinating tasks and integrating both human and fiscal resources
2. Using functions of planning, organizing, supervising, staffing, evaluating, and negotiating
3. Clarifying organizational structure
4. Evaluating client care outcomes and providing feedback
5. Coping with organizational complexity

B. Functions of management: managers have four basic functions—*planning, organizing, leading,* and *controlling*; these functions are known as the management process

    1. Planning (and setting direction) function

        a. Set goals and decide course of action through an inductive process

        b. Gather data and look for patterns

        c. Build relationships and linkages to help explain things

        d. Create visions and strategies for what the organization will look like in the future

    2. Organizing function (includes aligning people)

        a. Identify work to be accomplished and goals to be achieved

        b. Hire the right person for the right work

        c. Create interdependence by getting people to move in the same direction

        d. Delegate authority by talking to anyone who can help implement the vision and strategies and to anyone who can block implementation

        e. Coordinate work of others

    3. Leading function (includes getting others to believe the message)

        a. Influence others to get the job done

        b. Keep the message clear

        c. Communicate with integrity and trustworthiness

        d. Mold the culture and maintain morale

        e. Insist on consistency between words and deeds

    4. Controlling function

        a. Set standards for accomplishing organizations goals and activities

        b. Determine the means to measure performance and make sure that quality lapses are spotted immediately

        c. Evaluate performance

        d. Provide feedback

C. Skills for effective management

    1. Planning

    2. Problem solving

    3. Communicating

    4. Delegating

    5. Managing change

D. The Nurse Manager Leadership Collaborative (NMLC)

    1. The American Organization of Nurse Executives (AONE), American Association of Critical-Care Nurses (AACN), and Association of PeriOperative Registered Nurses (AORN) formed an alliance known as NMLC to assist in nurse manager leadership development

    2. The NMLC Learning Domain Framework contains key components of nurse manager leadership development (see Figure 2-1)

        a. The Science—Managing Business

        b. The Art—Leading the People

        c. The Leader Within—Creating the Leader Within Yourself

Figure 2-1

Nurse Manager Leadership
Collaborative Learning
Domain Framework

Source: Nurse Manager
Leadership Collaborative
(NMLC) (comprised of American
Organization of Nurse
Executives [AONE], the
American Association of
Critical-Care Nurses [AACN],
and the Association of
PeriOperative Registered
Nurses [AORN]) Learning
Domain Framework. http://www
.aone.org/aone/resource/NMLC/
nmlcLEARNING.html. Reprinted
by permission.

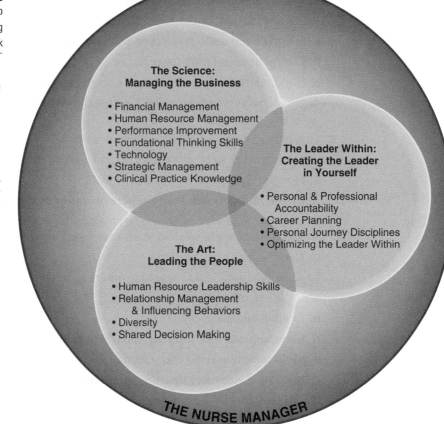

IV. THEORIES OF LEADERSHIP AND MANAGEMENT

A. Trait theory

1. Began during the early 1900s
2. Is sometimes called the "great man theory"
3. Individuals in key positions demonstrate certain personal qualities or traits
4. Focus is on the leader, not followers or the situation
5. Sought to identify inborn traits of successful leaders
6. Attempted to specify a universal set of leadership characteristics
7. Provided a benchmark by which most leaders continue to be judged
8. A menu of traits was developed, but no one trait or combination of traits was found to be acceptable

B. Leadership traits are often classified into three categories: intelligence, personality, and abilities; potential leaders possess and exhibit common traits:

1. Dominance
2. Aggressiveness
3. Ambition
4. High need to achieve
5. Self-confidence

► **Practice to Pass**

Describe two differences between the terms *leadership* and *management.*

6. Tolerance of others' viewpoints

7. Orderly thinking

8. Flexibility

C. Behavioral theories

1. Began in the early 1930s

   a. Focused on abilities and behaviors of leaders, including what leaders do

   b. Personal traits provide only one portion of leader capacity

   c. Leadership evolves through education, training, and life experiences

2. Four types of leadership styles:

   a. **Autocratic leadership**:

      1) Authoritarian and directive

      2) Individuals are motivated by power, authority, and need for approval

      3) Leader makes decisions for the group

      4) Assumes individuals are externally motivated

      5) Uses coercion and punishment

      6) Is most effective when used during an emergency or crisis

   b. **Democratic leadership**:

      1) Is consultative

      2) Assumes individuals are motivated by internal drives and impulses

      3) Leader desires active participation of others in decisions

      4) Leader desires to get tasks done

      5) Uses participation and majority rule for goal setting

   c. **Laissez-faire leadership**:

      1) Is nondirective and permissive

      2) Assumes individuals are motivated by internal drives and impulses

      3) Leaves the individual to make decisions about how to complete work

      4) The leader provides no direction or facilitation; uses hands-off approach

   d. **Bureaucratic leadership**:

      1) Is an inflexible approach

      2) Assumes that individuals are motivated by external forces

      3) Leader trusts neither followers nor self to make decisions

      4) Relies on organizational policies and rules to identify goals and direct work flow

3. Behavioral style of leadership includes initiating structure (task orientation) and consideration (people orientation) to achieve goals, as identified in Ohio State Leadership Studies

   a. Managers use initiating-structure behaviors to organize and define work goals, work patterns and methods, channels of communication, and roles

   b. Managers use consideration behaviors to show mutual trust, respect, friendship, warmth, and rapport between leader and followers

D. The managerial grid

1. Explains how managers move individuals toward goals based on concerns for work and people

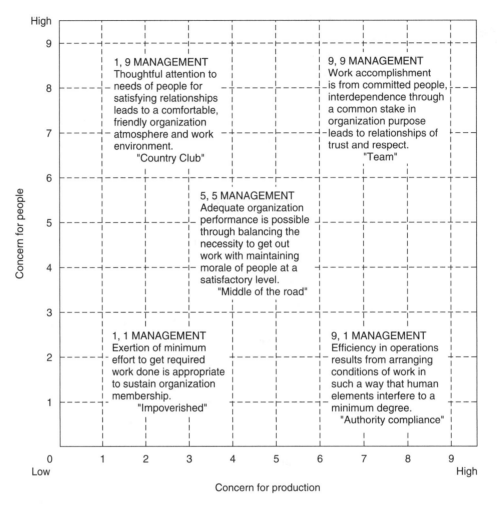

Figure 2-2

The managerial grid.

Source: Leadership Dilemmas—Grid Solutions, by R. R. Blake and A. A. McCanse, 1991, Austin, TX: Grid International. Copyright Elsevier (1991).

2. This behavioral leadership model was developed by Robert Blake and Jane Mouton

3. There are five leadership styles based on the concern for people and the concern for production that can be plotted into four quadrants of two-dimensional grid (see Figure 2-2)

    a. Impoverished management style (1,1): low concern for people, exertion of minimum effort to get required work done

    b. Authority compliance or task management style (9,1): high concern for production, low concern for people or efficiency in operations; minimizes interference of human elements

    c. Country club style (9,1): high concern for people, low concern for tasks or attention to needs of people, providing a comfortable, friendly atmosphere

    d. Middle of the road style (5,5): moderate concern for both tasks and people; balances need to get work done while maintaining morale at satisfactory level

    e. Team management style (9,9): high concern for both tasks and people; accomplishes work through committed people

E. Contingency theories

    1. Leaders adapt style according to the situation at hand

    2. Leader behavior ranges accordingly, from authoritarian to permissive

        a. Crisis situations often call for an authoritarian style to maintain command and control

        b. Problem-solving or consensus building calls for a participatory style to gain commitment and to respect followers' ideas and input

    3. Management style and organizational structure are also influenced by various aspects of the environment called contingency factors

    4. There is no one best way to lead; therefore, leaders must be able to base leadership style upon organizational environment, task to be achieved, and characteristics of their followers in order to be most effective

    5. Two examples of contingency models: Fiedler contingency theory and situational leadership theory

        a. Fiedler contingency theory

            1) Leadership effectiveness is based on "situational contingency," which is a result of interaction of two factors, known as leadership style and situational favorableness

            2) Leadership effectiveness is related to how best the leader's style (task-oriented or relationship-oriented) matches the current situation

            3) Fiedler identifies three situational factors that impact a leader's effectiveness:

                a) Manager-follower relationship (good to poor): if relations are good, the manager enjoys loyalty and support from followers

                b) Task structure (high to low): if the task is well-defined or standard procedures are followed

                c) Manager power (strong to weak): the ability of the leader to use legitimate power of position to reward or punish accordingly

            4) Task-leadership style is best used for high and low structured situations; relationship leadership style is more effective for intermediate situations

        b. Situational leadership theory considers the follower's readiness and willingness to perform a designated task; there are four leadership styles used according to readiness and ability of follower to perform task:

            1) The telling/directing style is used for followers who are unable and unwilling or insecure about performing an assigned task

            2) The selling/coaching style is used for followers who are unable but willing or confident in performing a task

            3) The participating/supporting style is used for followers able and willing and have confidence in performing a task

            4) The delegating/monitoring style used for followers who are fairly sophisticated in performance of the task and who are willing and able to perform the task; the follower is in charge of the situation and the leader lends support as needed

F. Contemporary theories

    1. Today's leaders realize the necessity of achieving organizational goals through effective and collaborative relationships built on trust and integrity; contemporary theories illustrate that the leader is only one component in the complexity of leadership

2. Quantum leadership
   a. The leader is viewed as an influential facilitator; followers assume an active role in decision-making
      1) Leadership is a shared activity
      2) Information is freely disseminated to followers and clients
      3) Leaders are expected to be expert communicators and to possess strong interpersonal skills
   b. Followers are equitable and accountable partners in client care outcomes
   c. Quantum leadership evolves from concepts of chaos theory
      1) Reality is constantly shifting
      2) Levels of complexity are constantly changing
      3) Movement reverberates throughout the system
      4) Roles are fluid and outcome oriented

3. Charismatic leadership: leaders have powerful personal qualities, such as charm, persuasiveness, personal power, self-confidence, extraordinary ideas, and strong convictions
   a. The leader's personality arouses affection and emotional commitment
   b. The leader's personality drives and advances the organization's vision, mission, and goals

4. **Transactional leadership**
   a. Is built on principles of social exchange
      1) Individuals engage in social interactions; they expect to give and receive rewards
      2) The exchange process between leaders and followers is economic
      3) Leaders are most successful when they understand and meet the needs of followers
      4) The social exchange between leader and follower continues until the exchange of performance and reward is no longer valuable
   b. Uses incentives to enhance follower loyalty and performance
      1) Is aimed at maintaining equilibrium or status quo
      2) Follower performs work according to policies and procedures
      3) It maximizes self-interests and personal rewards
      4) It fosters interpersonal dependence

5. **Transformational leadership**
   a. Emphasizes interpersonal relationships
   b. Is not concerned with the status quo
   c. Focuses on merging motives and values
   d. Generates followers' commitment to the leader's vision
   e. Fosters follower's inborn desires to pursue higher values and ideals
   f. Encourages followers to exercise leadership
   g. Inspires followers
   h. Uses power to instill the belief that followers can accomplish exceptional things

6. Relational leadership: acknowledges the importance of relationships as a cornerstone of effective leadership

   a. Connective relationships allow for better coordinated and integrated client care services in a caring, noncompetitive manner

   b. Connective leaders encourage collaboration and interpersonal skills to broker alliances

7. Shared leadership: is founded on principles of empowerment, participation, and transformational leadership

   a. No one person or leader possesses all knowledge and ability

   b. Elements of shared leadership include relationships, dialogues, partnerships, and understanding boundaries

   c. Different issues call for different responses

   d. Allows for appropriate leadership to emerge in relation to current problems and issues as they arise

8. **Servant leadership** begins with a focus on others and their specific strategies

   a. Focuses on desire to serve others

   b. Focuses on and utilizes desired leadership traits

   c. Believes the best of people

   d. Devoted to making people the best they can be

V. NURSING MANAGEMENT ROLE

A. **Includes being in a formal management position within the healthcare institution**

B. **Has the following functions:**

1. Establishes objectives and goals for one's area of responsibility and communicates with persons responsible for attaining them

2. Organizes and analyzes tasks, activities, decisions, and relationships needed and divides them into manageable tasks

3. Motivates and communicates with individuals responsible for various tasks through teamwork

4. Strives for excellence in **clinical practice** of nursing and delivery of client care on the selected unit or area within the healthcare institution

5. Manages human, fiscal, and other resources needed for clinical nursing practice and client care

6. Facilitates development of licensed and unlicensed nursing and healthcare personnel

7. Ensures institutional compliance with professional, regulatory, and government standards of care

8. Provides strategic planning as related to unit(s) or area(s), department, and organization as a whole

9. Facilitates cooperative and collaborative relationships among disciplines/departments to ensure the delivery of effective, quality client care

Figure 2-3

Levels of Leadership

Source: Fundamentals of Nursing (p. 121), by R. F. Craven & C. J. Hirnle, 2007, New York: Lippincott Williams & Wilkins. Reprinted by permission.

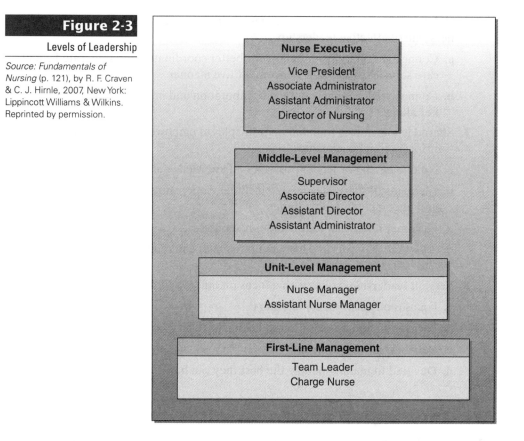

VI. LEVELS OF MANAGEMENT

A. **A nurse manager must accomplish the work of the organization**

B. **Work emerges from roles and functions of the job**

C. **Each organization develops differing levels of management and titles for management staff**

D. **Most healthcare organizations use leadership titles:** nurse executives, nurse managers, and charge nurses (see Figure 2-3)

1. First-Level Manager or Unit Manager: responsible for day-to-day activities or tasks of a specific work group; manager directs professional and ancillary staff members

2. Middle-Level Manager: responsible for supervising first-level managers and acting as a liaison between first-level manager and upper-level manager

3. Upper-Level Manager or Executive: responsible for developing strategic goals and direction for the organization

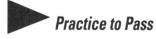

Practice to Pass

Describe how the nurse leader might understand similarities between the management process and the problem-solving process.

VII. ESSENTIAL CHARACTERISTICS OF AN EFFECTIVE MANAGER

A. **A nurse manager must:**

1. Be results or outcome oriented

2. Use problem solving, critical thinking, and team building when confronting clinical, economic, and personnel issues on daily basis

3. Be responsible for interpreting, enforcing, and supervising the unit/organization's policy, procedures, and regulations

B. Nurse manager scope of responsibility

1. Clinical excellence: ensuring high-level quality nursing care delivery

2. Provide for organization, coordination, and control of human, fiscal, and other resources

3. Strategic development and planning

   a. Ensure compliance with professional, regulatory, and governmental requirements and standards

   b. Provide for cross-discipline (or interdisciplinary) collaborative practice

C. Influence and power

1. Nurse leader must have ability to influence attitudes, actions, and behaviors of others to promote change and enhance the culture of the organization

2. Power is the potential ability to influence others

3. Power is based upon an individual's honor, respect, loyalty, and commitment

D. Nurse leader power requires:

1. Knowing about strengths and talents of followers

2. Knowing personal and professional values and visions

3. Demonstrating interpersonal competence

4. Knowing how to enlarge one's sphere of influence and connectedness

E. Types of power

1. Reward power: ability of the leader to provide rewards or incentives

2. Coercive power: ability of the leader to withhold or punish

3. Legitimate power: granted to an individual who occupies a specific position within an organization

4. Expert power: recognition of leader's knowledge, experience, and expertise

5. Referent power: respect and regard for the leader's character and talents

6. Charismatic power: ability to inspire and attract others

F. Using power

1. Nurse leaders apply their power base and use power effectively within their sphere of influence to make decisions and build consensus

2. Power never is abused or misused, but seeks to use:

   a. Persuasion over coercion

   b. Patience over impatience

   c. Compassion over confrontation (see Box 2-2 for rules on using power)

G. Competencies of the nurse manager

1. Critical thinking: a composite of knowledge, attitudes, and skills; ability to assess situation by asking open-ended questions about facts and assumptions that underlie it and use personal judgment and problem-solving ability in deciding how to deal with it

2. Problem solving: using a systematic process to solve a problem

3. Decision making: a purposeful and goal-directed effort using a systematic process to choose among options

Box 2-2	**1.** Use the least amount of power you can to be effective in your interactions with others.

Rules for Using Power

1. Use the least amount of power you can to be effective in your interactions with others.

2. Use power appropriate to the situation.

3. Learn when not to use power.

4. Focus on the problem, not the person.

5. Make polite requests, never arrogant demands.

6. Use coercion only when other methods don't work.

7. Keep informed to retain your credibility when using your expert power.

8. Understand you may owe a return favor when you use your connection power.

Source: E. J. Sullivan. (2004). *Becoming influential: A guide for nurses* (p. 35). Upper Saddle River, NJ: Prentice Hall. Reprinted by permission.

    4. Team building: supporting the efforts and work of a number of people associated together by specific tasks or activities

    5. Delegation: achieving performance of care outcomes for which an individual is accountable and responsible by sharing activities with others who have appropriate authority to accomplish the work

    6. Collaboration: an interdisciplinary type of problem solving that forms an equal power base on the client's behalf

    7. Professional and staff development: promoting further professional growth in work-related knowledge, skills, and abilities

    8. Change agent: an individual with formal or informal legitimate power whose purpose is to initiate, champion, and direct the change process

    9. Managing human and fiscal resources (people and money) to achieve outcomes that are consistent with the organization's mission and purpose

Case Study

As a nurse manager of an emergency department located in a large urban center, you have been notified of a five-alarm fire in a nearby housing complex. You have been informed by emergency medical services (EMS) to expect several casualties, including clients with full-thickness burns.

1. Describe the most appropriate leadership style to manage this crisis.

2. Explain why leadership development is important for nurses even if they are not in a formal management position in a healthcare organization, especially in an emergency situation.

3. Describe the core elements of the management process that would be used today by nurses or nurse managers in healthcare organizations.

4. Discuss the essential leadership characteristics that would be critical for this nurse leader to demonstrate during this emergency.

5. Discuss the types of power bases the nurse leader would apply in this emergency situation.

For suggested responses, see page 235.

POSTTEST

1 A nurse has been employed by a healthcare facility for 20 years. The nurse is knowledgeable, has excellent ideas, and actively participates in meetings. The nurse manager submits the nurse's name for an agency award to reward which type of leadership exemplified by the nurse?

1. Informal
2. Formal
3. Charismatic
4. Compassionate

2 A nurse manager delegates some tasks to the charge nurse, such as assisting with the development of the schedule, evaluations, employment, and termination of staff. The charge nurse is promoted to nurse manager of a surgical unit. The new nurse manager is aware that which type of leadership is inherent in the new position?

1. Informal
2. Formal
3. Compassionate
4. Charismatic

3 A nurse leader reinforces the healthcare agency's vision of client-centered care. The manager supports the clinical environment by doing which of the following? Select all that apply.

1. Putting the nurses' needs first
2. Putting clients' needs first
3. Enhancing quality care
4. Focusing on early client discharge
5. Focusing on safety

4 A staff nurse mentors new nurses and provides advice and guidance for staff. The nurse accepts voluntary tasks and jobs. The nurse manager identifies that this nurse uses which form of leadership?

1. Formal
2. Informal
3. Democratic
4. Laissez-faire

5 The new nurse manager plans to engage in which of the following actions as part of the role expectations of this new position?

1. Plan, organize, and supervise
2. Delegate and coordinate daily unit tasks
3. Restructure the organization
4. Critique the mission of the organization

6 A nurse manager assists other staff to support the agency's client-centered vision by installing a client conference room. The manager demonstrates which function of the management process?

1. Planning and setting direction
2. Organizing and aligning people
3. Getting others to believe the message
4. Controlling

7 A charge nurse often provides guidance to the staff and helps with problem solving as challenges arise. The charge nurse uses which strategy to develop staff members?

1. Personal attention
2. Role modeling
3. Precepting
4. Mentoring

8 A nurse manager who is confident, committed, and ambitious is implementing which managerial theory as a guide to personal leadership style?

1. Behavioral theory
2. Trait theory
3. Contemporary theory
4. Contingency theory

9 A nurse leader analyzes data on the number of urinary tract infections in clients on a medical unit. This leader uses which function of management?

1. Planning and setting direction
2. Organizing and aligning people
3. Getting others to believe in the message
4. Controlling

POSTTEST

10 The nurses on a clinical nursing unit are frustrated with the number of client falls on the unit during the last 3 months and a plan needs to be developed to reduce the unit's fall rate. The staff have voiced a number of ideas on how to accomplish this. Which situational leadership style would be best for the nurse leader to use in this situation to support staff in meeting this goal?

1. Telling/directing style
2. Selling/coaching style
3. Participating/supporting style
4. Delegating and monitoring style

➤ *See pages 44–46 for Answers and Rationales.*

ANSWERS & RATIONALES

Pretest

1 **Answer: 3** A leader uses charisma and social skills to exert power and influence over others. Leaders embrace change and get their followers to adopt change. One of the key characteristics of a leader is to facilitate others in changing their behaviors when appropriate. Of the positions listed, the one that involves working with nursing staff in the ways described in the question is the nurse manager. Nurse managers are also expected to have leadership abilities in addition to management skills. **Cognitive Level:** Application **Client Need:** Safe Effective Care Environment: Management of Care **Integrated Process:** Nursing Process: Analysis **Content Area:** Leadership/Management **Strategy:** Review all the options and choose the option that is the best fit for the description. Consider that case managers, chief operating officers, and chief financial officers may persuade others to buy into the agency's vision and mission, but the question specifically asks for a nurse leader. The closest fit is the nurse manager. **References:** Finkelman, A. W. (2006). *Leadership and management in nursing.* Upper Saddle River, NJ: Pearson Education, pp. 2–26; Sullivan, E. J., & Decker, P. (2005). *Effective leadership and management in nursing* (6th ed.). Upper Saddle River, NJ: Pearson Education, pp. 43–58.

2 **Answers: 1, 2, 3** Empowerment of nurses may be accomplished through decentralized decision making and representation of nurses on organizational committees. Nurses want their voices heard in the workforce. Empowerment is gained through contribution of opinions. Empowerment can also be gained through processes that analyze indicators specific for nursing in conjunction with the correction of clinical errors, all of which focus on client safety. It is not necessary to create additional positions (option 4) or forums that focus on negative aspects of the organization (option 5). **Cognitive Level:** Application **Client Need:** Safe Effective Care Environment: Management of Care **Integrated**

Process: Nursing Process: Implementation **Content Area:** Leadership/Management **Strategy:** Note that options 1, 2, and 3 demonstrate various forms of empowerment. However, option 4 presents as a barrier. Option 5 includes forums, but does not include a productive strategy to empower nurses. The critical word in the stem is *empowering.* Look for the options that address empowerment. **References:** Finkelman, A. W. (2006). *Leadership and management in nursing.* Upper Saddle River, NJ: Pearson Education, pp. 2–26; Sullivan, E. J., & Decker, P. (2005). *Effective leadership and management in nursing* (6th ed.). Upper Saddle River, NJ: Pearson Education, pp. 43–58.

3 **Answers: 1, 2, 4, 5** Nurse leaders show compassion toward their employees (option 1) and remain loyal to their employees and employers (option 2). The organization's mission (option 4), values, and goals drive nurse leaders. Leaders often analyze processes and change them accordingly (option 5). Although leaders are loyal to employees, their actions are not necessarily employee-driven. **Cognitive Level:** Application **Client Need:** Safe Effective Care Environment: Management of Care **Integrated Process:** Nursing Process: Implementation **Content Area:** Leadership/Management **Strategy:** First, recall that leaders have traits of being compassionate, loyal individuals to select options 1 and 2. Since not all decisions made by a leader are driven by employees, eliminate option 3. Recall next that effective leaders are driven by the agency's mission to select option 4. Finally, consider that leaders are process oriented to select option 5. **References:** Finkelman, A. W. (2006). *Leadership and management in nursing.* Upper Saddle River, NJ: Pearson Education, pp. 2–26; Sullivan, E. J., & Decker, P. (2005). *Effective leadership and management in nursing* (6th ed.). Upper Saddle River, NJ: Pearson Education, pp. 43–58.

4 **Answers: 1, 3, 5** A nurse leader possesses power and influence (option 1) to get others to change their behaviors. In addition, leaders are motivational (option 3);

they influence others to achieve the organization's goals. Their actions, values, and beliefs are consistent (option 5). In other words, they treat their employees fairly. Good leaders embrace change and get others to change when indicated, making options 2 and 4 incorrect. **Cognitive Level:** Application **Client Need:** Safe Effective Care Environment: Management of Care **Integrated Process:** Nursing Process: Assessment **Content Area:** Leadership/Management **Strategy:** Recall that leaders are powerful individuals who influence change in others. Leaders embrace change and transform others through change. With this in mind, eliminate options 2 and 4 as incorrect. Select the remaining options 1, 3, and 5 after recalling that these are consistent with leadership characteristics. **References:** Finkelman, A. W. (2006). *Leadership and management in nursing.* Upper Saddle River, NJ: Pearson Education, pp. 2–26; Sullivan, E. J., & Decker, P. (2005). *Effective leadership and management in nursing* (6th ed.). Upper Saddle River, NJ: Pearson Education, pp. 43–58.

5 **Answer: 4** Nurse managers use personal attention, role modeling, precepting, and mentoring to develop nurses professionally. In this question, the leader offers clinical advice to staff nurses and provides learning opportunities; both are congruent with mentoring (option 4) through support and guidance. Personal attention can occur without assisting in the development of staff (option 1). Role modeling consists of demonstrating behaviors for others to emulate (option 2). Precepting is a formal process of orientation to a job or role (option 3). **Cognitive Level:** Application **Client Need:** Safe Effective Care Environment: Management of Care **Integrated Process:** Nursing Process: Implementation **Content Area:** Leadership/Management **Strategy:** The goal here is to select the best specific answer to the question. Options 1, 2, and 3 could be plausible, but the best option is 4. This leader uses mentoring to develop staff. Use the "best choices" principle to make the correct selection. **References:** Finkelman, A. W. (2006). *Leadership and management in nursing.* Upper Saddle River, NJ: Pearson Education, pp. 2–26; Sullivan, E. J., & Decker, P. (2005). *Effective leadership and management in nursing* (6th ed.). Upper Saddle River, NJ: Pearson Education, pp. 43–58.

6 **Answer: 1** In this case, the leader is given formal power and authority to schedule the work of employees and reprimand staff if needed (option 1). This leader has legitimate authority. Shared leadership (option 4) is based on distributing leadership (informal leadership [option 2] in some cases) to other members of the team. Shared leadership and informal leadership are not addressed in this question. Compassionate leadership (option 3) is not addressed in this case.

Cognitive Level: Comprehension **Client Need:** Safe Effective Care Environment: Management of Care **Integrated Process:** Nursing Process: Analysis **Content Area:** Leadership/Management **Strategy:** Eliminate options 3 and 4 first because the question does not provide data to support compassionate leadership and shared leadership. Note that the leader is granted authority; therefore, one could deduce this leader has power that comes formal leadership. Use the "best choices" principle to select formal leadership (option 1) over informal leadership (option 2). **References:** Finkelman, A. W. (2006). *Leadership and management in nursing.* Upper Saddle River, NJ: Pearson Education, pp. 2–26; Sullivan, E. J., & Decker, P. (2005). *Effective leadership and management in nursing* (6th ed.). Upper Saddle River, NJ: Pearson Education, pp. 43–58.

7 **Answer: 1** A good leader gains the respect of the staff by providing rewards and supporting personal goals (option 1). This action shows the staff the leader respects them. The "country club" style of leadership (option 2) is primarily social in nature and does not necessarily facilitate respect from staff. While socialization (option 4) helps identify with the staff (option 3), it does not show the staff that the nurse leader values them. **Cognitive Level:** Application **Client Need:** Safe Effective Care Environment: Management of Care **Integrated Process:** Nursing Process: Implementation **Content Area:** Leadership/Management **Strategy:** Recall that the "country club" leader is a very social leader and option 4 also implies socialization, so rule out options 2 and 4. While identifying with employees is important (option 3), staff members want to feel respected. Thus, the best of the two remaining options is 1, which specifically addresses respect. Use the "best choices" principle to make the correct selection. **References:** Finkelman, A. W. (2006). *Leadership and management in nursing.* Upper Saddle River, NJ: Pearson Education, pp. 2–26; Sullivan, E. J., & Decker, P. (2005). *Effective leadership and management in nursing* (6th ed.). Upper Saddle River, NJ: Pearson Education, pp. 43–58.

8 **Answers: 2** The nurse manager is organizing and aligning people (option 2). Identifying goals for the unit keeps the staff on task and focused. People work best and show satisfaction with their work when they are given tasks that allow them to flourish and grow professionally and personally. Characteristics of controlling (option 4), planning and setting direction (option 1), and getting others to believe the message (option 3) are not addressed in this scenario. **Cognitive Level:** Application **Client Need:** Safe Effective Care Environment: Management of Care **Integrated Process:** Nursing Process: Implementation **Content Area:** Leadership/

Management **Strategy:** Look at the critical words *suited to their work ability* in the stem. Note that option 2 includes the term *align* in the answer, which is congruent with these critical words. Consider that although planning and setting direction may seem plausible, option 2 is a closer match. Options 3 and 4 do not apply to the stem and therefore must be eliminated. **References:** Finkelman, A. W. (2006). *Leadership and management in nursing.* Upper Saddle River, NJ: Pearson Education, pp. 2–26; Sullivan, E. J., & Decker, P. (2005). *Effective leadership and management in nursing* (6th ed.). Upper Saddle River, NJ: Pearson Education, pp. 43–58.

9 **Answer: 2** This nurse leader has been given a formal title of leadership. Informal leadership (option 2) occurs when the nurse does not have the title and power to accompany the influence the nurse has. Charisma and compassion (options 3 and 4) are not forms of leadership; they are, however, characteristics of good leaders. **Cognitive Level:** Comprehension **Client Need:** Safe Effective Care Environment: Management of Care **Integrated Process:** Nursing Process: Analysis **Content Area:** Leadership/Management **Strategy:** The question specifically asks for a type of leadership, which leads you to eliminate options 3 and 4 first . Consider that formal leaders are commissioned with a title while informal leaders have no title to choose option 2 over option 1. **References:** Finkelman, A. W. (2006). *Leadership and management in nursing.* Upper Saddle River, NJ: Pearson Education, pp. 2–26; Sullivan, E. J., & Decker, P. (2005). *Effective leadership and management in nursing* (6th ed.). Upper Saddle River, NJ: Pearson Education, pp. 43–58.

10 **Answer: 3** Nurse leaders should be driven by client care outcomes (option 3). Organizational changes are based on specific client indicators that are analyzed and scrutinized. Policies and procedures may be affected by the restructure but changes are guided by evidence-based practice. Although nurse safety (option 1) is considered in individual unit design, this is not the primary reason for restructuring the units. Rewarding success (option 2) is not addressed in the question. **Cognitive Level:** Application **Client Need:** Safe Effective Care Environment: Management of Care **Integrated Process:** Nursing Process: Planning **Content Area:** Leadership/Management **Strategy:** Identify what the question is asking then make the correct choice. Eliminate option 2 first because rewarding success does not fit the question. Next consider that although nurse safety is important (option 1), the restructure of units will not be based on this. Finally eliminate policy and procedure revision because these might follow restructuring, but not be the

driving force for it. The only option left is improving client care outcomes. **References:** Finkelman, A. W. (2006). *Leadership and management in nursing.* Upper Saddle River, NJ: Pearson Education, pp. 2–26; Sullivan, E. J., & Decker, P. (2005). *Effective leadership and management in nursing* (6th ed.). Upper Saddle River, NJ: Pearson Education, pp. 43–58.

Posttest

1 **Answer: 1** Informal leaders (option 1) do not hold an official title in the organization, but demonstrate profound efficiency influencing others. Formal leaders (option 2) have legitimate power and the ability to reward and punish. Charismatic leaders (option 3) empower their employees, foster participation in decision making, and attempt to transform individuals. Compassionate leaders (option 4) are driven by the needs of employees. **Cognitive Level:** Application **Client Need:** Safe Effective Care Environment: Management of Care **Integrated Process:** Nursing Process: Implementation **Content Area:** Leadership/Management **Strategy:** Think about the types of leadership. The two types of leadership listed are informal and formal, making options 3 and 4 incorrect. The nurse has not been granted an official title of leadership, making informal leadership correct. Use the "best choices" principle to make the correct selection. **References:** Finkelman, A. W. (2006). *Leadership and management in nursing.* Upper Saddle River, NJ: Pearson Education, pp. 2–26; Sullivan, E. J., & Decker, P. (2005). *Effective leadership and management in nursing* (6th ed.). Upper Saddle River, NJ: Pearson Education, pp. 43–58.

2 **Answer: 2** Formal leaders have legitimate power of the position held and the ability to reward and punish (option 1). Charismatic leaders (option 4) empower their employees, foster participation in decision making and attempt to transform individuals. The needs of the employees drive compassionate leaders (option 3). Informal leaders (option 2) do not hold an official title in the organization, but demonstrate profound efficiency influencing others. This leader moved from being an informal leader to a formal leader after demonstrating key characteristics essential in leadership. **Cognitive Level:** Application **Client Need:** Safe Effective Care Environment: Management of Care **Integrated Process:** Nursing Process: Analysis **Content Area:** Leadership/Management **Strategy:** The best way to answer this question is to reflect on the definitions of informal and formal leaders and apply that information to the question. Recognize that the new manager has an official title of leadership to make the correct selection. **References:**

Finkelman, A. W. (2006). *Leadership and management in nursing.* Upper Saddle River, NJ: Pearson Education, pp. 2–26; Sullivan, E. J., & Decker, P. (2005). *Effective leadership and management in nursing* (6th ed.). Upper Saddle River, NJ: Pearson Education, pp. 43–58.

3 **Answers: 2, 3, 5** Putting clients' needs first (option 2) supports the agency's vision and improves the quality of care (option 3) provided to clients. Option 1 is incorrect because it is opposite in focus to option 2. In providing safe care (e.g., medications, treatments, assessments) to clients, the nurse leader supports the vision of client-centered care. All of these aspects of care must be provided to clients in a safe manner (option 5). Focusing on early discharge (option 4) is incorrect because it may or may not support the vision of client-centered care. **Cognitive Level:** Application **Client Need:** Safe Effective Care Environment: Management of Care **Integrated Process:** Nursing Process: Planning **Content Area:** Leadership/Management **Strategy:** Eliminate option 1 first because it does not address the agency's vision of client-centered care. Next, eliminate option 4 because it may or may not improve client outcomes depending on individual client status and needs. Select each of the remaining options after noting the critical words *client-centered care* in the question. **References:** Finkelman, A. W. (2006). *Leadership and management in nursing.* Upper Saddle River, NJ: Pearson Education, pp. 2–26; Sullivan, E. J., & Decker, P. (2005). *Effective leadership and management in nursing* (6th ed.). Upper Saddle River, NJ: Pearson Education, pp. 43–58.

4 **Answer: 2** The staff nurse uses mentorship to provide leadership to peers and exhibits leadership skills through accepting additional tasks, both of which are informal leadership activities since the nurse does not have a formal (designated) position of leadership. Democratic leadership (option 3) involves participation and ruling by majority. Laissez-faire leadership (option 4) allows very little direction of staff and peers. **Cognitive Level:** Application **Client Need:** Safe Effective Care Environment: Management of Care **Integrated Process:** Nursing Process: Assessment **Content Area:** Leadership/Management **Strategy:** Note the critical words *staff nurse* in the question, which supports the definition of an informal leader rather than a formal leader. Look for the best answer that specifically answers the question. Options 3 and 4 may seem plausible, but the question does not provide any information leading one to believe the nurse is democratic or laissez-faire. **References:** Finkelman, A. W. (2006). *Leadership and management in nursing.* Upper Saddle River, NJ: Pearson Education, pp. 2–26; Sullivan, E. J., & Decker, P.

(2005). *Effective leadership and management in nursing* (6th ed.). Upper Saddle River, NJ: Pearson Education, pp. 43–58.

5 **Answer: 1** The roles of a nurse manager include planning and setting the direction of the unit through data collection and analysis. The role of the nurse manager continues with the organization of staff by identifying goals. Nurse managers must also sell the message to staff. Finally, managers must control activities on the unit through the implementation of standards and conducting evaluations. A charge nurse could delegate and coordinate daily unit tasks (option 2). It is beyond the scope of the nurse manager's role to restructure the organization (option 3) or critique the mission of the organization (option 4). **Cognitive Level:** Application **Client Need:** Safe Effective Care Environment: Management of Care **Integrated Process:** Nursing Process: Planning **Content Area:** Leadership/Management **Strategy:** Eliminate options 3 and 4 immediately because they are performed typically by an executive-level administrative team (such as chief executive officer, chief financial officer, chief nurse officer, vice presidents, etc.). Eliminate option 2 next because, although the manager may delegate some tasks, the wording of this option is more appropriate to a charge nurse. As an opposite strategy, select option 1 over option 2 because it is a broad statement that encompasses the functions of the nurse manager. **References:** Finkelman, A. W. (2006). *Leadership and management in nursing.* Upper Saddle River, NJ: Pearson Education, pp. 2–26; Sullivan, E. J., & Decker, P. (2005). *Effective leadership and management in nursing* (6th Ed.). Upper Saddle River, NJ: Pearson Education, pp. 43–58.

6 **Answer: 3** This nurse leader is successful in assisting staff to buy-in to a client-centered vision by providing a visible area in the environment that is conducive to implementing this vision. This is a function of leading and getting others to believe the message that client-centered care is important. Planning and setting direction (option 1) has already been accomplished with the focus on client-centered care. Controlling (option 4) and organizing people (option 2) are not addressed in this scenario. **Cognitive Level:** Comprehension **Client Need:** Safe Effective Care Environment: Management of Care **Integrated Process:** Nursing Process: Implementation **Content Area:** Leadership/Management **Strategy:** The question does not provide information to support planning, setting direction, organizing, aligning people, and controlling. The only option that fits is 3. Use the "best choices" principle to make the correct selection. **References:** Finkelman,

A. W. (2006). *Leadership and management in nursing.* Upper Saddle River, NJ: Pearson Education, pp. 2–26; Sullivan, E. J., & Decker, P. (2005). *Effective leadership and management in nursing* (6th ed.). Upper Saddle River, NJ: Pearson Education, pp. 43–58.

7 **Answer: 1** The definition of personal attention includes providing support and problem solving. Role modeling is the encouragement of self-management and assessment along with openness. Precepting includes training staff. In mentoring, the leader shares skills with the staff. **Cognitive Level:** Application **Client Need:** Safe Effective Care Environment: Management of Care **Integrated Process:** Nursing Process: Planning **Content Area:** Leadership/Management **Strategy:** The goal here is to select the specific answer to the question. Note that options 2, 3, and 4 could be plausible, but the best option is 1. The leader uses personal attention to develop staff. Use the "best choices" principle to make the correct selection. **References:** Finkelman, A. W. (2006). *Leadership and management in nursing.* Upper Saddle River, NJ: Pearson Education, pp. 2–26; Sullivan, E. J., & Decker, P. (2005). *Effective leadership and management in nursing* (6th ed.). Upper Saddle River, NJ: Pearson Education, pp. 43–58.

8 **Answer: 2** The trait theory suggests leaders possess key characteristics that increase their likelihood of effective leadership. Ambition, commitment, and self-confidence are all traits common to good leaders. Behavioral theories (option 1) are based on the actions of the leader. Leaders who use contingency theories (option 4) adjust their leadership style based on the current situation. Contemporary leadership (option 3) is based on the premise of collaboration and building relationships. **Cognitive Level:** Comprehension **Client Need:** Safe Effective Care Environment: Management of Care **Integrated Process:** Nursing Process: Implementation **Content Area:** Leadership/Management **Strategy:** The stem describes characteristics of a leader. All options may seem plausible, but trait theory is based on the premise that leaders possess specific characteristics. Option 2 specifically answers the question. The other options are not strongly linked to the stem. **References:** Finkelman, A. W. (2006). *Leadership and management in nursing.* Upper Saddle River, NJ: Pearson Education, pp. 2–26; Sullivan, E. J., & Decker, P. (2005). *Effective leadership and management in nursing* (6th ed.). Upper Saddle River, NJ: Pearson Education, pp. 43–58.

9 **Answer: 1** The nurse leader is gathering data and looking for patterns to help identify causes and solutions of urinary tract infections on the unit. Data collection is consistent with planning and setting direction. Analyzing these data allow the nurse leader to possibly set directions for the future of the unit. The other three options are not addressed in this scenario. **Cognitive Level:** Comprehension **Client Need:** Safe Effective Care Environment: Management of Care **Integrated Process:** Nursing Process: Planning **Content Area:** Leadership/Management **Strategy:** The stem does not provide any information that support options 3 and 4. While organizing is plausible, aligning people does not fit, making this option incorrect. The best choice is option one. Identify critical words in the question or stem to select the right answer. **References:** Finkelman, A. W. (2006). *Leadership and management in nursing.* Upper Saddle River, NJ: Pearson Education, pp. 2–26; Sullivan, E. J., & Decker, P. (2005). *Effective leadership and management in nursing* (6th ed.). Upper Saddle River, NJ: Pearson Education, pp. 43–58.

10 **Answer: 4** Four leadership styles can be used according to readiness and ability of followers to perform a task. A telling/directing style (option 1) is used for followers unable and unwilling or insecure about performing assigned task. A selling/coaching style (option 2) is used for followers unable but willing or confident in performing task. A participating/supporting style (option 3) is used for followers that are able and willing and have confidence in performing task. A delegating/monitoring style (option 4) is used for followers fairly sophisticated in task and willing and able to perform task; the followers are in charge of the situation and the leader lends support as needed. **Cognitive Level:** Application **Client Need:** Safe Effective Care Environment: Management of Care **Integrated Process:** Nursing Process: Implementation **Content Area:** Leadership/Management **Strategy:** Read the situation carefully and consider the definitions of each of the situational leadership styles identified in the question. Because in this case the nurses understand the problem and are willing to solve it, option 4 is the best choice. **References:** Finkelman, A. W. (2006). *Leadership and management in nursing.* Upper Saddle River, NJ: Pearson Education, pp. 2–26; Sullivan, E. J., & Decker, P. (2005). *Effective leadership and management in nursing* (6th ed.). Upper Saddle River, NJ: Pearson Education, pp. 43–58.

ANSWERS & RATIONALES

References

American Association of Colleges of Nursing. (2002). *Hallmarks of the professional nursing practice environment.* Washington, DC: Author.

American Association of Colleges of Nursing. (1999). *Faculty shortages intensify nation's nursing deficit.* Issue Bulletin. Washington, DC: Author.

Association of Nurse Executives. *Nurse Manager Leadership Collaborative (NMLC) Learning Domain Framework.* Retrieved August 30, 2007, from http://www.aone.org/aone/resource/NMLC/nmlc

Association of Nurse Executives. *Principles and Elements of a Healthful Practice/Work Environment.* Retrieved August 30, 2007, from http://www.aone.org/aone/pdf/PrinciplesandElementsHealthfulWorkPractice.pdf

Bennis, W. (1989). *On becoming a leader.* Reading, MA: Addison-Wesley.

Blake, R. R., & Mouton, J. S. (1985). The managerial grid III. Houston, TX: Gulf Publishing.

Conforti, M. (2000). Archetypal dynamics of leadership: Recognizing patterns in the organization. *The Inner Edge, 3*(5), 10–12.

Covey, S. R. (1992). *Principled-centered leadership.* New York: Simon & Schuster.

Craven, R. F., & Hirnle, C. J. (2007). *Fundamentals of nursing* (5th ed.). Philadelphia: Lippincott Williams & Wilkins.

Fiedler, F. A. (1967). *A theory of leadership effectiveness.* New York: McGraw-Hill.

Finkelman, A. W. (2006). *Leadership and management in nursing.* Upper Saddle River, NJ: Pearson Education.

Greenleaf, R. K. (1991). *The servant as leader.* Indianapolis: The Robert K. Greenleaf Center.

Kerfoot, K. (2000). On leadership: Leading from the inside out. *Nursing Economics, 18*(6), 6–7.

Mathena, K. A. (2002). Nursing manager leadership skills. *Journal of Nursing Administration, 32*(3), 136–142.

Mowinski Jennings, B., Scalzi, C. C., Rodgers, J. D., & Keane, A. (2007). Differentiating nursing leadership and management competencies. *Nursing Outlook, 55*(4), 169–175.

Porter-O'Grady, T. & Malloch, K. (2002). *Quantum leadership: A textbook of new leadership.* Gaithersburg, MD: Aspen.

Sullivan, E. J., & Decker, P. J. (2005). *Effective leadership and management in nursing.* Upper Saddle River, NJ: Pearson Education.

Ward, K. (2002). A vision for tomorrow: Transformational nursing leaders. *Nursing Outlook, 50*(3), 121–126.

Yoder-Wise, S. (2007). *Leading and managing in nursing* (4th ed.). St. Louis, MO: C.V. Mosby.

3 The Essentials of Ethics

Chapter Outline

Ethics versus Morals

Ethical Theories

Ethical Principles

Professional and Ethical Behavior

Types of Ethical Dilemmas

Model for Ethical Decision Making

American Nurses Association (ANA) Code of Ethics

Objectives

➤ Define the terms ethics and morals.

➤ Explain three ethical theories.

➤ Describe an ethical dilemma.

➤ Discuss three ethical issues in nursing practice.

➤ Identify the steps of the ethical decision-making process.

Review at a Glance

autonomy ability of an individual to determine his or her own course of action, also called self-determination

beneficence a duty to help others to further their important and legitimate interests by promoting good consequences

code of ethics a set of guidelines for professional practice that contains the values of the profession

confidentiality the ability to hold secret the confidences to which one is entrusted

deontology a principle-based theory that examines the moral significance of an act and contemplates the rightness or wrongness of the act itself

distributive justice a type of justice in which there is a fair and equitable distribution of limited resources and material benefits among members of society

ethics a branch of philosophy dealing with broad issues of morality, moral problems, and moral judgments and issues of human conduct, including actions considered to be right and wrong

ethical dilemma a situation in which various courses of action are suggested by competing moral options, none of which are completely satisfactory

ethical theory a model of moral values that provides approaches for identifying ethical choices

fidelity the act of keeping one's promises or commitments

informed consent a willingness to accept a particular intervention based on clear information about viable treatment options and their risks and benefits

justice a principle that treats all people equally and fairly

nonmaleficence an obligation to do no harm

values standards of choice that provide meaningful direction to an individual or group

values clarification a conscious process for identifying and ranking the importance of one's personal values

veracity truthfulness or power of perceiving and conveying truth

utilitarianism an ethical action referring to pleasure or utility, any source of happiness, good, benefit, or advantage, or any means of preventing pain, evil, or unhappiness

PRETEST

1 A nurse is newly assigned to the care of a client who has not been involved in the plan of care and instead, decisions have been made for the client. The nurse is concerned that which principle is of greatest concern in this client's situation?

1. Maleficence
2. Deontology
3. Autonomy
4. Beneficence

2 A nurse manager observes a staff nurse access a client's financial records. When asked about this behavior, the nurse responded, "As a nurse, I have a right to know the client's financial status." What is the best response of the nurse manager?

1. "You are not planning for this client's discharge."
2. "This is a breach in the client's confidentiality."
3. "What is your purpose in accessing the financial record?"
4. "While partial access is necessary, access to the client's financial record is not necessary."

3 A 15-year-old teenager confides in a nurse that she is ready to engage in sexual activity with her boyfriend. How should the nurse respond?

1. "Unfortunately, I'll have to tell your mother about this."
2. "We can make an appointment with a gynecologist."
3. "How do you plan to pay for your doctor's visit?"
4. "Have you had any conversations with your parents about this?"

4 A client scheduled for cardiac catheterization in two hours requests more information about the risks and benefits of the procedure. The nurse calls the cardiologist who demands that the nurse provide the client with the information and tell the client to sign the consent. What is the nurse's best response?

1. "This is inappropriate; this client deserves this information from you."
2. "Informed consent is the physician's responsibility. When are you coming in?"
3. "I will refer this case to the medical director for further input and guidance."
4. "My legal role in informed consent is to act as a witness, not to provide information about the procedure and its risks and benefits."

PRETEST

5 State boards of nursing protect the public from in-competent nurses. The safety of the public is secured by which of the following? Select all that apply.

1. National licensure examination
2. Practice regulation
3. Definition of practice by each state
4. Differentiated education
5. Continuing education credits

6 A client who is scheduled for surgery has signed the consent. The client is in the preoperative area of the operating room and tells the nurse that he has decided not to have the surgery. What is the best response by the nurse?

1. "You have signed the consent, you must have the surgery."
2. "You have the right to refuse the surgical procedure."
3. "You may refuse the surgical procedure. Can you share your concerns with me?"
4. "I'll have the surgeon speak to you at once."

7 A client is who is about to receive preoperative medication before surgery expresses doubts about the surgery and tells the nurse she is thinking about not having the surgery. In considering what reply to make to the client, the nurse determines that which nursing role is of highest priority at this time?

1. Advocate
2. Care manager
3. Direct caregiver
4. Educator

8 A nursing assistant asks a nurse, "Why is a national examination required to get a license as a nurse?" What is the nurse's best response?

1. "The national licensure exam identifies whether nurses are safe or unsafe to practice."
2. "The national licensure exam tests the physical skills that nurses must have to practice."
3. "The national licensure exam helps the state boards of nursing track the success of their nursing programs."
4. "The national licensure exam filters out weak nursing students just before they graduate."

9 A nurse wonders about the morality of an individual who had an abortion. What should the nurse recall about morals? Select all that apply.

1. Morals are influenced by environmental factors.
2. Morals are unchanging, private, and personal.
3. Morals are principles of right conduct.
4. Morals are applied to daily life circumstances.
5. Morals require deep religious connections.

10 A chief executive officer (CEO) decides to provide health maintenance organization (HMO) services to employees to provide follow-up care for chronic conditions. Approximately 70% of the employees have some form of chronic conditions that require follow-up medical services. However, employees who do not have chronic illnesses do not benefit from this service and must continue to pay for all preventive services. A nurse employee concludes that which ethical theory most likely guided the CEO's decision?

1. Deontology
2. Utilitarianism
3. Justice
4. Beneficence

➤ *See pages 59–62 for Answers and Rationales.*

I. ETHICS VERSUS MORALS

    A. Nurse leaders have an obligation to address ethical problems or dilemmas as they arise and to resolve them; the following are key approaches to addressing and solving ethical issues:

        1. Understanding the foundations of ethical practice

        2. Developing astute ethical decision-making skills

        3. Realizing ethical issues are common in clinical nursing practice and healthcare

    B. *Ethics:* a system of moral rules and principles that becomes the standard for professional conduct

        1. Reflects "should" behavior; identifies what should be done to live with others in civil society

        2. Involves a process of analyzing appropriateness and effects of human action

        3. Is a science that addresses principles of right and wrong, good and bad

        4. Is a formal process used to assess right conduct

        5. Is professionally and publicly stated

    C. Morals: established rules of conduct in situations where decisions about right and wrong must be made

        1. Reflect what is done

        2. Provide standards of behavior that guide actions of an individual or social group

    D. Morality: an individual's personal standard of what is right and wrong in conduct, character, and attitude

        1. Involves principles and rules of right conduct

        2. Is private and personal

        3. Implies a commitment to principles and values that are applied to daily life circumstances

> **▶ Practice to Pass**
>
> Describe how personal morality is different from professional ethics.

II. ETHICAL THEORIES

    A. *Ethical theory:* model of moral values that provides:

        1. Structure for clarifying and examining the moral basis for one's professional duties

        2. Obligations

        3. Judgments

        4. Actions in situations where moral conflict emerges

    B. Types of ethical theories

        1. Consequence-based: focus on the rightness of an action based on the consequences produced

        2. Utilitarianism: a consequentialist theory that focuses on providing benefits to achieve the greatest good and least harm for the greatest number

           a. Ethical action: any source of happiness, good, benefit, or advantage, or any means of preventing pain or unhappiness

           b. Pleasure or pain are subjective feelings and require people to define for themselves what might be a positive or negative action

3. **Deontology:** a principle-based theory that focuses on duties or means rather than on an end goal
   a. Looks at the inherent moral significance of an act
   b. Considers rightness and wrongness of the act itself
4. Character ethics: are relationship based; focuses on traits of a person that promote goodwill; traits can be cultivated through moral reasoning

III. ETHICAL PRINCIPLES

A. **Ethical principle:** a concept that guides decision making in clinical practice and in life in general; a foundation that the nurse leader uses in all types of decision making
   1. Includes general, broad philosophical concepts
   2. Provides a foundation of moral rules and specific responses to actions/situations
   3. Without principles to guide healthcare ethics (see Box 3-1), clinical care decisions are determined based on personal values and emotions

B. **Ethical principles important to nursing practice**
   1. **Autonomy:** a principle that affirms the ability of an individual to determine his or her own course of action, also called self-determination
      a. An autonomous person decides a personal course of action that is defined by personal values and is a self-chosen plan
      b. This principle is based on the concept that human beings are capable of making independent choices
   2. **Beneficence:** a principle in which an individual helps others to further their important and legitimate interests by promoting good consequences
      a. There is a duty to weigh the possible good against the possible harm of each action
      b. Nursing actions and interventions often have both harmful and beneficial consequences and so must be considered carefully
   3. **Justice:** a principle in which there is an obligation to treat all people fairly
      a. **Distributive justice:** fair and equitable distribution of limited resources and material benefits among all citizens of society
      b. The principle of justice in healthcare suggests that clients with the same diagnosis and needs should receive the same care; refers to equality in allocation of resources
      c. This is not always possible because some resources are scarce, such as organs for donation or healthcare dollars
   4. **Nonmaleficence:** a principle in which there is an obligation to do no harm
      a. Harm can be deliberate

Box 3-1	**Beneficence**—Doing or promoting good.
Principles of Healthcare Ethics	**Nonmaleficence**—Avoiding doing harm.
	Autonomy—Maintaining independence and self-direction.
	Justice—Fairness or treating all clients equally and fairly.
	Ethical rules seek to guide healthcare decision making and may also include veracity, fidelity, privacy, and confidentiality.

b. Risk of harm can be limited

c. Unintentional harm may occur in the course of healthcare treatment

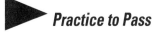 **5. Veracity:** truthfulness or power of perceiving and conveying the truth

a. Nurses tell the truth and do not intentionally deceive or mislead

b. Clients have the right to full and accurate information about their health status and treatment

6. Fidelity: the principle of respecting, maintaining, and carrying out promises one makes; nurses and nurse leaders are expected to be:

a. Respectful toward clients, staff, and other health professionals

b. Competent in clinical supervision and clinical skills

c. Able to implement quality standards

d. Able to protect clients from incompetent, illegal, or unethical practice

e. Able to honor agreements made in the course of the nurse-client relationship

C. Values

1. Values are defined as the attitudes, ideals, and beliefs that one uses to guide behavior; they are freely chosen and are influenced by upbringing and life experiences

2. Values often emerge from an individual's:

a. Culture

b. Ethnic background

c. Religion

d. Social traditions

e. Family and peer group

3. Values influence behavior by:

a. Acting as an internal control for behavior

b. Manifesting in patterns of behavior

D. Personal values: standards of choice that provide meaningful direction to an individual

E. Professional values: core professional values (see Table 3-1) define good practice, are affirmed by the professional organization, are acquired during socialization into professional nursing, and include:

1. A strong commitment to service

2. A belief in the dignity and worth of each person

3. A commitment to education

Practice to Pass

Define at least three principles of healthcare ethics.

Table 3-1	Value	Definition
Definitions of the Five Core Professional Nursing Values	Human Dignity	Respect for the inherent worth and uniqueness of individuals and populations
	Integrity	Acting in accordance with an appropriate code of ethics and accepted standards of practice
	Autonomy	The right to self-determination
	Altruism	A concern for the welfare and well-being of others
	Social Justice	Upholding moral, legal, and humanistic principles

Source: American Association of Colleges of Nursing. (1998). *The essentials of baccalaureate education: For professional nursing practice.* Washington, DC: Author. Reprinted by permission.

F. *Values clarification:* a conscious process for identifying and ranking the importance of one's personal values
   1. No single set of values is right for everyone
   2. Values can be retained or change over a lifetime
   3. Values often reflect personal growth

G. **The valuing process includes three important domains:**
   1. Cognitive: reflecting upon alternatives resulting in freely chosen beliefs
   2. Affective: choosing cherished beliefs
   3. Behavioral: incorporating chosen beliefs into behaviors, affirming them to others, and consistently repeating them

IV. PROFESSIONAL AND ETHICAL BEHAVIOR

A. **Professional and ethical behavior is often established by expectations set by nurse leaders, the healthcare organization, and nursing staff**

B. **Ethical behavior is having relevant facts available as evidence pointing toward a decision and having relevant knowledge to apply those facts**

C. **Ethical decision making**
   1. Nurse leaders must make decisions at times that challenge the values that they may personally cherish
   2. Values reflect ideals, standards, principles, beliefs, objects, and behaviors that give meaning and direction to life
   3. The process of clarifying values assists the nurse leader in making decisions

D. ***Ethical dilemma***
   1. A difficult moral problem that involves two or more mutually exclusive, morally correct courses of action
   2. Nurse leaders may confront a variety of ethical dilemmas arising from:
      a. Situations that involve conflicting values
      b. Competing moral claims
      c. Weighing benefits against burdens
      d. Weighing good against harm
   3. What is right in one situation may be subjectively different for each individual

V. TYPES OF ETHICAL DILEMMAS

A. **Nurses and other healthcare professionals are continually confronted with ethical dilemmas**
   1. Dilemmas often have no clear resolution or solution
   2. Dilemmas involve high emotion and are often more difficult to resolve than other problems associated with treatment and nursing care
   3. Dilemmas require time and deep reflection and sometimes lead to uncomfortable feelings and anxiety
   4. There is often lack of agreement in seeking ethical solutions because of differing personal values among healthcare professionals involved in the ethical dilemma

Box 3-2	**Dilemmas involving peers/professionals**

Common Ethical Dilemmas

- Should a baby with multiple severe anomalies be resuscitated?
- Should a 95-year-old client be given the ICU bed?
- How should a suspected drug-abusing registered nurse be confronted?
- Should nurses with a right-to-life perspective be mandated to care for clients seeking abortions?

Dilemmas involving clients

- Whether to resuscitate a client who has no advance directive.
- Nurses' responsibilities when clients refuse blood transfusions or surgery.
- Should a client be restrained because he is wandering the halls?
- Should a client be given medication because he is loud and abusive?

Dilemmas involving institutional issues

- Which hospital should have a cardiac department or pediatric ICU?
- How should clients without health insurance be cared for?

B. Ethical dilemmas in nursing often call for making a choice between two or more unsatisfactory alternatives; an action taken by the nurse leader may be considered good but not necessarily right; consensus is difficult to reach and some may be unsatisfied by the decision that is reached

C. Examples of situations that might lead to ethical dilemmas (see also Box 3-2):

1. Cost containment issues: how to balance cost-saving constraints of managed care against healthcare needs of people with limited resources

2. End-of-life care: how to decide who can be transferred from a critical care bed so that it is available for sicker person

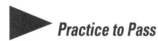

Practice to Pass

Have you been faced with an ethical dilemma? Are you satisfied with the way you handled your part? Describe how you would resolve your ethical dilemma.

3. Situations related to **informed consent**: a willingness to accept a particular intervention based on clear information about viable treatment options and their risks and benefits

4. Incompetent, unethical, or illegal practice of colleagues

5. Access to care for clients

6. Breaches of **confidentiality** (the ability to hold secret the confidences to which one is entrusted)

7. Issues in the care of clients with human immunodeficiency virus (HIV) or acquired immunodeficiency syndrome (AIDS)

8. Organ transplantation

9. Reproductive choices and therapies

10. End-of-life pain management issues

11. Use of advanced directives

VI. MODEL FOR ETHICAL DECISION MAKING

A. Nurse leaders are involved in collective or individual decisions; therefore, they need to know the steps in the ethical decision making process; these steps are not intended to be rigid (see Box 3-3)

Box 3-3	Ethical dilemmas often result if there are conflicting choices and it is difficult to determine which is the best choice because either one will not solve all of the problems.

How to Resolve an Ethical Dilemma

1. Start by identifying the feelings of all those who are involved in the situation.
2. Describe all the known facts and issues surrounding the situation.
3. Identify any and all alternative choices in the situation, looking toward what outcomes support the goals for the client's treatment plan.
4. Seek to clarify who is accountable for each part of the client's plan.
5. Be sure to check to see that all those involved have completed their components the plan.
6. Ensure that any consequences of the plan are resolved. If not, the ethical dilemma may be presented to the institution's ethics committee where recommendations for resolution may be sought.

B. **Ethical decision making:** a process in which ideas are thoroughly examined to determine the best solution in a difficult situation; it requires nurse leaders to make accurate assessments, thoughtful reflections, and constant evaluations; ethical problems are complex and common in clinical nursing practice

C. **Steps in ethical decision making:**
   1. Clarify the ethical dilemma/identify problem
   2. Gather additional data as needed
   3. Identify potential options and ethical principles that support each option
   4. Assist others in decision making
   5. Select the most appropriate course of action to address the ethical dilemma
   6. Evaluate the results of the choice of action

VII. AMERICAN NURSES ASSOCIATION (ANA) CODE OF ETHICS

A. A *code of ethics* is described as an implied contract through which a group or profession informs society of the rules and principles of how it will function
   1. It informs new professionals of ethical positions accepted by other members of the profession and guides professional behavior
      a. The code is a set of principles shared by members of profession
      b. It reflects professional moral judgment over time
      c. It serves as standard for professional action
      d. It sets a standard that is higher than the legal standard
   2. The *Code of Ethics for Nurses with Interpretive Statements* (ANA) is latest version of nursing's ethical code

B. **ANA Code of Ethics for Nurses**
   1. Is a 9-point code that helps nurses to understand that clients, families, groups, and/or communities are their first obligation
   2. A nurse leader must seek to ensure that provisions of the code are integrated into nursing care

3. The ANA Code commits to following values:
   a. Client dignity
   b. Privacy
   c. Safety
   d. Fair and equal treatment of clients
   e. Client advocacy
   f. Maintenance of professional competency
   g. Responsibility
   h. Accountability
   i. General maintenance and well-being of the nursing profession

C. **Purpose of the Code of Ethics**
   1. To provide a decision-making framework for solving ethical problems and offer ways of resolving them
   2. A nurse leader can role model ethical principles and ensure that frontline staff adhere to ethical conduct in practice settings
   3. A nurse leader can create an ethically principled environment that seeks to uphold standards of conduct set by the code
   4. A nurse leader has the responsibility to create an ethical climate in the workplace that allows staff nurses to experience congruence among caring for clients, fulfilling organizational mission, and having a supportive work environment
   5. Creating an ethical work climate has the following benefits:
      a. Increases employee morale
      b. Enhances organizational commitment
      c. Fosters an engaged and retained workforce
      d. Contributes to quality client care outcomes
      e. Improves overall organizational success

D. **Ethics committees:**
   1. Are interdisciplinary committees that help healthcare organizations develop ethical guidelines
   2. Review ethical dilemmas or situations referred by healthcare professional members
   3. Write, review, or revise the institutional policy on ethical considerations
   4. Educate staff and the community about ethical and moral issues
   5. Have as a function to deliberate without prejudice on basis of what is justifiable and what serves the rights and well-being of individual clients
   6. Nurse leaders play active role on ethics committees and are critical members

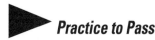

Practice to Pass

Read and Review the Code of Ethics for Nurses. Explain why nurse leaders would need to be familiar with the Code.

Case Study

As the nurse manager of the Pediatric Intensive Care Unit (ICU), a staff nurse has just informed you about giving an accidental medication overdose to an assigned 5-year-old client. The parents notice their child is very drowsy and ask for an explanation about their child's condition. The staff nurse replies, "There is nothing to worry about." What do you do?

1. Explain the values that influence your decision about the appropriate action to take.

2. State the ethical dilemma described in this situation.

3. State the problem inherent in this situation.

4. Discuss the ethical decision-making process you would use in resolving the issue.

5. What approach would you use in the future regarding medication errors involving your assigned staff?

For suggested responses, see pages 235–236.

POSTTEST

1. A nurse responds to a combative client by hitting the client on the legs. The nurse manager bases disciplinary action solely on the nurse's response to the client. The chief nurse officer (CNO) who is reviewing the case concludes that the nurse manager used which ethical principle to discipline the nurse?

1. Deontology
2. Utilitarianism
3. Justice
4. Beneficence

2. A client who is terminally ill with cancer has a choice of three treatment options. The healthcare provider decides the client will benefit from one option and leaves the client out of the decision-making process. The staff nurse on the unit considers whether to contact the Ethics Committee after concluding that the healthcare provider has breached which ethical principle?

1. Beneficence
2. Nonmaleficence
3. Justice
4. Autonomy

3. The clinical rule for a nursing school is that students who arrive late to clinical must function in a nursing assistant role for the day. An instructor upholds the rule for student A, but does not uphold the rule for student B. Student B concludes that the instructor has breached which ethical principle?

1. Justice
2. Deontology
3. Utilitarianism
4. Fidelity

4. A client who has right hemiparesis calls for assistance to go to the bathroom. The nurse who answers the call bell completes a few additional tasks on the way to the client's room. The client becomes impatient, attempts to go to the bathroom, and falls. Upon learning of this incident, the nurse manager uses which statement to discuss the appropriate ethical principle with the nurse?

1. "This incident directly challenges your veracity with clients."
2. "This incident indicates that you have a lack of respect for your clients."
3. "This incident exemplifies that you have failed to act in a manner consistent with beneficence to the client."
4. "This incident shows that you have little regard toward fidelity to your client."

5 A nurse seeking to uphold which ethical principle would allow a client who has residual deficits from a stroke to complete as much of the bath as possible while remaining at the bedside to provide assistance when needed?

1. Justice
2. Veracity
3. Autonomy
4. Fidelity

6 In a healthcare system, the average length of stay (LOS) for clients who have Medicaid health insurance is two days shorter than clients with private insurance. This issue has been referred to the Ethics Committee of the hospital. A nurse representative on this committee makes which statement to identify the best ethical principle that might be applied to this case?

1. "This practice is not treating some clients well, so what we are dealing with in this case is an issue of beneficence."
2. "Some clients were not aware that other clients were able to remain in the hospital longer, so we are faced with an issue of veracity."
3. "We are supposed to be acting in the best interests of our clients and so therefore the clearest issue is a breach of fidelity."
4. "Some clients are being treated differently from others, and therefore this case is clearly about the issue of justice."

7 It is discovered that a healthcare provider has been adding charges to clients' bills for services that were never rendered. When this matter is referred to the hospital Ethics Committee, the nurse representative considers that which ethical principles may be at issue in this case? Select all that apply.

1. Justice
2. Beneficence
3. Veracity
4. Fidelity
5. Nonmaleficence

8 A nurse leader uses education and socialization to guide leadership decisions. This nurse leader has made a choice to be guided by which of the following in the decision-making process?

1. Culture
2. Values
3. Purpose
4. Preference

9 A nurse is time-oriented and persistent in getting tasks done. The nurse manager notes these qualities in the employee and recognizes that these characteristics emerge from the nurse's: (Select all that apply.)

1. Culture.
2. Family group.
3. Academic preparation.
4. Occupation.
5. Spirituality.

10 A nurse seeking to maintain ethical personal behavior would focus on doing which of the following in clinical practice? Select all that apply.

1. Use standard methods of practice
2. Use ethical principles
3. Evaluate personal morals
4. Refer ethical decisions to the appropriate committee
5. Familiarize oneself with ANA Code of Ethics

➤ *See pages 62–64 for Answers and Rationales.*

ANSWERS & RATIONALES

Pretest

1 Answer: 3 This client has not provided any input into the plan of care, which takes away the client's autonomy. Autonomy allows a client to determine the course of treatment or action by healthcare providers. Beneficence addresses the duty to promote good consequences for clients, whereas nonmaleficence is the duty to cause no harm to clients. Deontology is focused on the moral significance of an action.
Cognitive Level: Comprehension **Client Need:** Safe Effective Care Environment: Management of Care **Integrated Process:** Nursing Process: Analysis **Content Area:** Leadership/Management **Strategy:** Determine the best answer. Recall that the definitions of maleficence, deontology, and beneficence do not address the lack of

autonomy this client experiences. The main issue is the lack of autonomy. Identify the core issue to prevent selection of incorrect distracters. **References:** Finkelman, A. W. (2006). *Leadership and management in nursing.* Upper Saddle River, NJ: Pearson Education, pp. 275–302; Sullivan, E. J., & Decker, P. (2005). *Effective leadership and management in nursing* (6th ed.). Upper Saddle River, NJ: Pearson Education, pp. 67–80.

2 **Answer: 3** The nurse manager should first determine the nurse's purpose in accessing the client's financial record. The question does not address whether the nurse is planning specific discharge needs for the client. Accessing the client's financial record is a breach in confidentiality only if the nurse does not need to know the client's financial status. Financial information includes types of insurance and income, all of which are necessary in planning home care needs for clients. **Cognitive Level:** Application **Client Need:** Safe Effective Care Environment: Management of Care **Integrated Process:** Communication and Documentation **Content Area:** Leadership/Management **Strategy:** In this scenario, start with assessment. Option 1 implies nurses do not plan discharges; this is incorrect. Option 2 presupposes the nurse has breached confidentiality regulations. The stem of the question does not clearly identify a breach. Option 4 is a premature conclusion. Option 3 allows further investigation into this matter. Use the "best choices" principle to make the correct selection. **References:** Finkelman, A. W. (2006). *Leadership and management in nursing.* Upper Saddle River, NJ: Pearson Education, pp. 275–302; Sullivan, E. J., & Decker, P. (2005). *Effective leadership and management in nursing* (6th ed.). Upper Saddle River, NJ: Pearson Education, pp. 67–80.

3 **Answer: 4** Option 4 allows the nurse to assess whether the teenager has spoken to her parents about sexual behavior, and it opens the door to communication. The nurse should not discuss this with the teenager's mother (option 1); the teenager has a right to confidentiality. Option 2 (gynecologist) and option 3 (payment) do not address the affective need the teenager expresses. **Cognitive Level:** Application **Client Need:** Safe Effective Care Environment: Management of Care **Integrated Process:** Communication and Documentation **Content Area:** Leadership/Management **Strategy:** Note first that option 1 is incorrect because it is a fallacy. Eliminate options 2 and 3 next because they do not address the affective need of the client. Identify the core issue. Option 4 is the best choice. Use communication concepts and the process of elimination to select the correct response. **References:** Finkelman, A. W. (2006). *Leadership and*

management in nursing. Upper Saddle River, NJ: Pearson Education, pp. 275–302; Sullivan, E. J., & Decker, P. (2005). *Effective leadership and management in nursing* (6th ed.). Upper Saddle River, NJ: Pearson Education, pp. 67–80.

4 **Answer: 4** The nurse should keep the dialogue professional, but should also remind the physician of the legal responsibilities surrounding informed consent. While option 2 may seem feasible, it sounds like a directive coming from the nurse. Before referring this case to the medical director, the nurse should first talk to the physician about his or her responsibilities to the client. **Cognitive Level:** Application **Client Need:** Safe Effective Care Environment: Management of Care **Integrated Process:** Communication and Documentation **Content Area:** Leadership/Management **Strategy:** Use communication concepts and the process of elimination to select the correct response. Options 1, 2, and 3 could potentially lead to unnecessary conflict. Option 4 is the best choice because it explicitly states the legal facts without further embellishment. **References:** Finkelman, A. W. (2006). *Leadership and management in nursing.* Upper Saddle River, NJ: Pearson Education, pp. 275–302; Sullivan, E. J., & Decker, P. (2005). *Effective leadership and management in nursing* (6th ed.). Upper Saddle River, NJ: Pearson Education, pp. 67–80.

5 **Answers: 1, 2, 3, 5** Each nursing graduate must apply to take the national licensure examination with the appropriate state board of nursing. The state board regulates nursing practice and provides a definition of practice in each state. Some states require that practicing nurses take continuing education courses to maintain competency in practice. **Cognitive Level:** Comprehension **Client Need:** Safe Effective Care Environment: Management of Care **Integrated Process:** Nursing Process: Analysis **Content Area:** Leadership/Management **Strategy:** Identify critical words in the question or stem to select the right answer(s). Options 1, 2, 3, and 5 are all strategies that protect the public from unsafe practice. Option 4 stands out. Differentiated education does not protect the public. **References:** Finkelman, A. W. (2006). *Leadership and management in nursing.* Upper Saddle River, NJ: Pearson Education, pp. 275–302; Sullivan, E. J., & Decker, P. (2005). *Effective leadership and management in nursing* (6th ed.). Upper Saddle River, NJ: Pearson Education, pp. 67–80.

6 **Answer: 3** Option 3 is correct because it reiterates that the client does not have to go through with the surgery, and it allows the nurse to assess factors such as barriers or obstacles and fears. Signing the consent does not

mean the client must have the surgery (option 1); the client may withdraw the consent for surgery at any time. The nurse should inform the surgeon (option 4), but the nurse should first assess the reason the client does not want to have the surgery. Option 2 states a fact but does not allow the nurse to assess the reason for refusal of surgery.
Cognitive Level: Application **Client Need:** Safe Effective Care Environment: Management of Care **Integrated Process:** Communication and Documentation **Content Area:** Leadership/Management **Strategy:** Eliminate option 1 first because it is incorrect; it's false information. Option 2 is correct, but it does not assess the client's refusal of the surgical procedure. Option 4 is passive. Option 3 is true, and it follows up with a statement of assessment, which is the critical need at this time. Use communication concepts and the process of elimination to select the correct response. **References:** Finkelman, A. W. (2006). *Leadership and management in nursing.* Upper Saddle River, NJ: Pearson Education, pp. 275–302; Sullivan, E. J., & Decker, P. (2005). *Effective leadership and management in nursing* (6th ed.). Upper Saddle River, NJ: Pearson Education, pp. 67–80.

7 **Answer: 1** The highest priority of the nurse at this time is to fulfill the role of client advocate. Although the nurse is a direct caregiver and may also be a care manager, these are not the priority. The role that is critical to this scenario is the role of an advocate, in which the nurse lets the client know the decision to have surgery belongs to the client. The nurse may also utilize the role of educator to help allay any unfounded concerns, but this role would become important only after the nurse fulfills the role of advocate.
Cognitive Level: Application **Client Need:** Safe Effective Care Environment: Management of Care **Integrated Process:** Nursing Process: Planning **Content Area:** Leadership/Management **Strategy:** Become familiar with the roles of the registered nurse. In this case, the only answer is advocate. Consider that the nurse needs to act in the client's best interests and wishes in such a case to help you choose easily from the available options. **References:** Finkelman, A. W. (2006). *Leadership and management in nursing.* Upper Saddle River, NJ: Pearson Education, pp. 275–302; Sullivan, E. J., & Decker, P. (2005). *Effective leadership and management in nursing* (6th ed.). Upper Saddle River, NJ: Pearson Education, pp. 67–80.

8 **Answer: 1** The national licensure exam determines minimal competency and safe practice in individuals who have graduated from an accredited school of nursing. It is not administered before graduation (option 4). It

does not test the physical skills a nurse must have to practice (option 2). State boards of nursing review the national licensing examination (NCLEX®) exam results of each school of nursing and track the success of nursing programs, but this is not a primary reason for licensure (option 3). The primary reason is to determine minimal competency of nurses in an effort to protect the public.
Cognitive Level: Application **Client Need:** Safe Effective Care Environment: Management of Care **Integrated Process:** Communication and Documentation **Content Area:** Leadership/Management **Strategy:** The core issue of this question is an understanding of the purpose of the licensing examination. Eliminate option 4 first because one must be a graduate of a nursing program to be eligible to take the test. Eliminate option 2 next because the test does not directly measure physical skills; it is a cognitive test rather than a performance test. Finally, eliminate option 3 because although true, it does not explain *why* the national exam is *required for licensure*. Note that option 1 is correct because it succinctly answers the question and the statement is true. **References:** Finkelman, A. W. (2006). *Leadership and management in nursing.* Upper Saddle River, NJ: Pearson Education, pp. 275–302; Sullivan, E. J., & Decker, P. (2005). *Effective leadership and management in nursing* (6th ed.). Upper Saddle River, NJ: Pearson Education, pp. 67–80.

9 **Answers: 1, 3, 4** Morals are personal standards of right and wrong conduct. They are private and personal but may change from one developmental stage to another. Morals are applied to daily life circumstances and may not have any religious connections.
Cognitive Level: Knowledge **Client Need:** Safe Effective Care Environment: Management of Care **Integrated Process:** Nursing Process: Analysis **Content Area:** Leadership/Management **Strategy:** In this question, look for options that represent correct statements. Options 1, 3, and 4 are correct statements, while options 2 and 5 are incorrect statements. **References:** Finkelman, A. W. (2006). *Leadership and management in nursing.* Upper Saddle River, NJ: Pearson Education, pp. 275–302; Sullivan, E. J., & Decker, P. (2005). *Effective leadership and management in nursing* (6th ed.). Upper Saddle River, NJ: Pearson Education, pp. 67–80.

10 **Answer: 2** The utilitarian theory provides benefits based on the greatest good and least harm for the greatest number. In this case, 70% of employees will benefit from follow-up services while the other 30% will have the same deductibles and monthly payments. Deontological theorists look at the moral significance of an action and evaluate the rightness and wrongness of the behavior (option 1). Justice on the other hand, is an issue of fairness (option 3). The other 30% of employees could argue that the decision by the CEO is not just because it does not change their monthly insurance premiums and provide them with any additional services. While this event is beneficial, it does not provide the same services for all employees (option 4).

Cognitive Level: Application **Client Need:** Safe Effective Care Environment: Management of Care **Integrated Process:** Nursing Process: Evaluation **Content Area:** Leadership/Management **Strategy:** Recall definitions associated with ethical terminology and choose the option that best fits the scenario. Consider that beneficence and justice clearly do not fit the scenario. Based on the definition of deontology, determine that it does not fit the scenario either. The best and only choice is option 2. Identify critical information in the question such as *70%* and *30%* to select the correct answer. **References:** Finkelman, A. W. (2006). *Leadership and management in nursing.* Upper Saddle River, NJ: Pearson Education, Inc., pp. 275–302; Sullivan, E. J., & Decker, P. (2005). *Effective leadership and management in nursing* (6th ed.). Upper Saddle River, NJ: Pearson Education, Inc., pp. 67–80.

Posttest

1 Answer: 1 In this case, the nurse manager has used the deontological approach, in which the manager examines the rightness and wrongness of the nurse's response to the combative client. Utilitarianism is focused on providing the greatest good and least harm for the greatest number; this principle has no bearing on this incident. The stem specifically asks for the ethical principle the nurse manager demonstrates, so beneficence does not apply to the manager's response to the nurse. However, it does apply to what should be the appropriate nurse's response to the client. Justice may be applied, but the question asks for the principle the manager demonstrates.

Cognitive Level: Comprehension **Client Need:** Safe Effective Care Environment: Management of Care **Integrated Process:** Nursing Process: Evaluation **Content Area:** Leadership/Management **Strategy:** Recall the various ethical principles and choose the option that best fits the scenario. The stem does not provide information to support the utilitarianism principle. Justice and beneficence clearly do not fit the scenario. The best choice is option 1. Use the "best choices" approach to make the correct selection. **References:** Finkelman, A. W. (2006). *Leadership and management in nursing.* Upper Saddle River, NJ: Pearson Education, pp. 275–302; Sullivan,

E. J., & Decker, P. (2005). *Effective leadership and management in nursing* (6th ed.). Upper Saddle River, NJ: Pearson Education, pp. 67–80.

2 Answer: 4 The healthcare provider violated the client's autonomy (option 4) by not allowing the client to make a decision that affects the client's care. Justice (option 3) involves treating all people fairly, and there is no indication the healthcare provider treats clients unfairly. The healthcare provider is attempting to provide a service to the client that the client will benefit from, which is consistent with beneficence (option 1). The healthcare provider is not trying to harm the client, so nonmaleficence (option 2) is not applicable to this case.

Cognitive Level: Comprehension **Client Need:** Safe Effective Care Environment: Management of Care **Integrated Process:** Nursing Process: Analysis **Content Area:** Leadership/Management **Strategy:** Recall the various ethical principles and their definitions. Note that the question does not provide data to support options 1, 2, and 3. Identify the core issue of the question to assist you in making the correct choice. **References:** Finkelman, A. W. (2006). *Leadership and management in nursing.* Upper Saddle River, NJ: Pearson Education, pp. 275–302; Sullivan, E. J., & Decker, P. (2005). *Effective leadership and management in nursing* (6th ed.). Upper Saddle River, NJ: Pearson Education, pp. 67–80.

3 Answer: 1 The instructor does not treat all students fairly. Deontology (option 2) applies the rightness or wrongness of a single act, and this scenario involves a comparison between two sets of actions. Utilitarianism (option 3) is focused on providing the greatest good and least harm for the greatest number and does not apply to this scenario. Fidelity (option 4) is the duty to keep promises and is not applicable to the situation described.

Cognitive Level: Comprehension **Client Need:** Safe Effective Care Environment: Management of Care **Integrated Process:** Nursing Process: Analysis **Content Area:** Leadership/Management **Strategy:** Identify that the core issue is inconsistency in upholding rules, an issue of justice (fairness). Recall the definitions of the various principles to realize that the only applicable option is 1. The stem does not provide supporting data for options 2, 3, and 4. **References:** Finkelman, A. W. (2006). *Leadership and management in nursing.* Upper Saddle River, NJ: Pearson Education, pp. 275–302; Sullivan, E. J., & Decker, P. (2005). *Effective leadership and management in nursing* (6th ed.). Upper Saddle River, NJ: Pearson Education, pp. 67–80.

4 Answer: 3 Beneficence is the duty to help others by promoting good consequences. The nurse who completes other activities en route to the client's room knowing the client needs assistance is not acting in a beneficent manner. The nurse's behavior may have indirectly caused the fall. Respect (option 2) is the acknowledgment of a person's self-worth and dignity and does not apply directly in this case. Veracity (option 1) is truthfulness and fidelity (option 4) is keeping one's promise to a client; both do not apply to this scenario. **Cognitive Level:** Application **Client Need:** Safe Effective Care Environment: Management of Care **Integrated Process:** Communication and Documentation **Content Area:** Leadership/Management **Strategy:** Identify the core issue of the question, which is that the nurse has willfully failed to take adequate care of the client. Next, recall the definitions of various ethical principles. Note that beneficence addresses the core issue, while veracity, respect, and fidelity are ethical principles that are not addressed in the stem of the question. **References:** Finkelman, A. W. (2006). *Leadership and management in nursing.* Upper Saddle River, NJ: Pearson Education, pp. 275–302; Sullivan, E. J., & Decker, P. (2005). *Effective leadership and management in nursing* (6th ed.). Upper Saddle River, NJ: Pearson Education, pp. 67–80.

5 Answer: 3 Autonomy promotes client dignity and self-worth by allowing clients self-determination and decision making. The principle of justice (option 1) implies all clients are treated fairly. The principle of veracity is conveying the truth to clients (option 2). Fidelity is the duty to keep promises (option 4). **Cognitive Level:** Comprehension **Client Need:** Safe Effective Care Environment: Management of Care **Integrated Process:** Nursing Process: Planning **Content Area:** Leadership/Management **Strategy:** The critical word in the stem is *participation*. Recall the definition of the various ethical principles and note that participation in care best matches option 3. Options 1, 2, and 4 are not addressed in the question. Use the "best choices" principle to make the correct selection. **References:** Finkelman, A. W. (2006). *Leadership and management in nursing.* Upper Saddle River, NJ: Pearson Education, pp. 275–302; Sullivan, E. J., & Decker, P. (2005). *Effective leadership and management in nursing* (6th ed.). Upper Saddle River, NJ: Pearson Education, pp. 67–80.

6 Answer: 4 The point to consider is why clients with Medicaid are being discharged two days earlier than clients who have private insurance. This question points to the principle of justice, a duty to treat all clients fairly. Beneficence (option 1), the duty to promote good consequences, could be applied if outcomes were added to this question. Veracity or truthfulness (option 2) and fidelity or faithfulness to the client's interests (option 3) are not applicable in this case.

Cognitive Level: Application **Client Need:** Safe Effective Care Environment: Management of Care **Integrated Process:** Communication and Documentation **Content Area:** Leadership/Management **Strategy:** Identify the core issue, disparity in care between two groups. Considering the definitions of all options, justice fits best. Beneficence, promoting good consequences, is too broad for this scenario. Option 4 is more specific. Based on definitions of veracity and fidelity, these two options are inapplicable. **References:** Finkelman, A. W. (2006). *Leadership and management in nursing.* Upper Saddle River, NJ: Pearson Education, pp. 275–302; Sullivan, E. J., & Decker, P. (2005). *Effective leadership and management in nursing* (6th ed.). Upper Saddle River, NJ: Pearson Education, pp. 67–80.

7 Answers: 1, 3, 4 In this case, a client was not provided a service, but was charged for the service nonetheless. Truthfulness and fidelity are applicable in this case. The provider was supposed to provide the service (fidelity) and be truthful (veracity). Furthermore, this client was not treated fairly and so justice is also an issue (option 1). Nonmaleficence and beneficence (options 2 and 5) are not applicable in this case because the focus is not on the harm or good that came to the client as a result of the care delivered.

Cognitive Level: Application **Client Need:** Safe Effective Care Environment: Management of Care **Integrated Process:** Nursing Process: Analysis **Content Area:** Leadership/Management **Strategy:** First consider that promoting good consequences (beneficence) does not apply. Using the same line of thought, eliminate maleficence because there is no indication that harm was caused to the client's health. The cores issues are truth, fairness, and keeping one's promises. Identify the core issues to select the correct option. **References:** Finkelman, A. W. (2006). *Leadership and management in nursing.* Upper Saddle River, NJ: Pearson Education, pp. 275–302; Sullivan, E. J., & Decker, P. (2005). *Effective leadership and management in nursing* (6th ed.). Upper Saddle River, NJ: Pearson Education, pp. 67–80.

8 Answer: 2 Values are beliefs about a person's worth, ideas, or actions. They tend to influence decisions, both professional and personal. Values emerge from culture, religion, social traditions, and family. Purpose (option 3) is the reason for the action and preference (option 4) represents choice; neither are applicable to the question as stated. Culture (option 1) is the environment that leaders create to facilitate goal accomplishment. **Cognitive Level:** Analysis **Client Need:** Safe Effective Care Environment: Management of Care **Integrated Process:** Nursing Process: Planning **Content Area:** Leadership/

Management **Strategy:** First consider the definition of the various terms in the options. Education and socialization in this case do not represent culture, so eliminate option 1 first. Leaders are influenced by culture, but in this case the leader uses socialization and education as a guide, which are values. Options 3 and 4 do not answer the question because purpose and preference are vaguer terms that do not fit the question as stated. Consider that socialization and education represent values of the leader to make the correct selection. **References:** Finkelman, A. W. (2006). *Leadership and management in nursing.* Upper Saddle River, NJ: Pearson Education, pp. 275–302; Sullivan, E. J., & Decker, P. (2005). *Effective leadership and management in nursing* (6th ed.). Upper Saddle River, NJ: Pearson Education, pp. 67–80.

9 **Answers: 1, 2** Culture and family (options 1 and 2) shape the traits and characteristics of human beings. Culture can influence religion (option 5), but spirituality is a broader term than religion. Time orientation and persistence are characteristics needed for academic success and occupational excellence, but do not occur as a direct result of academic preparation or occupation (options 3 and 4).

Cognitive Level: Comprehension **Client Need:** Safe Effective Care Environment: Management of Care **Integrated Process:** Nursing Process: Analysis **Content Area:** Leadership/Management **Strategy:** Religion, culture, and family group all fit together as elements that influence time orientation. Spirituality is broader than religion and as such must be eliminated. Next, note that academic

preparation and occupation are not associated with time orientation and can therefore be eliminated. Use the "best choices" principle to make the correct selection. **References:** Finkelman, A. W. (2006). *Leadership and management in nursing.* Upper Saddle River, NJ: Pearson Education, pp. 275–302; Sullivan, E. J., & Decker, P. (2005). *Effective leadership and management in nursing* (6th ed.). Upper Saddle River, NJ: Pearson Education, pp. 67–80.

10 **Answers: 2, 3, 5** The use of ethical principles will keep the nurse aware of issues that affect ethical behavior in the workplace. Nurses should evaluate and reevaluate their personal morals; this action forces them to become aware of biases that may affect ethical decision making. The ANA Code of Ethics is a set of principles that serves as a standard of professional action.

Cognitive Level: Application **Client Need:** Safe Effective Care Environment:Management of Care **Integrated Process:** Nursing Process: Planning **Content Area:** Leadership/Management **Strategy:** Look at the options that are similar, such as options 2, 3 and 5. These address the core issue of the question and can be selected. Note that option 1 does not address ethical decision making and that option 4 is a passive strategy, which will enable you to eliminate both of these choices. **References:** Finkelman, A. W. (2006). *Leadership and management in nursing.* Upper Saddle River, NJ: Pearson Education, pp. 275–302; Sullivan, E. J., & Decker, P. (2005). *Effective leadership and management in nursing* (6th Ed.). Upper Saddle River, NJ: Pearson Education, pp. 67–80.

References

American Association of Colleges of Nursing. (1998). *The essentials of baccalaureate education: For professional nursing practice.* Washington, DC: Author.

American Nurses Association. (2006). *The Code of Ethics for Nurses with interpretive statements.* Retrieved July 2007 from http://nursingworld.org/ethics/code/ethicscode150.htm.

Beauchamp, T. L., & Childress, J. F. (2001). *Principles of biomedical ethics* (5th ed.). New York: Oxford University.

Cohen, S. (2004). The new manager's guide to surviving and thriving. *Nursing Management, 36*(4), 20–21.

Cooper, R. W., Frank, G. L., Gouty, C. A., & Hansen, M. C. (2002). Key ethical issues encountered in healthcare organizations. *Journal of Nursing Administration, 32*(6), 331–337.

Doane, G., Pauly, B., Brown, H., & McPherson, G. (2004). Exploring the heart of ethics education. *Nursing Ethics, 11*(3), 240–253.

Drew, S. (2004). Ethical decision making in practice: A triage decision. *Nursing Outlook, 27*(1), 18–20.

Finkelman, A. W. (2006). *Leadership and management in nursing.* Upper Saddle River, NJ: Pearson Education.

Perkel, L. K. (2002). Nurse executives' values and leadership behavior. *Nursing Leadership Forum, 6*(4), 100–107.

Redman, B. A., & Fry, S. T. (2003). Ethics and human rights issues experienced by nurses in leadership roles. *Nursing Leadership Forum, 7*(4), 501–556.

Shirely, M. R. (2005). Ethical climate in nursing practice: The leader's role. *Journal of Nursing Administration. Healthcare, Law, Ethics, and Regulation, 7*(2), 59–67.

Sullivan, E. J. & Decker, P. (2005). *Effective leadership and management in nursing* (6th ed.). Upper Saddle River, NJ: Pearson Education.

Woods, M. (2005). Nursing ethics education: Are we really delivering the good(s)? *Nursing Ethics, 12*(1), 5–18.

Safety First: Legal Rights and Responsibilities

4

Chapter Outline

Board of Nursing

Nurse Practice Acts

Types of Laws

Criminal and Civil Law

Nursing Practice and Tort Liability

Categories of Negligence

Malpractice

Good Samaritan Law and Client's Rights

Incident Reports and Irregular Occurrences

Nursing Care Reporting Requirements

Advance Directives

Use of Restraints

Federal Legislation and Nursing Practice

Objectives

➤ Define the term *nurse practice acts*.

➤ Describe the four primary sources of law that affect nursing practice.

➤ Describe the terms *malpractice* and *negligence*.

➤ Identify the categories of negligence.

➤ Explain client rights including confidentiality and informed consent.

➤ Define the key aspects of incident reports and irregular occurrences.

➤ Explain the use of client restraints.

➤ Explore the issue of nurse impairment.

NCLEX-RN® Test Prep

Use the CD-ROM enclosed with this book to access additional practice opportunities.

Review at a Glance

administrative law a law created by the administrative or executive branch of government, including a multitude of agencies, empowered to define terms, establish standards, and guide interpretation of statutes

advance directive a set of instructions given by a competent adult about personal choices concerning future treatment should he or she become incapacitated

Americans with Disabilities Act a federal law to end discrimination against disabled individuals

Board of Nursing an administrative agency of state government that administers the state's Nurse Practice Act

civil law a law that protects the rights and responsibilities of private individuals

Client Self-Determination Act a federal law that mandates healthcare facilities receiving Medicare or Medicaid funds give clients information on admission about their rights under state law to make informed medical decisions, including their right to make advance directives

confidentiality an individual's right to privacy of records and personal information

common law or case law a body of judicial decisions made when cases are taken to court

corporate liability the responsibility of an organization for its own wrongful conduct

criminal law a law that applies to conduct considered offensive to the public or society as whole

do-not-resuscitate (DNR) a medical order that is also called "no code," in which the client will not be resuscitated in the event of cardiac or respiratory arrest

durable power of attorney also called **healthcare proxy**; a person authorized by the client to make medical decisions if the client becomes incapable of doing so

Emergency Medical Treatment (or Active Labor) Act a law that applies to all hospitals with emergency departments that participate in Medicare and Medicaid and to their physicians on staff; it requires appropriate treatment of any emergency department client including medical screening examination, treatment, and stabilization of a client if that client has an emergency medical condition and is in unstable condition

felony a crime of a serious nature, punishable by a prison term

Good Samaritan statute a law that provides immunity for acts that might otherwise result in a claim of negligence provided those acts are provided free of charge to aid in an emergency

incident a situation in which there is deviation from the routine operation of a facility

incident report an agency form that contains date, time, and location of incident; facts of occurrence; client assessment; direct quotes from client; treatment received and other actions taken; family members notified; names of witnesses; suspected cause of incident; follow-up action taken

informed consent the client's right to voluntarily consent to or refuse treatment, based on understandable information about risks, benefits, and alternatives to the proposed treatment

licensure a mandatory process through which a government agency grants an individual or institution the right to provide certain services; a license is a credential provided by state statute that authorizes qualified individuals to perform designated skills and services

living will a client's statement of medical care or treatment wished for in the event of a terminal illness or if the client becomes permanently unconscious

malpractice improper or unethical conduct or unreasonable lack of skill by someone holding a professional or official position to denote negligent or unskillful performance of duties when professional skills are obligatory

misdemeanor a criminal act, such as altering a client's medical record or violating client's rights, that is less serious than a felony

negligence a tort that focuses on an individual's conduct, rather than his or her state of mind or intent

nurse practice act a collection of statutes or laws that govern the practice of nursing in a particular state; includes the definition of nursing, requirements for licensure (initial and renewal), exceptions to practice act, actions or conditions that can result in loss or limitation of license, and an administrative structure that implements and administers the practice act

respondeat superior a legal principle that allows the court to hold an employer responsible for the actions of its employees when performing services for the organization

Safe Medical Devices Act a federal law mandating reporting to the Food and Drug Administration (FDA) of device-related incidents by hospitals, home care agencies, and other healthcare organizations

statutory law a set of laws or acts enacted by the legislative branch of government at the federal, state, or local level

tort a civil wrong by one person against a person or the property of another

PRETEST

1 The nursing unit educator explains to a group of new nurse orientees that the nursing shortage has impacted medical cases in which of the following ways in society?

1. It has led to an increase in medical errors due to under-staffing.
2. It has reduced autonomy and independence of individual nurses.
3. It has raised to a new level the need for delegation to unlicensed personnel.
4. It has led to refined narrow definitions of liability.

2 Which of the following is the best measure for the professional nurse to use in reducing personal liability for malpractice litigation?

1. Offer an expression of regret to the client when you make an error.
2. Maintain a clear and open line of communication with each client.
3. Adhere to professional national standards of care.
4. Develop policies to ensure adequate client assessment.

3 After an incident occurred that involved the use of a medical device and the incident resulted in serious injury to a client, the nurse manager explains to staff that the report will forwarded to which federal agency?

1. Food and Drug Administration (FDA)
2. Centers for Disease Control and Prevention (CDC)
3. Centers for Medicare and Medicaid Services (CMMS)
4. National Institute of Health (NIH)

4 On admission to the hospital a client gives the nurse a document naming an individual to make choices in the case of the client becoming incapacitated. The document also includes the client's end-of-life wishes. The nurse communicates during intershift report that the client has a copy of which document in the medical record?

1. Living will
2. Durable power of attorney
3. Last will and testament
4. Do-not-resuscitate order

5 A nurse accidentally administers an overdose of a medication that subsequently leads to the client's death. The nurse understands that this is a sentinel event that may have financial consequences under which of the following types of laws?

1. Constitutional law
2. Administrative law
3. Civil law
4. Statutory law

6 A nurse wrongfully administers a large dose of insulin by the intravenous push (IVP) route, which causes complications for the client and an extended hospital stay. The nurse anticipates that the client may file which of the following claims against the nurse to cover the additional expenses incurred?

1. Intentional tort
2. Breach of duty
3. Tort
4. *Respondeat superior*

7 A nurse manager lives in a state that does not allow Licensed Practical Nurses/Licensed Vocational Nurses (LPN/LVNs) to administer intravenous push (IVP) medications. A charge nurse gives in to time pressures and allows two LPN/LVNs to give IVP medications. The nurse manager is aware that which agency will take action after being notified of this incident?

1. American Nurses Association (ANA)
2. National League for Nursing (NLN)
3. Joint Commission for Accreditation of Health Care Organizations (JCAHO)
4. State Board of Nursing (BON)

8 The state Board of Nursing disciplines a nurse with a public reprimand. How should the nurse interpret this disciplinary action?

1. The nurse does not have an infraction against his or her nursing license.
2. The nurse is not allowed to practice in the state the incident occurred.
3. The nurse must practice only in public hospitals.
4. The nurse may practice, but has an infraction against his or her nursing license.

9 A nurse smells alcohol on the breath of a nurse coworker. The nurse's behavior is consistent with a state of intoxication. The nurse witnessing the coworker's behavior reports this to the nursing supervisor, understanding that this incident may be reported to which organization?

1. American Nurses Association (ANA)
2. State Board of Nursing (BON)
3. American Nurses Credentialing Center (ANCC)
4. National League for Nursing (NLN)

10 A nurse uses a new intravenous pump for the first time. The client receives too much intravenous (IV) fluid and develops heart failure. The nurse manager concludes that which type of law benefits the client in this case?

1. Constitutional law
2. Administrative law
3. Statutory law
4. Tort

➤ *See pages 82–84 for Answers and Rationales.*

I. *BOARD OF NURSING*

A. Definition
1. An administrative agency of each state government; each state has a Board of Nursing organized within the executive branch of state government
2. The board's responsibility is administration of the state nurse practice act for registered nurses (RNs) and for licensed practical/vocational nurses (LPNs/LVNs)

B. Functions
1. Establishes educational and professional standards of licensure
2. Conducts examinations, registers, and licenses applicants
3. Conducts investigations of violations of statutes and regulations
4. Issues citations and holds disciplinary hearings for possible suspension or revocation of licenses
5. Imposes penalties following disciplinary hearings
6. Formulates regulations to implement the state's Nurse Practice Act.

II. *NURSE PRACTICE ACT*

A. Definition: A series of statutes enacted by each state legislature to regulate practice of nursing in that state

B. Statutes provide for the following:
1. Definition of the practice of nursing
2. Requirements for licensure (initial and renewal)
3. Exceptions to the practice act
4. Actions or conditions that can result in loss or limitations of license
5. An administrative structure to implement and administer the practice act

    6. Actions that nurses can take independently

    7. Actions that require a physician's or advanced practice nurse's order before completion

  C. In the United States (U.S.), most nurse practice acts are similar in content and hold a professional nurse legally responsible for licensure requirements and regulations of practice as defined by the state in which he or she is practicing

  D. Nursing process: there is legal authority to apply nursing process mandated by society through the license given to professionals

    1. Nurses need general knowledge of law

    2. Laws provide foundation to understand:

      a. Rights

      b. Privileges

      c. Responsibilities that exist between nurses and clients, nurses and other providers, and nurses and employers

III. TYPES OF LAWS

  A. Introduction

    1. A variety of laws act as principles to govern society

    2. Laws require citizens to uphold standards and behave in accordance with guidelines of complex state and federal statutes, regulations, court decisions, and legal procedures

  B. Laws affecting nursing practice

    1. Constitutional law: a document that sets forth the fundamental body of law that establishes the overall structure and powers of government (of a state or the nation and the rights of citizens under that government)

      a. The Constitution determines individual rights and responsibilities

      b. The Constitution protects client's rights to self-determination, including rights to make informed choices and refuse treatments

      c. The Constitution contains a three-part system of government: legislative, executive, and judicial, with each part having a role in law-making functions

    2. Statutory law

      a. Consists of statutes enacted by the legislative branch of government at federal, state, or local level

      b. A nurse practice act is an example of a state statute authorizing the practice of nursing enacted within the standards of the Constitution of each state

    3. Administrative law

      a. A specialized area of law created by administrative or executive branch of government including a multitude of agencies empowered to define terms, establish standards, and guide interpretation of statutes

      b. A state board of nursing is example of an administrative agency

      c. Administrative agencies implement the statutes and enact regulations defining terms, establishing standards, and guiding interpretations of statutes

      d. The nurse practice act is the statute upheld by state board of nursing

    4. Common law (or case law)

        a. A body of judicial decisions made when cases are taken to court

        b. Common law often addresses gaps in law or questions of interpretation

        c. Nursing malpractice cases are sometimes decided on the basis of precedent, meaning that a lower court will follow the decision of a higher court in the same jurisdiction

C. *Licensure*

    1. A mandatory process through which a government agency grants an individual or institution the right to provide a certain service

    2. The state functions respond to local requirements for service, cultural norms, and regional resources

    3. Each state is authorized to license professionals and institutions under its constitutional power to protect the health and welfare of its citizens

    4. The type of credential provided by state statutes authorizes qualified individuals to perform designated skills and services

    5. All U.S. nurses take the same licensing examination (National Council Licensure Examination) after completing a required educational program

    6. Nurses in good standing can obtain licensure by reciprocity in other states because the licensing examination is nationwide

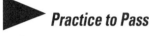

Practice to Pass

Explain what is the best way nurses can reduce potential liability and protect their license.

IV. CRIMINAL AND CIVIL LAW

A. *Criminal law*

    1. Consists of conduct considered offensive to the public or society as a whole

        a. A criminal action is defined as an action brought by the state against an individual for breaking the law (committing a crime)

        b. The crime can be either a **misdemeanor** (minor offense) or a **felony** (a major offense punishable by a prison term)

        c. Nurses can be charged for such felonies as manslaughter, negligent homicide, assault, diversion of narcotics, and insurance fraud

    2. Civil law involves the rights and responsibilities of private individuals

        a. They are designed to provide monetary compensation to individuals for harm caused to themselves or their property

        b. Nurse can be involved in a variety of civil cases including personal injury lawsuits, worker's compensation claims, malpractice actions, and divorce and custody proceedings

B. Nurses need to be familiar with criminal and civic law and how each of these types of laws impacts professional nursing practice

V. NURSING PRACTICE AND TORT LIABILITY

A. *Tort*

    1. A civil wrong by one person against another person or the property of another

    2. Nurses encounter this type of civil action most often

    3. It is pursued by both the board of nursing and the state prosecutor

4. In order to be pursued in court, an injury or harm constituting the basis of the claim must have been suffered by plaintiff; the person harmed by tort may sue the wrongdoer

5. The goal of a tort case is to obtain money damages (or injunction) against the bad actor, known as the tort feasor

   a. The plaintiff in a tort case, or injured party, may recover in damages all lost wages past and future, mental anguish, medical expenses past and future, disability, pain and suffering, and any other reasonable expenses that naturally flow from the wrongful conduct

   b. Outcomes include compensation for harm in money damages including past and future economic damages—medical bills, lost wages, and future medical bills as well as past and future noneconomic damages for pain and suffering

B. Intentional tort

1. A civil wrong with the intent to do a specific act or achieve a specific result

2. The person committing the intentional act must or should have known that outcome would occur; there are several types of intentional torts:

   a. Assault: threatening or attempting to make contact with a person without his or her consent

   b. Battery: an assault that is carried out

   c. False imprisonment: restraining another person without legal justification or his or her consent

   d. Fraud: a purposeful misrepresentation that causes harm to another

3. The proximate cause is decided upon the facts at hand in each particular case; another popular test for causation is called the "but for" test and refers to idea that negligence will lie where injury would not have occurred but for the defendant's negligent act or omission

4. The standard of conduct: in medical malpractice cases this is defined as that degree of skill ordinarily possessed and used by a reasonably competent practitioner in that area, under the same or similar circumstances

VI. CATEGORIES OF *NEGLIGENCE:* THE MAJOR REASONS THAT A MALPRACTICE LAWSUIT MAY BE FILED (SEE BOX 4-1):

A. Failure to follow standards of care, including failure to:

1. Perform a complete admission assessment or design the plan of care

2. Adhere to standardized protocols or institutional policies and procedures

3. Follow a physician's verbal or written orders

B. Failure to use equipment in a responsible manner, including failure to:

1. Follow manufacturer's recommendations for operating equipment

2. Check equipment for safety prior to use

3. Place or position equipment properly during treatment

4. Learn how equipment functions

C. Failure to communicate, including failure to:

1. Notify the physician or other healthcare provider in a timely manner when conditions warrant

Box 4-1 **Knowing the Elements of Negligence**	Negligence is misconduct or practice that is below the standard expected of an ordinary, reasonable, and prudent person. Therefore, the nurse leader is responsible for knowing the elements of negligence: 1. Negligent conduct by the nurse places a client at risk for harm. 2. Negligent conduct includes a situation where the nurse has a duty toward the client. This duty requires that the nurse have a relationship with the client that involves providing care and following an acceptable standard of care. 3. Negligent conduct occurs when a nurse fails to fulfill his or her duty (breach of duty). This conduct includes a duty or standard of care that the nurse did not observe.

2. Listen to a client's complaint and act on it
3. Communicate effectively with a client
4. Seek higher medical authorization for treatment

D. **Failure to document, including failure to:**
1. Record a client's progress and response to treatment
2. Record client's injuries
3. Record important nursing assessment information
4. Record physician's medical orders
5. Document information or telephone conversations with physicians, including time, content of communication between nurse and physician, and actions taken

E. **Failure to assess and monitor, including failure to:**
1. Complete a shift assessment
2. Implement the plan of care
3. Observe the client's ongoing progress
4. Interpret the client's signs and symptoms

F. **Failure to act as client advocate, including failure to:**
1. Question discharge orders when the client's condition warrants
2. Question incomplete or illegible medical orders
3. Provide a safe environment for the client

VII. MALPRACTICE

A. **Description**
1. An improper or unethical conduct or unreasonable lack of skill by someone in a professional or official position; or the negligent or unskillful performance of duties when professional skills are required
2. This is the form of negligence that addresses the negligent conduct of professionals
3. Occurs when there is a violation of the professional standard of care that results in injury to client

B. **Malpractice is frequently defined from a variety of sources:**
1. State nurse practice act
2. Institutional policies
3. Federal guidelines
4. JCAHO standards

Malpractice in nursing includes negligence that involves the presence of six elements:

1. Duty involves the relationship a nurse has with a client and follows acceptable standards of care.

2. Breach of duty involves the nurse failing to follow or observe the standard of care.

3. Foreseeability involves the connection between the nurse's action and injury suffered by the client.

4. Causation involves harm that occurred as a direct result of the nurse's failure to follow the standard of care.

5. Harm or injury involves the client sustaining some type of harm or injury as a result of the breach of duty owed.

6. Damages involve the nurse being held liable for the damages caused by the injury.

C. Four elements must be present for malpractice to have occurred (see Box 4-2):

1. *Duty owed the client* involves how nurses conducts themselves when engaging in client care activities; nurses have a legal duty to act as an ordinary, prudent, reasonable professional would act during client care, meaning they would take precautions against creating undue risk of injury to clients; the duty to care involves two important elements: it must be demonstrated that a duty was indeed owed the client and the scope of that duty must be proven.

2. *Breach of duty* is a deviation from the standard of care owed the client; for example, something was done that should have not been or nothing was done when something should have been

3. *Injury* or actual harm has come to the client, including physical, financial, or emotional injury that resulted from the breach of duty owed the client

4. *Causation injury* must have been incurred directly as a result of the breach of duty owed the client; explained in two ways:

   a. *Cause-in-fact*, in which the breach in duty owed caused the injury

   b. *Proximate cause* seeks to determine the extent to which or how far the liability of the client's injury is the consequence of negligent activity

D. Majority of payments in malpractice suits involving nurse negligence occur with nonspecialized registered nurses who have problems with:

1. Monitoring: failing to monitor the client during post-operative recovery

2. Treatment: using equipment incorrectly

3. Medication: improper medication administration

4. Obstetrics: failing to adequately monitor fetal heart rate during labor

5. Surgery: failing to provide for the client's safety prior to or during surgery

E. Several factors are known to contribute to an increase in the number of malpractice cases against professional nurses:

1. Delegation

2. Early discharge

3. Nursing shortage

4. Advances in technology

5. Increased autonomy and responsibility

6. Better-informed consumers

7. Expanded legal definitions of liability

F. Nurse liability

1. Nurses, physicians, hospitals, clinics, and other employers may be held liable for negligent acts of their employees

2. The *respondeat superior* doctrine does not support acts of gross negligence or acts outside the scope of employment; it holds the employer responsible for actions of an employee when performing activities and services for the organization

G. *Corporate liability* **states that an organization is responsible for its own wrongful conduct; it includes a duty to:**

1. Hire, supervise, and maintain qualified and competent staff who are adequate in number

2. Provide, inspect, repair, and maintain reasonably adequate equipment

3. Maintain safety in the physical plant, building, and environment

4. Maintain policy and procedure for reporting incompetent, unethical, and illegal practice

VIII. GOOD SAMARITAN LAW AND CLIENT'S RIGHTS

A. *Good Samaritan statutes* **help protect and provide immunity to nurses and other health professionals for acts that might otherwise result in negligence cases**

1. If a nurse provides emergency care and intervention away from his or her worksite, the law protects him or her from allegations of negligence

2. Laws vary state by state

3. The nurse must always act in good faith and receive no compensation for services provided

4. The nurse must understand that gross negligence and criminal wrongdoing are not protected

B. Client rights: nurses have an obligation to be aware of, respect, and support each client's freedom to exercise his or her rights

1. **Confidentiality**: any and all information concerning the client's prognosis, diagnosis, and treatment must be kept confidential by all those providing treatment, unless the client authorizes its release to a third party

   a. The nurse has a right to know information concerning any assigned client's prognosis, diagnosis, and treatment (including HIV status)

   b. HIV-related information is highly sensitive and receives additional protection under law; specific written consent is needed for release of this information to third parties

   c. Nurses should not discuss a client's condition in public places such as:

      1) Elevators

      2) Restrooms

      3) Parking lots

      4) Cafeterias

Practice to Pass

You have just been assigned to a postoperative female client who has left the post-anesthesia care unit (PACU) awake and oriented. As you receive this client onto the general surgical unit, she complains about the intravenous infusion and informs you that she has decided not to have the next bag of solution started. What are your obligations to the client at this time? Explain what steps you will take as this client refuses medical treatment.

2. **Informed consent**: the right of a client to be given sufficient understandable information about risks, benefits, and alternatives to proposed treatments to enable the client to voluntarily consent or refuse treatment

    a. Informed consent is needed for any and all invasive procedures or one that may endanger the client's health

    b. A valid informed consent requires that sufficient information is given to the client

    c. The consent must be voluntary and the client must have the capacity to decide (client understands information given and can evaluate it and make a decision)

    d. Information given to client must include:

        1) A description of the nature and purpose of the procedure or treatment

        2) Alternatives to the procedure or treatment

        3) Associated risks and hazards

        4) Anticipated benefits of the procedure or treatment

    e. Children under age 18 in most states do not have the legal capacity to provide consent for medical or surgical procedures

        1) Parents must give consent

        2) Exceptions to parental consent:

            a) Minors who are married or emancipated in a court of law

            b) Minors serving in armed services

            c) Minors who are pregnant or HIV-positive

    f. Adults who are unable to grant consent because of confusion or memory loss may require a court-appointed guardian or another individual on their behalf to provide informed consent

    g. A health professional who treats a client without consent or against the client's wishes may face allegations of assault and battery, lack of informed consent, or violation of the client's bill of rights

    h. In an emergency, consent may be obtained via telephone depending on the organization's policy; telephone consent must be verified and requires two healthcare providers on the telephone to ascertain permission from the person granting consent

    i. A physician performing a procedure is responsible for obtaining the client's informed consent

    j. A nurse may be asked to witness the client's signature on consent, which includes:

        1) Consent was voluntary

        2) The client's signature is authentic

        3) The client has the capacity to understand information given

    k. If a language barrier exits, an interpreter must be obtained

    l. If the nurse cannot assess that a client understands the procedure, he or she must not sign as a witness

IX. INCIDENT REPORTS AND IRREGULAR OCCURRENCES

A. ***Incident***: a deviation from the routine operation within a healthcare organization

    1. All nurses must be familiar with agency policy and procedure for reporting, investigating, and taking corrective action when incidents occur

    2. All serious incidents must be reported immediately

    3. The nurse leader must be immediately contacted by telephone and informed about the incident

    4. A written report must be completed within 24 hours

    5. Prompt reporting can identify any danger to client safety and allow for an immediate response

    6. Examples of incidents include:

        a. A client fall

        b. A medication error (the most common source of liability and number one cause of client mortality and morbidity)

        c. Administration of incorrect blood product by blood type

    7. Put client needs first to reduce the frequency of errors and incidents

        a. Establish a culture of safety

        b. Identify problem areas

        c. Share findings

        d. Seek feedback to motivate change

        e. Speak up and help prevent errors

B. ***Incident report:*** is a specific form of required documentation that is used as an agency's internal risk management tool; it includes:

    1. Date

    2. Time

    3. Location of incident

    4. Facts of the occurrence

    5. Client assessment

    6. Direct quotes from the client

    7. Treatment provided at the time of the incident

    8. Family members notified

    9. Names of witnesses

    10. Suspected cause of the incident

    11. Follow-up actions taken

C. Preventing incidents and occurrences by creating a safe client environment

    1. Provide a formalized orientation program for nursing staff

    2. Validate competency through job descriptions, client care policies, expected conduct, and supervised clinical experience

    3. Provide recurring hands-on safety training with returns demonstrations in:

        a. Appropriate hand-washing

        b. Medication safety processes

        c. Client identification

    4. Promote a blame-free reporting system in the organization

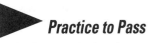

Practice to Pass

As the nurse leader of a 25-bed medical unit, you have just completed nursing grand rounds. On your way back to the nursing station, you overhear a certified nursing assistant (CNA) speaking in a loud voice and using abusive language to an elderly client. The client is screaming for the CNA to stop touching her and let her be. What action, if any, should you take?

> *!* ⬛ **D. Incident reports are confidential to the healthcare facility**
>
> 1. Incident reports describe adverse events that occur within a healthcare organization; incident reports are *not* part of the client's medical record
> 2. Nurses are not required and should not make reference to an incident report in their documentation; instead record the facts of the situation, client assessment data, interventions, and client response
> 3. Nurses are not allowed to copy any information from the incident report for their personal use
> 4. Copying such material is a breach of confidentiality and violation of the healthcare organization's policy

X. NURSING CARE REPORTING REQUIREMENTS

A. Nurses are mandated by law to report to state authorities any and all situations where client safety or public safety is at risk (see Box 4-3 for a variety of internet resources useful to nurses regarding legal practice of nursing)

B. Nurses are mandated reporters in cases of suspected abuse or neglect

1. Abuse: mistreatment of a person's physical, mental, or moral well-being
2. Neglect: failing to provide necessary physical, medical, surgical, or emotional care of a person, causing harm to health and well-being
3. Nurses who have reasonable cause to suspect elder abuse must report that information to the required state agency
4. Nurses who have reasonable cause to suspect abuse of any child under age 18 must report that information to the appropriate state agency and local police department
5. Failure to file a report will, in some states, subject the nurse to fine and disciplinary action
6. All assessment data or other nursing observations consistent with suspected abuse or neglect should be recorded in the client's medical record

! ⬛ **C. Impaired co-workers:** nurses who witness impaired or incompetent peers or co-workers must report their observations to their employer

1. The state nurse practice act may require that a report be made to the state board of nursing

Box 4-3	
Helpful Internet Resources	Licensure, certification information: www.ajn.org
	Certification, malpractice insurance information: www.nursingnet.org
	Health law (including court decisions): www.busph.bu.edu
	Health care practice: www.healthcarepractice.com
	Medical-Legal Consulting Institute: www.legalnurse.com/cer/cer_l.html
	National Council of State Boards of Nursing: www.ncsbn.org
	American Nurses Association: www.nursingworld.org
	Find Law: www.findlaw.com
	'Lectric Law Library: www.lectlaw.com
	The Nurse Advocate: www.nurseadvocate.org
	U.S. Department of Justice: www.usdoj.org

Practice to Pass

You have been called in as an expert witness because of your personal knowledge about a client case in your hospital. Explain what your rights and obligations are in regard to this legal action.

2. This is a confidential report prepared by the nurse leader and must include:

   a. Date

   b. Time

   c. Witnesses

   d. Observed behavior and action

   e. Adverse consequences to client or staff

D. **Communicable diseases:** nurses are required to report certain communicable diseases to state and local agencies and health department:

   1. Tuberculosis (TB)

   2. Human immunodeficiency virus (HIV) or acquired immunodeficiency syndrome (AIDS)

   3. Certain sexually transmitted infections (STIs)

   4. Chickenpox (varicella)

   5. Hepatitis

XI. *ADVANCE DIRECTIVE*

A. **Is a document that provides instructions about choices concerning future treatment made by a competent adult should he or she become incapacitated**

B. **Clients have two choices for treatment directives:**

   1. **Living will**: client's statement of desired medical care or treatment when in a terminal state or permanently unconscious; states life support systems and treatments the client does not want utilized in care

   2. **Durable power of attorney (or healthcare proxy)**: designates a person authorized by the client to make medical decisions if the client is incapable of doing so; in some states, a healthcare proxy acts when the client lacks decision-making capacity, regardless of severity of illness or injury

   3. An advance directive must be in writing, signed by the individual, and witnessed by two people who are not heirs, relatives, or healthcare providers currently treating the client

   4. An advance directive can be revoked any time, verbally or in writing by the client

   5. An advance directive becomes part of client's record and health providers are legally obligated to follow its instructions

C. *Client Self-Determination Act* **(1991):** mandates that healthcare facilities receiving Medicare and Medicaid funds give clients information on admission about their rights under state law to make informed medical decisions, including their right to make advance directives

D. *Do-not-resuscitate (DNR)* **order:** also called "no code"; means that client will not be resuscitated

   1. DNR decisions are legally made with client's informed consent

   2. DNR decisions pursuant to an advance directive will be found in the client's medical record

XII. USE OF RESTRAINTS

A. **Nurses are responsible and must be sufficiently knowledgeable about agency's policies and procedures for use of physical restraints, including the medical record forms used for documentation of a restrained client and associated safety measures**

1. Protective devices are a type of restraint used in a variety of healthcare settings to prevent clients from:
   a. Falling
   b. Wandering
   c. Removing invasive devices
2. Restraints are primarily used to protect client safety and/or the safety of others
3. Using restraints restricts a client's movement and might pose a hazard if not properly applied
4. Nurses are responsible for maintaining client safety at all times and therefore should frequently assess the restrained client according to agency policy

B. **The Federal Omnibus Budget Reconciliation Act of 1987 regulates the use of restraints in long-term care facilities with respect to:**
1. Arm restraints
2. Leg restraints
3. Hand mittens
4. Safety vests
5. Geri chairs

XIII. FEDERAL LEGISLATION AND NURSING PRACTICE

A. **The *American with Disabilities Act* (1990) is designed to end discrimination against disabled individuals**
1. Disability: a physical or mental impairment that limits one or more major life activities; includes a(an):
   a. Physiological disorder
   b. Cosmetic disfigurement
   c. Anatomical loss
   d. Learning disability
   e. Mental illness
2. Nurses must be aware of services available within their health organizations and be prepared to assist in providing services to clients and families
3. Courts have held healthcare providers accountable for making reasonable efforts to meet the needs of clients and families

B. ***Emergency Medical Treatment (or Active Labor) Act:*** called anti-dumping act statute, this is a federal law enacted in 1986 and pertains to all hospitals with emergency departments that participate in Medicare and Medicaid reimbursement, and to the physicians on their medical staff
1. Requires an appropriate medical screening examination
2. Requires treatment of any emergency room client
3. Requires treatment and stabilization of client, if client has emergency medical condition and is unstable; clients may refuse this examination and treatment
4. Unstable clients with an emergency condition may not be discharged unless they refuse treatment
5. Any hospital or physician who violates this law may be fined up to $50,000

<table>
<tr><td>

Box 4-4

Safety Measures for Nursing Practice

</td><td>

- Ask for a job description upon employment and know key responsibilities.
- Know where to locate organizational policies and procedure manual and be sure to know the policies.
- Introduce self to clients and be sure to know clients by name.
- When in doubt about a client procedure, ask for validation or clarification.
- When unsure about a written or verbal order, ask for clarification before proceeding to carry it out.
- Be alert and oriented to environment to prevent accidents before they happen.
- Maintain clinical competence and retool whenever necessary.
- Accept assignments for which you are prepared.
- Properly document all nursing care.
- Know own practice limits.

</td></tr>
</table>

C. **The National Practitioner Data Bank (NPDB), created by the Health Quality Improvement Act of 1986, provides a central repository for information on adverse disciplinary actions and malpractice payments**

1. Contains names of licensed health professionals who have had malpractice payment made on their behalf or have had adverse action taken against them

2. Information on settlements made either by healthcare organizations or insurance companies in malpractice payment must be reported to NPDB

3. Hospitals are required to request information from the data bank on advanced practice nurses who have been granted clinical privileges or belong to the medical staff such as nurse midwives, nurse anesthetists, and nurse practitioners

D. *Safe Medical Devices Act:* is a federal law mandating reporting to the FDA of device-related incidents by hospitals, home care agencies, and other healthcare organizations

1. Any medical device that causes or contributes to the death or serious injury or illness to a client is a reportable incident

2. The purpose of this law is to assist in early detection of device problems

3. Nurses are key reporters in device-related incidents and must follow organizational policy for reporting incidents

4. Failure to report can lead to civil fines up to $15,000 for a single violation or one million dollars for a series of violations

E. **See Box 4-4 for suggestions to maintain safety in a variety of client care environments**

Case Study

As the nurse manager on a 22-bed surgical unit, you become aware that a staff nurse has been signing out narcotics ordered for assigned clients and keeping the narcotics for personal use.

1. Explain what law the staff nurse's behavior violated.

2. Discuss how you would handle this situation.

3. Describe how this incident could affect nursing licensure.

See page 236 for suggested responses.

POSTTEST

1 A newly licensed nurse is explaining to a potential applicant to nursing school how nursing practice is regulated. The nurse identifies which of the following as a state statute that constitutes statutory law?

1. Nurse practice act
2. State board of nursing
3. Good Samaritan law
4. Active Labor Act

2 A nurse does not use a moist heating pad (K-pad) correctly, and a client with diabetic neuropathy of the legs suffers a burn injury. The nurse contacts the professional insurance carrier, fearful of which type of legal consequence to this level of care?

1. *Respondeat superior*
2. Defamation
3. Wrongful injury
4. Malpractice

3 A college student who is contemplating transferring into the nursing major asks a neighbor, who is a nurse, about "this NCLEX® exam I keep hearing about." The nurse explains that this test is the National Council Licensing Examination, which is designed to ensure which of the following?

1. Nurses are competent to function in critical care units.
2. Nurses function at an expert level.
3. Nurses are competent in providing safe care.
4. Baccalaureate nurses are able to practice at an advanced level.

4 A nurse is caught stealing narcotic pain medications. The nurse manager reports this incident to which of the following regulating bodies?

1. State board of nursing
2. American Nurses Association
3. National League for Nursing
4. Department of Health and Environmental Control

5 A nurse wrongfully administers potassium by the intravenous push (IVP) route and the client experiences cardiac arrest and cannot be resuscitated. The nurse manager counsels the nurse that which types of law are likely to be applied in this case? Select all that apply.

1. Criminal law
2. Statutory law
3. Civil law
4. Common law
5. Administrative law

6 The nurse completes an application for renewal of nurse licensure but accidentally does not mail it out. Which agency should the nurse contact when the nurse finds the unmailed application after the license expiration date has passed?

1. American Nurses Association (ANA)
2. National League for Nursing (NLN)
3. American Nurses Credentialing Center (ANCC)
4. State board of nursing (BON)

7 During a severe hurricane, accusations surface around healthcare providers who allegedly euthanized clients to make better use of limited resources. A nurse working in a facility that is a target of this accusation considers that these accusations could fall under: (Select all that apply.)

1. Common law.
2. Intentional tort.
3. Statutory law.
4. Administrative law.
5. Criminal law.

8 A nurse inserted a urinary drainage catheter without properly cleaning the client's perineal area according to agency policy and the directions on the prepackaged kit. Subsequently, the client developed urosepsis and died. The nurse understands that, in a court of law, these actions could be considered grounds for which of the following most specific charges?

1. Negligence
2. A tort
3. A criminal action
4. *Respondeat superior*

9 A nurse uses a new intravenous (IV) pump for the first time. The client receives too much intravenous fluid and develops heart failure. The nurse is aware that which type of negligence is involved in this case?

1. Standards
2. Equipment
3. Communication
4. Documentation

10 A state board of nursing mandates that Licensed Practical/Vocational Nurses (LPN/LVNs) are not permitted to draw blood specimens from central line devices. The nurse recognizes that this regulation is based on which type of law?

1. Constitutional law
2. Statutory law
3. Common law
4. Standard law

➤ *See pages 84–86 for Answers and Rationales.*

ANSWERS & RATIONALES

Pretest

1 Answer: 1 The nursing shortage, at a nursing unit level, can lead some nurses to take short cuts in practice to save time, but which in some cases can also lead to increased risk of medical error. Subsequently, clients suffer untoward effects. The nursing shortage has also required nurses to work extra shifts, which means nurses are making critical decisions while they are fatigued, again increasing the risk of errors. Client autonomy has increased within the last decade, making option 2 incorrect. Delegation to unlicensed personnel is appropriate as long as the delegated tasks are within the scope of practice of the unlicensed personnel (option 3). Definitions of liability have broadened rather than narrowed over time (option 4). **Cognitive Level:** Comprehension **Client Need:** Safe Effective Care Environment: Management of Care **Integrated Process:** Nursing Process: Implementation **Content Area:** Leadership/Management **Strategy:** Recognize first that options 2 and 4 are false statements to rule them out. Option 3 does not include whether delegation has increased or decreased, so that is eliminated next. This leaves you with option 1 as the best option. **References:** Finkelman, A. W. (2006). *Leadership and management in nursing.* Upper Saddle River, NJ: Pearson Education, pp. 275–302; Sullivan, E. J., & Decker, P. (2005). *Effective leadership and management in nursing* (6th ed.). Upper Saddle River, NJ: Pearson Education, pp. 67–80.

2 Answer: 3 Healthcare providers should remember to adhere to national standards of practice when providing care to clients. National standards provide a measurement of safe care. Offering apologies after an error has occurred (option 1) does not prevent errors and malpractice litigation. Clear communication (option 2) plays a role in reducing malpractice litigation, but it is not the best choice since poor adherence to standards is a greater issue. Developing policies to ensure adequate assessment (option 4) may help, but the nurse needs to know how to intervene once the assessment has been completed. **Cognitive Level:** Application **Client Need:** Safe Effective Care Environment: Management of Care **Integrated Process:** Nursing Process: Planning **Content Area:** Leadership/Management **Strategy:** Consider first that options 1 and 2 do not reduce liability. These measures are reactive and so these options are eliminated. While client assessment is important, adhering to national standards of care prevents errors. Identify the core issue of the question to eliminate incorrect distracters. **References:** Finkelman, A. W. (2006). *Leadership and management in nursing.* Upper Saddle River, NJ: Pearson Education, pp. 275–302; Sullivan, E. J., & Decker, P. (2005). *Effective leadership and management in nursing* (6th ed.). Upper Saddle River, NJ: Pearson Education, pp. 67–80.

3 Answer: 3 Facilities that receive Medicare and Medicaid funding must report sentinel events to the Centers of Medicare and Medicaid Services (CMMS). Adverse effects to medications would be reported to the FDA (option 1). Communicable diseases would be reported to the CDC (option 2). The NIH is a large organization that has many functions, some of which are research and setting clinical guidelines (option 4). **Cognitive Level:** Application **Client Need:** Safe Effective Care Environment: Management of Care **Integrated Process:** Teaching/Learning **Content Area:** Leadership/Management **Strategy:** This question requires knowledge of regulating bodies. Recall that healthcare agencies do not have to report incidents to the NIH and that medication–related incidents are reported to the FDA. Agencies do report incidence and prevalence of various diseases to the CDC. Note that the stem specifies injuries or death due to medical devices and recall that this information must be reported to CMMS. Identify critical words in the stem of the question to select the right answer. **References:** Finkelman, A. W. (2006).

Leadership and management in nursing. Upper Saddle River, NJ: Pearson Education, pp. 275–302; Sullivan, E. J., & Decker, P. (2005). *Effective leadership and management in nursing* (6th ed.). Upper Saddle River, NJ: Pearson Education, pp. 67–80.

4 **Answer: 2** The Durable Power of Attorney gives an individual the authority to make decisions on behalf of another; in addition, clients may choose to add their wishes to this document. A living will is a client's statement indicating the type of care he or she does or does not want should a terminal condition incapacitate the client. A last will and testament is a legal document that gives individuals the right to name others as possessors of property after the party has died. A do-not-resuscitate order is a physician order based on a client's decision to ***not*** be resuscitated; this is an informed decision. **Cognitive Level:** Application **Client Need:** Safe Effective Care Environment: Management of Care **Integrated Process:** Communication and Documentation **Content Area:** Leadership/Management **Strategy:** Critical words in the question are *naming an individual to make decisions.* Look at all options and decide which fits best. Option 3 is not applicable. Option 4 does not require an assigned person to make decisions on behave of the client. Option 1 may or may not include a durable power of attorney. The best option is 2. Use the "best choices" principle to make the correct selection. **References:** Finkelman, A. W. (2006). *Leadership and management in nursing.* Upper Saddle River, NJ: Pearson Education, pp. 275–302; Sullivan, E. J., & Decker, P. (2005). *Effective leadership and management in nursing* (6th ed.). Upper Saddle River, NJ: Pearson Education, pp. 67–80.

5 **Answer: 3** Civil law examines personal injuries inflicted by others in society, and in many cases, provides compensation for harm and injury. The nurse in this case could be sued for damages. Constitutional law does not address personal injuries, but examines the rights of clients. Administrative and statutory laws involve disciplinary action by the state board of nursing, but the client wouldn't collect compensation for damages incurred. **Cognitive Level:** Application **Client Need:** Safe Effective Care Environment: Management of Care **Integrated Process:** Nursing Process: Analysis **Content Area:** Leadership/Management **Strategy:** Consider that the issue of the question is negligence. Next, think about which law plays an important role in negligence and choose this option as the answer to the question. **References:** Finkelman, A. W. (2006). *Leadership and management in nursing.* Upper Saddle River, NJ: Pearson Education, pp. 275–302; Sullivan, E. J., & Decker, P. (2005). *Effective leadership and management in nursing* (6th ed.). Upper Saddle River, NJ: Pearson Education, pp. 67–80.

6 **Answer: 3** A tort falls under civil law and allows a plaintiff to file a suit to gain compensation for damages incurred. An intentional tort in this case would be difficult to prove because there must be intent to injure. Nurses are aware that some medications, when given incorrectly, can have detrimental effects and in the vast majority of cases, do not intend to give a medication that could be deadly. However, a malpractice claim must show duty, breach of duty, injury, and cause, and could be pursued by the client. *Respondeat superior* means the employer is also responsible for the act, but this is not filed against the nurse; it is filed against the healthcare organization. **Cognitive Level:** Application **Client Need:** Safe Effective Care Environment: Management of Care **Integrated Process:** Nursing Process: Analysis **Content Area:** Leadership/Management **Strategy:** Use knowledge of legal terms to select the correct answer. Use the "best choices" principle to make the correct selection. **References:** Finkelman, A. W. (2006). *Leadership and management in nursing.* Upper Saddle River, NJ: Pearson Education, pp. 275–302; Sullivan, E. J., & Decker, P. (2005). *Effective leadership and management in nursing* (6th ed.). Upper Saddle River, NJ: Pearson Education, pp. 67–80.

7 **Answer: 4** Each state Board of Nursing investigates and disciplines nurses who violate statutes and/or regulations. The ANA is the professional nursing organization. The NLN is a nursing organization that is open to public membership and is one accrediting body for schools of nursing. JCAHO is a voluntary accrediting organization for healthcare institutions. The ANA, NLN, and JCAHO do not have the authority to investigate or discipline nurses. **Cognitive Level:** Comprehension **Client Need:** Safe Effective Care Environment: Management of Care **Integrated Process:** Nursing Process: Analysis **Content Area:** Leadership/Management **Strategy:** Recall that the only option that regulates the practice of nurses is the board of nursing. This will help you to immediately eliminate each of the incorrect choices. **References:** Finkelman, A. W. (2006). *Leadership and management in nursing.* Upper Saddle River, NJ: Pearson Education, pp. 275–302; Sullivan, E. J., & Decker, P. (2005). *Effective leadership and management in nursing* (6th ed.). Upper Saddle River, NJ: Pearson Education, pp. 67–80.

8 **Answer: 4** This type of disciplinary action is minor; it allows the nurse to practice, but it also sends the message that the nurse must comply with all statutes and regulations deemed by the state board of nursing. The other options are incorrect interpretations of this finding. **Cognitive Level:** Application **Client Need:** Safe Effective Care Environment: Management of Care **Integrated Process:** Nursing Process: Analysis **Content Area:** Leadership/Management **Strategy:** Recognize that options 1 and 2 are false statements; rule them out first. Option 3 contains the term *only*, which makes it an unlikely answer. Option 4 makes it clear the nurse may practice, but the nurse has committed some action against regulations. Use the "best choices" principle to make the correct selection. **References:** Finkelman, A. W. (2006). *Leadership and management in nursing*. Upper Saddle River, NJ: Pearson Education, pp. 275–302; Sullivan, E. J., & Decker, P. (2005). *Effective leadership and management in nursing* (6th ed.). Upper Saddle River, NJ: Pearson Education, pp. 67–80.

9 **Answer: 2** All violations of state statutes and regulations regarding nursing practice must be reported to the organization that governs nursing practice, which is the state Board of Nursing. The ANA is the professional nursing organization. The NLN is a public organization for nurses that also is an accrediting body for some schools of nursing. The ANCC is a certification organization that is affiliated with the ANA.
Cognitive Level: Application **Client Need:** Safe Effective Care Environment: Management of Care **Integrated Process:** Nursing Process: Analysis **Content Area:** Leadership/Management **Strategy:** Recognize that the only correct option is the board of nursing because the other options do not regulate the practice of nursing. Identify the core issue to prevent selection of incorrect choices. **References:** Finkelman, A. W. (2006). *Leadership and management in nursing*. Upper Saddle River, NJ: Pearson Education, pp. 275–302; Sullivan, E. J., & Decker, P. (2005). *Effective leadership and management in nursing* (6th ed.). Upper Saddle River, NJ: Pearson Education, pp. 67–80.

10 **Answer: 4** The client could file a tort to receive punitive damages for the incident. Under statutory and administrative law, the state board of nursing can investigate the case and take disciplinary actions against the nurse; however, this does not benefit the client directly. Constitutional law does not apply.
Cognitive Level: Application **Client Need:** Safe Effective Care Environment: Management of Care **Integrated Process:** Nursing Process: Planning **Content Area:** Leadership/Management **Strategy:** Consider that the core issue of the question is what will benefit the client directly. The critical words in the question are *client benefit*. Eliminate constitutional law (option 1) immediately because it is not applicable. Note next that options 2 and 4 (administrative and statutory law) impact the nurse in this case. Using the process of elimination, the client would benefit most from filing a tort. **References:** Finkelman, A. W. (2006). *Leadership and management in nursing*. Upper Saddle River, NJ: Pearson Education, pp. 275–302; Sullivan, E. J., & Decker, P. (2005). *Effective*

leadership and management in nursing (6th ed.). Upper Saddle River, NJ: Pearson Education, pp. 67–80.

Posttest

1 **Answer: 1** The nurse practice act constitutes a state statute that falls under statutory law. This act allows nurses to practice in states in which they are licensed. The state board of nursing (option 2) is authorized by statute to enforce and uphold the nurse practice act. The Good Samaritan Law protects individuals who deliver care in an emergency without pay (option 3). The Active Labor Act is another name for the Emergency Medical Treatment Act (option 4), which requires an appropriate level of screening and treatment for clients that present to an emergency services department for treatment in an emergency.
Cognitive Level: Comprehension **Client Need:** Safe Effective Care Environment: Management of Care **Integrated Process:** Nursing Process: Analysis **Content Area:** Leadership/Management **Strategy:** Note that the focus of the question is law to help eliminate option 2, which is a regulating body. From there, note the association between the words *nursing practice* in the stem of the question and *nurse practice* in option 1 to choose correctly. **References:** Finkelman, A. W. (2006). *Leadership and management in nursing*. Upper Saddle River, NJ: Pearson Education, pp. 275–302; Sullivan, E. J., & Decker, P. (2005). *Effective leadership and management in nursing* (6th ed.). Upper Saddle River, NJ: Pearson Education, pp. 67–80.

2 **Answer: 4** This action could result in a malpractice case because the provider neglected to provide a standard of care to a client. "Wrongful injury" in option 3 is not a formal legal term. *Respondeat superior* (option 1) is a term that refers to the financial liability of an agency for its employee's actions. Defamation (option 2) is a charge in which one person makes false statements against the character of another individual.
Cognitive Level: Application **Client Need:** Safe Effective Care Environment: Management of Care **Integrated Process:** Nursing Process: Planning **Content Area:** Leadership/Management **Strategy:** Note that the core issue of the question relates to failure to uphold standards of practice. Note that the stem does not provide data to support options 1 and 2 and that option 3 is not a formal legal term to help you choose correctly. **References:** Finkelman, A. W. (2006). *Leadership and management in nursing*. Upper Saddle River, NJ: Pearson Education, pp. 275–302; Sullivan, E. J., & Decker, P. (2005). *Effective leadership and management in nursing* (6th ed.). Upper Saddle River, NJ: Pearson Education, pp. 67–80.

3 **Answer: 3** The National Council Licensing Examination (NCLEX®) determines if a graduate of a nursing program is minimally safe to practice at the novice level. It does not measure expert status (option 2); it measures safe practice in nurses who graduate from a nursing program with a diploma, associate degree, or baccalaureate degree. Critical care units are specialty units, and this examination does not measure a graduate nurse's ability to practice in a critical care unit.
Cognitive Level: Comprehension **Client Need:** Safe Effective Care Environment: Management of Care **Integrated Process:** Teaching/Learning **Content Area:** Leadership/Management **Strategy:** Recall the purpose of the NCLEX® licensing exam and note that options 1, 2, and 4 are false statements relative to this examination. Note the critical words *designed to ensure* in the stem of the question to select the statement of purpose as the correct answer. **References:** Finkelman, A. W. (2006). *Leadership and management in nursing.* Upper Saddle River, NJ: Pearson Education, pp. 275–302; Sullivan, E. J., & Decker, P. (2005). *Effective leadership and management in nursing* (6th ed.). Upper Saddle River, NJ: Pearson Education, pp. 67–80.

4 **Answer: 1** The state board of nursing has authority by the governor to discipline nurses for behavioral problems as well as drug problems. The board investigates any violations of state statutes and regulations. The other agencies listed do not get involved with the reprimand of nurses.
Cognitive Level: Application **Client Need:** Safe Effective Care Environment: Management of Care **Integrated Process:** Nursing Process: Planning **Content Area:** Leadership/Management **Strategy:** Recognize that options 2, 3, and 4 do not regulate the practice of nurses. This leaves option 1 as the only correct option. **References:** Finkelman, A. W. (2006). *Leadership and management in nursing.* Upper Saddle River, NJ: Pearson Education, pp. 275–302; Sullivan, E. J., & Decker, P. (2005). *Effective leadership and management in nursing* (6th ed.). Upper Saddle River, NJ: Pearson Education, pp. 67–80.

5 **Answers: 1, 3** Because of the impact on the heart of administering potassium IVP, there may be a criminal action against the nurse for this mistake. Criminal action involves the district attorney or solicitor's office. In addition, the client may file a civil claim where the client or the client's family could collect compensation for punitive damages.
Cognitive Level: Application **Client Need:** Safe Effective Care Environment: Management of Care **Integrated Process:** Nursing Process: Implementation **Content Area:** Leadership/Management **Strategy:** Think about which

laws play an important role in negligence, which is the issue of the question. Compare and contrast the definitions of each type of law to make the correct selection. **References:** Finkelman, A. W. (2006). *Leadership and management in nursing.* Upper Saddle River, NJ: Pearson Education, pp. 275–302; Sullivan, E. J., & Decker, P. (2005). *Effective leadership and management in nursing* (6th ed.). Upper Saddle River, NJ: Pearson Education, pp. 67–80.

6 **Answer: 4** Each state board of nursing issues licenses for nurses to practice. The board develops requirements for licensure and holds all nurses responsible for maintaining all requirements to practice. The ANA is the professional nursing organization. The NLN is a nursing organization that is open to public membership and is one accrediting body for schools of nursing. The ANCC is a certification center that is associated with the ANA.
Cognitive Level: Application **Client Need:** Safe Effective Care Environment: Management of Care **Integrated Process:** Nursing Process: Implementation **Content Area:** Leadership/Management **Strategy:** The only option that regulates the practice of nurses is the board of nursing. Identify the core issue to eliminate incorrect distracters and choose the correct option. **References:** Finkelman, A. W. (2006). *Leadership and management in nursing.* Upper Saddle River, NJ: Pearson Education, pp. 275–302; Sullivan, E. J., & Decker, P. (2005). *Effective leadership and management in nursing* (6th ed.). Upper Saddle River, NJ: Pearson Education, pp. 67–80.

7 **Answers: 2, 3, 4, 5** An intentional tort in this case could be possible if purpose and intent are identified. This action could also be considered criminal because of the intentional death of individuals. Statutory and administrative laws give the state board of nursing the authority to investigate allegations and take further disciplinary actions. Common law does not apply to this case.
Cognitive Level: Comprehension **Client Need:** Safe Effective Care Environment: Management of Care **Integrated Process:** Nursing Process: Analysis **Content Area:** Leadership/Management **Strategy:** The core issue of the question is knowledge of the various types of laws. Use knowledge of the definitions of each type of law to make the correct selections. **References:** Finkelman, A. W. (2006). *Leadership and management in nursing.* Upper Saddle River, NJ: Pearson Education, pp. 275–302; Sullivan, E. J., & Decker, P. (2005). *Effective leadership and management in nursing* (6th ed.). Upper Saddle River, NJ: Pearson Education, pp. 67–80.

8 **Answer: 1** In healthcare, negligence is referred to as a failure to provide a standard of care other nurses or healthcare providers give in similar situations.

Negligence is a form of tort (option 2); however, option 2 is too broad because the question asks for the most specific charge. Criminal action would be very difficult to prove, and the complainant may not be able to charge the healthcare organization with liability. Instructions for urinary drainage catheter insertion are clear. *Respondeat superior* means the employer is also responsible for the actions of employees, but this is not filed against the nurse; it is filed against the healthcare organization. **Cognitive Level:** Comprehension **Client Need:** Safe Effective Care Environment: Management of Care **Integrated Process:** Nursing Process: Analysis **Content Area:** Leadership/Management **Strategy:** The critical words in the question are *most specific charge*. Note that the stem does not provide data to support *respondeat superior*. The action is not considered criminal. Option 2 is too broad. Negligence specifically answers the question. Use knowledge of law to make the correct selection. **References:** Finkelman, A. W. (2006). *Leadership and management in nursing*. Upper Saddle River, NJ: Pearson Education, pp. 275–302; Sullivan, E. J., & Decker, P. (2005). *Effective leadership and management in nursing* (6th ed.). Upper Saddle River, NJ: Pearson Education, pp. 67–80.

9 Answer: 2 In this case, equipment is a critical part of the problem because the question states that the client received too much intravenous fluid via an IV pump that the nurse is not familiar with. Standards and documentation do not apply. Communication could be related if the nurse misunderstood directions for using the pump, but it is not the best choice because the equipment is at the center of the issue. **Cognitive Level:** Comprehension **Client Need:** Safe Effective Care Environment: Management of Care **Integrated Process:** Nursing Process: Analysis **Content Area:** Leadership/Management **Strategy:** Note that the stem of the question focuses on new equipment. The stem does not provide data to support options 1, 3, and 4. Unfamiliarity with equipment could lead the nurse to set the pump incorrectly and excess fluid could then be the cause of heart failure. Identify the core issue and connect the word *pump* in the question with the word *equipment* in the correct answer. **References:** Finkelman, A. W. (2006). *Leadership and management in nursing*. Upper Saddle River, NJ: Pearson Education, pp. 275–302; Sullivan, E. J., & Decker, P. (2005). *Effective leadership and management in nursing* (6th ed.). Upper Saddle River, NJ: Pearson Education, pp. 67–80.

10 Answer: 2 Constitutional law protects clients' constitutional rights to self-determination. Statutory law is a set of statutes enacted by a legislative branch of the government such as the state board of nursing and the nurse practice act, and applies to scope of practice and upholding standards of care. Administrative law protects the civil rights of individuals such as the age discrimination act. Common law is a document that sets forth the fundamental body of law that establishes the overall structure and powers of government. Standard law is not an official type of law. **Cognitive Level:** Application **Client Need:** Safe Effective Care Environment: Management of Care **Integrated Process:** Nursing Process: Planning **Content Area:** Leadership/Management **Strategy:** Read all options and select the best one. Identify critical words in the question or stem to select the right answer. The stem does not provide data to support options 1 and 3. Option 4 is not an official type of law; rule it out. **References:** Finkelman, A. W. (2006). *Leadership and management in nursing*. Upper Saddle River, NJ: Pearson Education, pp. 275–302; Sullivan, E. J., & Decker, P. (2005). *Effective leadership and management in nursing* (6th ed.). Upper Saddle River, NJ: Pearson Education, pp. 67–80.

References

Calfee, B. E. & Follows, J. M. (2000). Legal questions. *Nursing, 30*(12), 82–84.

Croke, E. (2003). Nurses, negligence, and malpractice. *American Journal of Nursing, 103*(9), 54–64.

Elisi, J. R., & Hartley, C. L. (2001). *Nursing in today's world: Challenges, issues, and trends*. New York: Lippincott.

Finkelstein, A. W. (2006). *Leadership and management in nursing*. Upper Saddle River, NJ: Pearson Education.

Lee, N. G. (2000). Proving nursing negligence. *American Journal of Nursing, 7*(11), 55–56.

Lin, L., & Liang, B. (2007). Addressing the nursing work environment to promote patient safety. *Nursing Forum, 42*(1), 20–30.

Murer, M. J. (2001). Ten resolutions to minimize liability. *Nursing Homes Long Term Care Management, 50*(4), 64–68.

Smetzer, J., & Navarra, M. B. (2007). Measuring change: A key component of building a culture of safety. *Nursing Economic$, 25*(1), 49–51.

Sullivan, E. J. & Decker, P. (2005). *Effective leadership and management in nursing* (6th ed.). Upper Saddle River, NJ: Pearson Education.

White, G. B. (2000). Informed consent. *American Journal of Nursing, 100*(9), 83.

ANSWERS & RATIONALES

The Details of Delegation

5

Chapter Outline

The Art of Delegation

Components of Delegation

Barriers to Delegation

Accountability and Liability

Responsibility and Authority

Care Team Functions of Delegation

Advantages and Disadvantages of Delegation

Five Rights of Delegation

Transcultural Delegation

Continuity of Care

Objectives

➤ Define the term *delegation*.

➤ Explain the process of delegation.

➤ Describe the meaning and implications of the terms *accountability*, *liability*, *responsibility*, and *authority* for clinical leadership.

➤ Explain the care team functions of delegation.

➤ Describe the advantages and disadvantages of delegation.

➤ Identify the five rights of delegation.

➤ Discuss why transcultural delegation is important to clinical leadership.

➤ Explain how continuity of care is maintained through delegation.

NCLEX-RN® Test Prep

Use the CD-ROM enclosed with this book to access additional practice opportunities.

Review at a Glance

accountability a process of reflecting legal liability for actions; holds individual nurses answerable for overall care of designated clients

authority right to instruct others to carry out orders and possession of power to expect compliance; derived from a person's rank or position within an organization

delegation use of personnel to accomplish a desired objective through allocation of authority and responsibility

continuity of care involves a variety of relationships between the client and members of the healthcare system including availability of information, availability or constancy of the clinician, usual source of care, and the goal of seamlessness in transitions from one care setting to another

liability responsibility for actions of oneself or for actions of those under one's supervision

overdelegation delegation of too much authority and/or too much responsibility to others; may occur when one becomes overwhelmed by a situation and loses control

responsibility a personal obligation to perform or deliver desired results so that the entire organization benefits

reverse delegation a team member's request that a nurse leader complete a task because of inability or unwillingness to perform the designated task or procedure

transcultural delegation processes of having personnel from diverse cultures perform duties that have different connotations in various cultures; nurse leaders have the ability to delegate nursing care that is appropriate and acceptable to clients even though this care is not a part of the caregiver's own belief system

underdelegation a situation in which the delegator does not think that team members can perform an assignment and instead completes the assignment or does not transfer full authority

PRETEST

1 A client experiences respiratory distress with shallow respirations at a rate of 32/minute. The client has assumed an orthopneic position and is pale and confused. Heart rate is 118 bpm and blood pressure is 90/40 mm Hg. Which task should the nurse delegate to the charge nurse?

1. Completion of a head-to-toe assessment
2. Insertion of a second IV line
3. Application of oxygen per protocol order
4. Paging of the respiratory therapist

2 A registered nurse (RN) delegates complicated wound care to a licensed practical/vocational nurse (LPN/LVN). The LPN/LVN has only changed this type of dressing once. Which component of delegation has the RN neglected?

1. Authority
2. Competency
3. Communication
4. Responsibility

3 A charge nurse begins the shift overwhelmed by many nursing care activities that need to be completed. The staff has been working short-handed for months, and the charge nurse has become reluctant to delegate nursing activities such as checking the code cart and performing narcotic counts to other qualified staff. When questioned by the nursing supervisor about insufficient delegation, the nurse explains that which barrier is of key concern at this time?

1. Inadequate support
2. Disorganization
3. Hostile environment
4. Incompetence

4 A nurse assists a client in room A with lunch. The charge nurse calls the nurse and reports the client in room C reports pain and is requesting pain medication. What is the nurse's best action?

1. Finish feeding client in room A, then medicate client in room C for pain.
2. Stop feeding client in room A and medicate client in room C for pain.
3. Finish feeding client in room A and ask charge nurse to medicate client in room C.
4. Ask charge nurse to feed client in room A while nurse medicates client in room C for pain.

5 The registered nurse (RN) has completed making client assignments for the shift and is preparing to delegate appropriate nursing care activities to the staff. Which tasks may the RN delegate to the certified nursing assistant (CNA)? Select all that apply.

1. Ambulating a client in the hallway
2. Recording intake and output from meal trays
3. Measuring and recording vital signs
4. Completing a skin risk assessment using the Braden scale
5. Recording a client's oxygen saturation measurements

6 After receiving intershift report on a medical nursing unit, the registered nurse (RN) prepares for the work of the day. Which of the following activities can the nurse delegate to a licensed practical/vocational nurse (LPN/LVN)? Select all that apply.

1. Irrigating a nasogastric tube on a client receiving tube feedings
2. Irrigating a clogged urinary drainage catheter on an older adult client
3. Rechecking vital signs on a post-surgical client with a previous BP of 98/60 mm Hg
4. Changing a dressing on a client admitted with an infected diabetic foot ulcer the previous day
5. Administering a unit packed red blood cells (RBCs) to a client with a hemoglobin of 10.2 grams/L

7 The care delivery system on a medical nursing unit is team nursing. On wing A, there is a registered nurse (RN) and licensed practical/vocational nurse (LPN/LVN) team to care for eight clients. Which tasks should the RN delegate to the LPN/LVN?

1. Vital signs and assessment on a postoperative client
2. Wound care and oral and intravenous (IV) medications for all clients
3. Vital signs and hygiene care on all eight clients
4. Assessments on two young, stable clients

8 A nurse delegates care of clients to the certified nursing assistant (CNA) and licensed practical/vocational nurse (LPN/LVN). Which tasks should the nurse assign to the CNA and LPN/LVN?

1. CNA—check vital signs; LPN—give oral meds to assigned clients
2. CNA—change noninfected dressing; LPN—administer intravenous piggyback (IVPB) medications
3. CNA—ambulate a client who had a stroke; LPN—assess two clients
4. CNA—take vital signs; LPN—complete all admission paperwork

9 A nurse prepares for the day, and makes a list of delegated tasks for the certified nursing assistant (CNA). Which task should the nurse delegate to the CNA?

1. Feed a client admitted with a stroke who has dysphagia
2. Monitor drainage from the chest tube of a client with hemothorax
3. Recheck vital signs on client whose blood pressure is 190/102 mm Hg
4. Turn and reposition a client with multiple sclerosis who has severe weakness

10 A registered nurse (RN) assesses a client and finds that the client uses accessory muscles to breathe and has a respiratory rate of 27/minute. Two hours previously, this client was eupneic with a respiratory rate of 18. What are the best actions for the nurse to take next?

1. Stay with client; call the certified nursing assistant (CNA) to bring pulse oximeter, and check the client's oxygen (O_2) saturation level
2. Obtain a pulse oximeter; check the client's O_2 saturation and ask the CNA to check vital signs
3. Obtain a pulse oximeter; check the client's O_2 saturation level; and solicit support from the charge nurse
4. Stay with the client; call the charge nurse for help; call the CNA to bring a pulse oximeter and vital signs monitor to the room

➤ *See pages 101–104 for Answers and Rationales.*

Box 5-1	1. Delegate only tasks for which you have responsibility.
Tools for Delegation	2. Transfer authority when you delegate responsibility.
	3. Be sure you follow state regulations, job descriptions, and agency policies when delegating.
	4. Follow the delegation process and key behaviors for delegating described in the chapter.
	5. Accept delegation when you are clear about the task, time frame, reporting, and other expectations.
	6. Confront your fears about delegation; recognize those that are realistic and those that are not.

Source: Sullivan, E. J., & Decker, P. J. (2005). *Effective leadership and management in nursing* (6th ed.). Upper Saddle River, NJ: Pearson Prentice Hall, p. 153. Reprinted by permission.

I. THE ART OF DELEGATION

A. *Delegation*
1. The use of nursing personnel to accomplish desired objectives through allocation of authority and responsibility
2. Nurse leaders must seek to entrust responsibility and authority to competent individuals and must be accountable for the results (see Box 5-1)
3. Delegation is a complex process and a crucial management skill
4. Delegation encompasses retaining accountability for the number and diversity of caregivers
5. It includes awareness of the amount of different knowledge and skill needed to provide care that benefits clients
6. It is used to accomplish nursing tasks in the most efficient way using appropriate resources

B. The National Council of State Boards in Nursing (NCSBN) defines delegation as transferring to a competent individual the authority to perform selected nursing tasks in selected situations

C. Delegation of nursing assignments
1. Nursing care assignments are delegated based on the competency of the delegate, including:
   a. Education level
   b. Knowledge level
   c. Skill level
   d. Job description/agency policy
2. Nurse leaders must be clear about the outcomes or expectations of each assigned nursing task or activity including:
   a. The standard of care
   b. The time frame for assignment completion
   c. Limitations regarding performance of the task
3. See Box 5-2 for strategies for effective delegation

<table>
<tr><td>**Box 5-2**

Learning Effective Delegation</td><td>Delegation is an act of transferring to a competent individual the authority to perform a selected nursing task in a selected situation.

1. Many nurse leaders and even staff nurses are often unable to perform all of the activities assigned to them. Thus, they must delegate some of these to unlicensed assistive personnel.

2. Make sure that the task being delegated is within the delegate's scope of practice and that the person has the competency to perform the task.

3. Give clear, concise, correct, and complete directions to the delegate.

4. Provide for ongoing feedback and evaluation.</td></tr>
</table>

Practice to Pass

Describe the essential skills required by the nurse leader in order to effectively delegate. What are some ways the nurse leader would implement effective delegation?

D. Why nurse leaders must delegate

1. No one person can do everything

2. Delegation allows for the most efficient way of utilizing appropriate resources

3. Delegation sparks interest and helps prevent nursing staff from becoming nonproductive and ineffective

4. Delegation builds teamwork and encourages staff to discover duties or tasks that best suit them and makes staff feel like they are part of the team regardless of position

5. Nurse leaders can delegate authority but cannot delegate responsibility

E. Three *Do Not Delegate* tasks for nurse leader to know:

1. Initial nursing assessment, subsequent assessments, and those requiring professional judgment

2. Nursing diagnoses, nursing care goals, and progress plans

3. Interventions requiring professional knowledge and skill

4. Be aware that the only phase of the nursing process that may be delegated to nonprofessional staff is implementation

II. COMPONENTS OF DELEGATION

A. Principles of delegation

1. Nurse leaders must understand that only authority can be delegated, not their responsibility

2. All delegated tasks must be clearly assigned and continuously clarified

3. If nurse leaders know their job responsibilities, they will know what can and cannot be delegated

4. The nurse leader must set clear parameters around how much authority is needed to accomplish a task, and delegate just enough authority to accomplish the assigned task successfully

5. The nurse leader should be sure the delegated task is completed as assigned and not handed back incomplete or unfinished

B. Components of delegation

1. Delegator: the person doing the delegating

2. Delegate: the person to whom an activity is delegated

3. The task or activity to be accomplished

Box 5-3
 	
Process of Delegation
Decision Making
	1. Assess the situation
	    a. Identify the needs of the client, consulting the plan of care
	    b. Consider the circumstances/setting
	    c. Assure the availability of adequate resources, including supervision
	2. Plan for the specific task(s) to be delegated
	    a. Specify the nature of each task and the knowledge and skills required to perform it
	    b. Require documentation or demonstration of current competence by the delegate for each task
	    c. Determine the implications for the client, other clients, and significant others
	3. Assure appropriate accountability
	    a. As delegator, accept accountability for performance of the task(s)
	    b. Verify that the delegate accepts the delegation and the accountability for carrying out the task correctly
	4. Supervise performance of the task
	    a. Provide directions and clear expectations of how the task(s) is to be performed
	    b. Monitor performance of the task(s) to assure compliance to established standards of practice, policies and procedures
	    c. Intervene if necessary
	    d. Ensure appropriate documentation of the task(s)
	5. Evaluate the entire delegation process
	    a. Evaluate the client
	    b. Evaluate the performance of the task(s)
	    c. Obtain and provide feedback
	6. Reassess and adjust the overall plan of care as needed

Source: National Council of State Boards of Nursing, Inc. (n.d.). Retrieved January 8, 2008, from www.ncsbn.org/cps/rde/xchg/ncsbn/hs.xsl/323.htm#Delegation_Decision-Making_Process. Reprinted by permission.

  C. Delegation process (see Box 5-3)
     1. Determine and identify the task and level of responsibility of each task
     2. Evaluate delegate's fit with assigned task
     3. Decide what level of supervision is needed and describe expectations
     4. Reach agreement on performance and outcome
     5. Provide continuous feedback, monitor performance, and adjust accordingly

III. BARRIERS TO DELEGATION

  A. Nurse leaders frequently experience barriers that impact their ability to delegate, including:
     1. A "Do it myself" attitude
     2. An inability to ask others or to organize/manage
     3. Feelings of uncertainty

    4. Fear of competition, liability, or loss of control

    5. Fear of decreased job satisfaction for delegates

B. Delegates may resist and sometimes refuse to accept delegated tasks because of:

    1. Inexperience

    2. Incompetence

    3. Disorganization

    4. Irresponsibility

    5. Situational barriers

C. The workplace itself may become a barrier to delegation because of:

    1. Inadequate support

    2. A hurried atmosphere

    3. Hostile management

IV. ACCOUNTABILITY AND LIABILITY

A. *Accountability*

    1. Occurs when professional nurse leader becomes legally liable for actions and is answerable for overall nursing care for designated clients

    2. The nurse leader makes sure that team members:

        a. Understand the job

        b. Accept the responsibility that the job entails

        c. Commit to deliver the desired results

B. *Liability*

    1. Responsibility for one's own actions and those that nurse leader supervises during delegation process

    2. The nurse leader is responsible for knowing all tasks that are:

        a. Within the scope of practice within state's nurse practice act

        b. Within the scope of practice of assigned nursing staff members

        c. Compatible with the competencies and abilities of nursing staff assigned to those tasks

Practice to Pass

Describe what is meant by standards of care. Discuss the reasons why the nurse leader would need to document when nursing staff deviate from the standard of practice.

C. Standards of care

    1. Standards of care are expected levels of performance

    2. They act as guidelines in providing nursing care

    3. Nurses who breach standards of care or assign tasks outside scope of practice of assigned staff may be found negligent; thus, standards of care are useful in malpractice situations and in cases where the nurse's license is at stake because of failure to uphold them

V. RESPONSIBILITY AND AUTHORITY

A. *Responsibility*

    1. There are qualifications for both the delegator and the delegate regarding the process of delegation (see Box 5-4)

    2. Both delegator and delegate have responsibilities regarding delegation

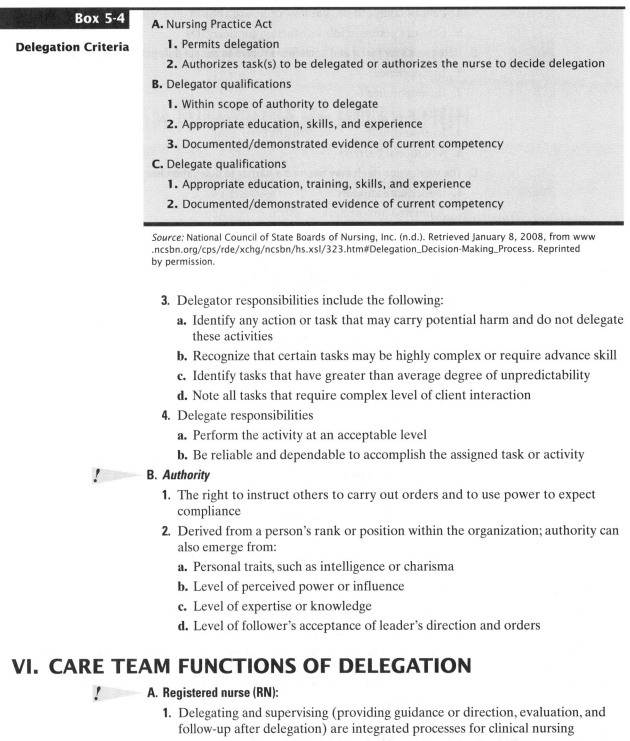

Box 5-4	**A.** Nursing Practice Act
Delegation Criteria	**1.** Permits delegation

A. Nursing Practice Act

1. Permits delegation

2. Authorizes task(s) to be delegated or authorizes the nurse to decide delegation

B. Delegator qualifications

1. Within scope of authority to delegate

2. Appropriate education, skills, and experience

3. Documented/demonstrated evidence of current competency

C. Delegate qualifications

1. Appropriate education, training, skills, and experience

2. Documented/demonstrated evidence of current competency

Source: National Council of State Boards of Nursing, Inc. (n.d.). Retrieved January 8, 2008, from www .ncsbn.org/cps/rde/xchg/ncsbn/hs.xsl/323.htm#Delegation_Decision-Making_Process. Reprinted by permission.

3. Delegator responsibilities include the following:

   a. Identify any action or task that may carry potential harm and do not delegate these activities

   b. Recognize that certain tasks may be highly complex or require advance skill

   c. Identify tasks that have greater than average degree of unpredictability

   d. Note all tasks that require complex level of client interaction

4. Delegate responsibilities

   a. Perform the activity at an acceptable level

   b. Be reliable and dependable to accomplish the assigned task or activity

B. *Authority*

1. The right to instruct others to carry out orders and to use power to expect compliance

2. Derived from a person's rank or position within the organization; authority can also emerge from:

   a. Personal traits, such as intelligence or charisma

   b. Level of perceived power or influence

   c. Level of expertise or knowledge

   d. Level of follower's acceptance of leader's direction and orders

VI. CARE TEAM FUNCTIONS OF DELEGATION

A. Registered nurse (RN):

1. Delegating and supervising (providing guidance or direction, evaluation, and follow-up after delegation) are integrated processes for clinical nursing

2. Know delegation rules

3. Know regulations of nurse practice act in state in which nursing is being practiced

4. Review delegation policies of the organization and job descriptions of nursing team members

5. Assess each client to be sure delegation is appropriate for his or her care

6. Ensure that the person to whom a task is delegated has competency to perform safely and effectively

7. Supervise the delegate to ensure the task is completed correctly and in a timely manner

B. Licensed practical/vocational nurse (LPN/LVN):

1. Determine which tasks may be delegated

2. Remember that the LPN/LVN works with an RN, who initiates the nursing care plan; the LPN/LVN may update the care plan

3. RN completes the initial assessment and validates assessment changes noted by LPN/LVN

4. RN initiates client teaching and evaluates the outcomes

5. LPN/LVN may not initiate client teaching with exception of using a standard care plan and may reinforce client teaching

6. It is important to know the legal limits of delegation to an LPN/LVN according to both state and organizational policy; IV administration regulations vary state to state; LPN/LVNs may initiate IVs on each state's standards and may or may not add medications to an IV or administer IV push or IV piggyback solutions

7. Determine the amount of judgment and experience required to perform a task or skill

8. Determine the LPN/LVN's capacity to perform the assigned task

C. Unlicensed assistive personnel (UAP):

1. Unlicensed personnel may not perform functions (even under direction of RN) that require a certain amount of scientific knowledge and technical skill

2. UAPs can:

    a. Implement care to meet specific client needs

    b. Monitor progress in client care through the feedback process

VII. ADVANTAGES AND DISADVANTAGES OF DELEGATION

A. Advantages

1. Delegator benefits by gaining more managerial and leadership time (higher efficiency) to accomplish other activities that cannot be delegated to staff

2. Delegate benefits by gaining new skills and abilities in accepting assigned tasks as well as the opportunity to demonstrate proficiency and self-confidence

3. Increases motivation of both delegator and delegate

4. Develops skills of both delegator and delegate

5. Allows for better distribution of work through group

B. Disadvantages

1. Ineffective delegation: nurse leaders can become ineffective delegators when:

    a. Tasks are not completed or are completed incorrectly

    b. Accepting one or more delegated tasks from team members

    c. Delegating too much authority or responsibility to team members

2. **Underdelegation:**

   a. Occurs when delegator does not think that team members can perform and complete the assignment or does not transfer full authority

   b. It is crucial to develop team members who can provide complete and comprehensive client care

   c. If unable to perform tasks, team members must be directed and equipped with training and appropriate skill development

3. **Reverse delegation:**

   a. Occurs when a team member requests that a nurse leader complete a task because of inability or unwillingness to perform the designated task or procedure

   b. Nurse leader needs to address this issue through use of competency-based orientation programs and in-service/staff development classes

4. **Overdelegation:**

   a. Occurs when delegator becomes overwhelmed by the situation and loses control by delegating too much authority and/or responsibility to delegate

   b. Tasks are delegated inappropriately; the nurse leader cannot successfully achieve goals if overwhelmed by numerous requests

   c. Each nurse leader must determine the ability of staff to take on the assigned request; balance requests after prioritizing the needs of unit staff and clients

   d. Tasks should not be delegated to LPN/LVNs or UAPs that are beyond their scope of practice

VIII. FIVE RIGHTS OF DELEGATION

A. The National Council of State Boards of Nursing (1995) has defined five rights of delegation

B. The five rights include the following (see Box 5-5):

1. Right task
2. Right circumstance
3. Right person
4. Right direction/communication
5. Right supervision

Practice to Pass

Explain why the nurse leader is accountable for the care given to assigned clients even if that care has been delegated to a staff nurse or UAP.

Box 5-5
Five Rights of Delegation

➤ **Right Task:** One that is delegable for a specific client.

➤ **Right Circumstances:** Appropriate client setting, available resources, and other relevant factors considered.

➤ **Right Person:** Right person is delegating the right task to the right person to be performed on the right person.

➤ **Right Direction/Communication:** Clear, concise description of the task, including its objective, limits, and expectations.

➤ **Right Supervision:** Appropriate monitoring, evaluation, intervention, as needed, and feedback.

Source: National Council of State Boards of Nursing, Inc. (n.d.). Retrieved January 8, 2008, from www.ncsbn.org/cps/rde/xchg/ncsbn/hs.xsl/323.htm#The_Five_Rights_of_Delegation. Reprinted by permission.

IX. *TRANSCULTURAL DELEGATION*

A. Definition

1. Process of having personnel from diverse cultures perform duties that have different connotations in various cultures

2. Nurse leaders have the ability to delegate nursing care that is appropriate and acceptable to clients even though this care is not a part of the caregiver's own belief system

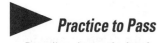

B. Important cultural phenomena to consider when delegating to team members from culturally diverse backgrounds:

1. Communication: is affected by cultural diversity in the workforce by dialect, volume, use of touch, context of speech, and kinesics, i.e., gestures, stance, and eye behavior

2. Space: Americans prefer interpersonal space between people for communication to be between 2 and 3 feet, whereas in other cultures this distance may be too close or too distant

3. Social support: an essential environmental aspect of any group or unit in providing support in an individual's life

4. Time: past, present, or future oriented; promptness is expected in American culture; in other cultures lateness of 15 minutes or more may be acceptable

5. Environmental influence: an individual's perception of influence over his or her environment; an individual who believes that he or she has internal influence over the environment is more likely to be autonomous in decision making

X. *CONTINUITY OF CARE*

A. Defined as multidimensional and describes a variety of relationships between clients and the healthcare delivery system, including:

1. Availability of information

2. Availability or constancy of the clinician

3. The usual source of care

4. The goal of seamlessness in transitions from one care setting to another

B. Continuity is also an important component in the delegation process

1. Not all relevant information about a client is included in the medical record; some information may be outdated or incorrect; other information is intentionally omitted or was simply never recorded

2. Nurse and/or unlicensed personnel may have an ongoing relationship with the client and may be able to recognize significant changes or client reports because of having a referent period (client is his or her own control)

3. Affect and body language are important and may be as valuable as clinical findings in identifying a significant clinical event

C. A continuous relationship between the client and nurse is thought to promote trust, a core part of the nurse-client relationship, and can itself be part of healing process

D. Continuum of care

1. Involves the client's health status and the roles of the nurse and unlicensed assistive personnel (UAPs)

Practice to Pass

Describe why continuity of nursing care is an essential component of the delegation process.

2. The following principles suggest how nurses and UAPs care for clients across the continuum of care:

   a. The client's health status influences who initiates, provides, and is accountable for the provision of care

   b. Care decisions may be made by the client or client surrogate; a surrogate is an individual appointed to act on the client's behalf

   c. Care may be provided by a licensed nurse and/or assistive personnel

   d. In non-healthcare systems, care is directed by the client or client surrogate

   e. Assistive personnel may function across the continuum of care

   f. A licensed nurse is not accountable for care decisions when a client contracts independently with assistive personnel

   g. A licensed nurse determines and is accountable for appropriateness of delegated nursing tasks

   h. A licensed nurse is ultimately responsible and accountable for management and provision of nursing care

   i. The values and experiences of clients and licensed nurses influence decision making

   j. Boards of nursing have accountability and authority for regulation of nursing practice

3. The continuum of care addresses the roles of licensed nurses and assistive personnel in relation to client health status and ability to direct own care

4. It is important that nursing seeks to protect the public and clearly defines the lines of authority and accountability among licensed nurses, assistive personnel, and clients to whom care is provided

E. Client's health status

1. Falls within a range of three levels of dependence: independent, partially dependent, and fully dependent

2. Independent status: a client with or without a health impairment who has the ability for self-care; a client at this level may initiate, accept, and direct health-related interventions

   a. Interventions may be provided by licensed nurses or assistive personnel; may or may not constitute the practice of nursing depending on circumstance and the state nurse practice act

   b. For a client without an identified health impairment, interventions may include general education and support to promote wellness, health maintenance, and disease prevention

   c. For a client with an identified health impairment, the nurse may also provide consultation, initiated by the client or nurse, to support and maintain the client's independent status

3. Partially dependent status: a client with self-care deficits who needs assistance in activities of daily living (ADLs) and/or health maintenance activities

   a. A nurse's primary responsibilities for partially dependent clients involve care coordination including consultation, needs assessment, health education, support, and other direct care activities; there is ongoing evaluation of care provided by self and others; and teaching and validating competencies of assistive personnel who perform care activities

      b. The client or nurse may direct care and often reflect upon the degree of self-care deficit and level of monitoring and interventions required by the nurse or assistive personnel

   4. Fully dependent status: a client's responsibility for care has been transferred to the licensed professional nurse within a healthcare system; the clients may or may not be competent or capable of participating in self-care

      a. The nurse is accountable for overall management of nursing care

Practice to Pass

Describe the care requirements when a client has a fully dependent status.

      b. When assistive personnel are used, they are authorized to perform care through the delegation process

      c. Nurses play an especially key role as client advocate when a client is fully dependent and cannot advocate for self in the healthcare environment

---

Case Study

As the nurse manager on the Labor, Delivery, Recovery and Postpartum Unit (LDRP), you have decided to gave the unit clerk responsibility for the unit's staffing, including finding replacements for sick calls because of a sudden influx of clients in active labor.

1. Identify the steps of the delegation process.

2. Differentiate the concepts of responsibility, accountability, and authority.

3. Explain the type of delegation that the nurse manager used in this situation.

4. Discuss whether the supervision was appropriate to the task by the nurse manager.

5. Did the nurse manager delegate appropriately to the unit clerk's abilities? Why or why not?

For suggested responses, see page 236.

POSTTEST

1 A licensed practical/vocational nurse (LPN/LVN) is assigned to the care of several clients. One client is receiving morphine via intravenous push (IVP) for left shoulder pain rated as 7 on a scale of 1 to 10. A second client has an order for oral digoxin (Lanoxin) and furosemide (Lasix) for congestive heart failure (CHF). A third client is stable and has vitamins ordered to improve wound healing. Which task should the LPN/LVN reverse delegate to a registered nurse (RN)?

1. Administration of IVP morphine for the client with pain
2. Administration of oral medications for the client with CHF
3. Administration of vitamins for the stable client with wounds
4. None, the LPN/LVN should administer all medications to these clients

2 A charge nurse makes assignments for the day. Which client should the registered nurse (RN) assign to the licensed practical/vocational nurse (LPN/LVN)?

1. A client with sickle cell anemia requiring pain medication every 3 hours
2. A four-day postoperative client with hypertension who will be discharged today
3. A 76-year-old client admitted three days ago with type 2 diabetes mellitus
4. A client who underwent repair of a fractured leg and pelvis who has a hemoglobin of 6.4 grams/dL

POSTTEST

❸ An applicant for a nurse manager position tours a nursing unit following an interview and finds one licensed practical/vocational nurse (LPN/LVN) performing wound care and venipunctures while another LPN/LVN is administering oral and parenteral medications. The registered nurses (RNs) are completing assessments. The charge nurse is administering IV push (IVP) and IV piggyback (IVPB) medications. The nurse applicant concludes that the unit utilizes which care delivery model?

1. Task
2. Operational
3. Primary
4. Team

❹ The nursing supervisor telephones a medical-surgical unit and informs the charge nurse that clients from the emergency department (ED) and operating room (OR) will be admitted to the unit. The ED is sending a client who has pneumonia and a history of diabetes mellitus (DM). The OR is sending two clients, one who had a total abdominal hysterectomy and another who underwent right hip replacement. How should the charge nurse assign these clients?

1. Assign a registered nurse (RN) on orientation to the postoperative client who underwent hip replacement.
2. Assign a skilled RN to the postoperative client with the hip replacement.
3. Assign a licensed practical/vocational nurse (LPN/LVN) to the client with pneumonia and DM.
4. Assign another LPN to the client who underwent abdominal hysterectomy.

❺ A client has residual deficits from a stroke two years ago and requires assistance with activities of daily living (ADLs). The client is treated for a urinary tract infection (UTI) with intravenous (IV) antibiotics and receives IV push (IVP) ketorolac (Toradol) for management of back pain. The client has wound care twice a day to an arterial leg ulcer. Which tasks should the licensed practical/vocational nurse (LPN/LVN) delegate to the certified nursing assistant (CNA) and charge nurse?

1. ADLs should be delegated to CNA; IV medications and wound care should be delegated to charge nurse.
2. ADLs should be delegated to CNA; IV medications should be delegated to charge nurse.
3. Wound care and ADLs should be delegated to CNA; IV medications should be delegated to charge nurse.
4. Wound care and ADLs should be delegated to CNA and antibiotics should be delegated to charge nurse.

❻ A charge nurse is floated to the rehabilitation unit because the usual charge nurse has a sick day, and the nurse observes the following. On each wing there is a registered nurse/licensed practical nurse (RN/LPN) or RN/certified nursing assistant (RN/CNA) pair that provides care for a group of eight clients. The nurse concludes that which care delivery system is being utilized on this unit?

1. Task
2. Primary
3. Paired
4. Team

❼ A nurse is assigned to the care of a client with an unsteady gait. The client is later found by the certified nursing assistant (CNA) lying on the floor; the client reports right hip pain. How should the nurse document this incident?

1. Complete an incident report and file a copy in the client's medical record.
2. Complete an incident report and document the fall in the client's medical record.
3. Record the incident in the client's chart and place a copy in the nurse's record.
4. Complete an incident report and give the client's caregivers a copy for their records.

8 An obstetric unit nurse floats to a medical unit to care for a group of acutely ill clients. The charge nurse should assign which group of clients to the float nurse?

1. A client with an old stroke; a client with a three-day-old total knee replacement; a 30-year-old client with pneumonia; and a 20-year-old client with an exacerbation of asthma
2. An 80-year-old client with dehydration; a 75-year-old client with atrial fibrillation; a 62-year-old postoperative client who underwent colectomy; and a 90-year-old client with a hip fracture
3. A client with an old stroke; a client with a 3-day-old hip replacement; a client with atrial fibrillation; and a postoperative client with a hysterectomy
4. A 30-year-old client with pneumonia; a 20-year-old client with an exacerbation of asthma; a postoperative client with a total hip replacement; and a postoperative client with a hysterectomy

9 A nurse receives a call from a client's son who is requesting specific information about the client's diagnosis for "insurance purposes." How should the nurse respond to the client's son?

1. "Your mother is doing a lot better; she'll be discharged within the next few days."
2. "You have no right to ask such questions about your mother's care."
3. "Privacy regulations preclude me from disclosing information about our clients."
4. "I can only provide you with your mother's surgical procedure, but that is all."

10 A registered nurse (RN) plans to delegate some responsibilities of client care to a licensed practical/vocational nurse (LPN/LVN) and a certified nursing assistant (CNA). Which task should the RN delegate to the LPN/LVN?

1. Assessment of a newly admitted client
2. Assessment of a postoperative client
3. Dry sterile dressing changes for a client with superficial wounds
4. Assistance of a client with ambulation and morning hygiene care

➤ *See pages 104–106 for Answers and Rationales.*

ANSWERS & RATIONALES

Pretest

1 **Answer: 2** This client's condition is deteriorating. The nurse has to work quickly to prepare this client for stat medication orders. When a client's condition is deteriorating, the nurse needs additional support, especially from experienced nurses. The assigned nurse at the bedside should apply oxygen (option 3) to improve oxygenation as the most immediate action (option 3). The assigned nurse should complete a head-to-toe assessment (option 1), since this nurse knows more about the client than other nurses on the unit and can best determine a change in status. The unit secretary could page respiratory therapist to the room stat for assistance. The charge nurse should be used to complete a secondary task within the RN's scope of practice such as starting

an intravenous line, which does not require in-depth knowledge of the client's condition. **Cognitive Level:** Application **Client Need:** Safe Effective Care Environment: Management of Care **Integrated Process:** Nursing Process: Planning **Content Area:** Leadership/Management **Strategy:** Note the client's condition and that there is some assessment data in the stem of the question to eliminate option 1. Recall that when a client is decompensating, a focused assessment rather than a complete assessment is indicated. Next, eliminate option 3 since the primary nurse should have applied oxygen immediately to treat the respiratory distress. Option 4 is a task for the unit secretary. In this case, option 2 is correct because it gives the assigned nurse an opportunity to provide direct care or to call the healthcare provider. Use knowledge of scope of practice and delegation to select the correct answer. **References:** Finkelman, A. W. (2006). *Leadership and management in nursing.* Upper Saddle River, NJ: Pearson Education, pp. 224–233; Sullivan, E. J., & Decker, P. (2005). *Effective leadership and management in nursing* (6th ed.). Upper Saddle River, NJ: Pearson Education, pp. 143–152.

2 Answer: 2 The RN did not consider the LPN/LVN's skills and knowledge of complicated dressing changes if the LPN/LVN had only completed complicated wound care once before. Thus, the RN did not consider competency (option 2). The LPN/LVN clearly has authority to change the dressing within the LPN/LVN scope of practice (option 1). Even when an RN has communicated the task (option 3), the RN retains responsibility for the delegated task (option 4).
Cognitive Level: Comprehension **Client Need:** Safe Effective Care Environment: Management of Care **Integrated Process:** Nursing Process: Implementation **Content Area:** Leadership/Management **Strategy:** Use knowledge of the concepts of scope of practice and delegation to select the correct answer. The RN gives the LPN/LVN authority to complete a task. The task is communicated to the LPN/LVN; however, responsibility for the task remains with the RN. Conclude that because the LPN/LVN may lack the necessary skills to complete the task properly, competency has been negated. **References:** Finkelman, A. W. (2006). *Leadership and management in nursing.* Upper Saddle River, NJ: Pearson Education, pp. 224–233; Sullivan, E. J., & Decker, P. (2005). *Effective leadership and management in nursing* (6th ed.). Upper Saddle River, NJ: Pearson Education, pp. 143–152.

3 Answer: 1 With insufficient numbers of healthcare workers, the nurse is handicapped in the ability to delegate because of inadequate support (option 1). The situation in the question does not imply the nurse or other staff are disorganized (option 2) or that the work environment is hostile (option 3). There is no evidence in the question that the nurse is incompetent (option 4), giving further support to option 1.
Cognitive Level: Application **Client Need:** Safe Effective Care Environment: Management of Care **Integrated Process:** Nursing Process: Planning **Content Area:** Leadership/Management **Strategy:** Note that the main theme of the question is inadequate numbers of staff. Next, note that question does not provide supporting data for disorganization, hostile environment, or incompetence. Use knowledge of delegation barriers and the process of elimination to select the correct answer. **References:** Finkelman, A. W. (2006). *Leadership and manage-*

ment in nursing. Upper Saddle River, NJ: Pearson Education, pp. 224–233; Sullivan, E. J., & Decker, P. (2005). *Effective leadership and management in nursing* (6th ed.). Upper Saddle River, NJ: Pearson Education, pp. 143–152.

4 Answer: 2 The nurse should stop feeding the client in room A and medicate the client in room C. While eating is a priority, it does not take precedence over an individual with pain. The client in pain is experiencing discomfort that should be addressed immediately. The activity of feeding the client in room A can be delegated, but it should be delegated to the appropriate person such as a nursing assistant. The charge nurse is busy overseeing the functions on the unit and feeding a client is not an appropriate activity for the nurse to reverse delegate to the charge nurse.
Cognitive Level: Application **Client Need:** Safe Effective Care Environment: Management of Care **Integrated Process:** Nursing Process: Implementation **Content Area:** Leadership/Management **Strategy:** Use knowledge of prioritization and delegation to select the correct answer. Eliminate option 1 immediately because it does not provide a timely resolution to address the client with pain. Eliminate option 4 next because it recommends the charge nurse feed the client, which is not good utilization of the charge nurse. Option 3 recommends the charge nurse medicate the client for pain, but the primary nurse, who knows the client's status best, should complete this task if possible. The nursing assistant could feed the client. Option 2 addresses the immediate need of the client with pain. **References:** Finkelman, A. W. (2006). *Leadership and management in nursing.* Upper Saddle River, NJ: Pearson Education, pp. 224–233; Sullivan, E. J., & Decker, P. (2005). *Effective leadership and management in nursing* (6th ed.). Upper Saddle River, NJ: Pearson Education, pp. 143–152.

5 Answers: 1, 2, 3, 5 The RN may delegate nursing care activities that are skill-based and within the scope of practice of the CNA. The CNA has been trained in procedures such as ambulating clients (option 1), recording intake and output (option 2), measuring and recording vital signs or oxygen saturation levels (options 3 and 5). A skin assessment (option 4) should be completed by the RN since it involves client assessment.
Cognitive Level: Application **Client Need:** Safe Effective Care Environment: Management of Care **Integrated Process:** Nursing Process: Implementation **Content Area:** Leadership/Management **Strategy:** Consider the nursing assistant's scope of practice when answering this question. Recall that skin assessment falls within the RN scope of practice to eliminate option 4, and choose the

remaining options 1, 2, 3, and 5 because they are all tasks that may be delegated to the CNA. Use knowledge of delegation and the process of elimination to select the correct answers. **References:** Finkelman, A. W. (2006). *Leadership and management in nursing.* Upper Saddle River, NJ: Pearson Education, pp. 224–233; Sullivan, E. J., & Decker, P. (2005). *Effective leadership and management in nursing* (6th ed.). Upper Saddle River, NJ: Pearson Education, pp. 143–152.

6 Answers: 1, 2 The scope of practice for LPNs/LVNs allows them to irrigate urinary catheters and feeding tubes. A BP of 98/60 is marginal on a postoperative client and follow-up assessment should be done by the RN (option 3). A client with an infected wound (option 4) should have the dressing changed by the RN for assessment of wound therapy effectiveness. The RN must administer blood products (option 5). In general, the RN should perform any task that may require assessment skills and critical thinking for problem solving. **Cognitive Level:** Application **Client Need:** Safe Effective Care Environment: Management of Care **Integrated Process:** Nursing Process: Implementation **Content Area:** Leadership/Management **Strategy:** Consider the LPN/LVN's scope of practice when answering this question. Recall that LPN/LVNs may complete skilled nursing activities but that the RN is responsible for client assessment. Use knowledge of delegation and the process of elimination to select the correct answer. **References:** Finkelman, A. W. (2006). *Leadership and management in nursing.* Upper Saddle River, NJ: Pearson Education, pp. 224–233; Sullivan, E. J., & Decker, P. (2005). *Effective leadership and management in nursing* (6th ed.). Upper Saddle River, NJ: Pearson Education, pp. 143–152.

7 Answer: 3 In this case, the delivery care system is team nursing. Because of the scope of practice and the RN's responsibility to problem solve and think critically, the RN should check vital signs and assess the postoperative client and both stable clients (options 1 and 4). The LPN/LVN may provide uncomplicated wound care and administer oral medications, but would not be responsible for complicated wound care or IV medication administration (option 2). Based on the concept of team nursing, the LPN/LVN will check vital signs and give bed baths (option 3). **Cognitive Level:** Application **Client Need:** Safe Effective Care Environment: Management of Care **Integrated Process:** Nursing Process: Implementation **Content Area:** Leadership/Management **Strategy:** Note that options 1 and 4 contain assessments of clients, which should be conducted by the RN. Based on the concept of team

nursing, the LPN will complete vital signs and bed baths. Use knowledge of delegation and scope of practice to choose the correct answer. **References:** Finkelman, A. W. (2006). *Leadership and management in nursing.* Upper Saddle River, NJ: Pearson Education, pp. 224–233; Sullivan, E. J., & Decker, P. (2005). *Effective leadership and management in nursing* (6th ed.). Upper Saddle River, NJ: Pearson Education, pp. 143–152.

8 Answer: 1 The scope of practice and most job descriptions for CNAs include measurement of vital signs. It is within the scope of practice for the LPN to administer oral medications. The best option is 1. In some facilities CNAs are allowed to change dressings; however, changing a client's dressing gives the RN the opportunity to assess the incision, and it is the RN's responsibility to assess the client (option 2). CNAs are allowed to ambulate clients, but LPNs should not assess clients (option 3) or complete all sections of admission paperwork on newly admitted clients (option 4). **Cognitive Level:** Application **Client Need:** Safe Effective Care Environment: Management of Care **Integrated Process:** Nursing Process: Implementation **Content Area:** Leadership/Management **Strategy:** Evaluate each option and recall that it is not within the scope of practice for the LPN/LVN to assess clients. Thus, options 3 and 4 may be eliminated first. Next, eliminate option 2 because the LPN/LVN could give medications by the oral route and some parenteral routes (such as subcutaneous or intramuscular), but not intravenous. Realize that option 1 is correct because those tasks fall within the LPN's and CNA's scope of practice. Use knowledge of delegation and scope of practice to select the correct answer. **References:** Finkelman, A. W. (2006). *Leadership and management in nursing.* Upper Saddle River, NJ: Pearson Education, pp. 224–233; Sullivan, E. J., & Decker, P. (2005). *Effective leadership and management in nursing* (6th ed.). Upper Saddle River, NJ: Pearson Education, pp. 143–152.

9 Answer: 4 Because of the risk for aspiration, the nurse should feed the client with dysphagia. The nurse should monitor drainage from a chest tube to assess the characteristics of the drainage. When a client has a high or low blood pressure, the nurse should recheck and assess the client for validity of information and changes in status. Of the four options, option 4 is the best choice. The CNA is qualified to turn and reposition a client with multiple sclerosis and severe weakness. **Cognitive Level:** Application **Client Need:** Safe Effective Care Environment: Management of Care **Integrated Process:** Nursing Process: Implementation **Content Area:** Leadership/Management **Strategy:** Recall that CNAs are

ANSWERS & RATIONALES

trained to perform simple nursing skills and procedures. Options 1, 2, and 3 all contain clients with some form of medical complexity, which should be addressed by a nurse. Option 4 is a weak client who needs help turning and repositioning in bed. Use knowledge of delegation and the process of elimination to select the correct answer. **References:** Finkelman, A. W. (2006). *Leadership and management in nursing*. Upper Saddle River, NJ: Pearson Education, pp. 224–233; Sullivan, E. J., & Decker, P. (2005). *Effective leadership and management in nursing* (6th ed.). Upper Saddle River, NJ: Pearson Education, pp. 143–152.

10 **Answer: 4** In this scenario, the client is in distress so the nurse should stay with the client and call for help from other members of the team (option 4). The charge nurse has expertise in handling emergencies, and the CNA can obtain necessary equipment for assessment. In emergencies or whenever a client is in distress, the nurse should perform measurements such as vital signs and O_2 saturation levels (options 1 and 2). The nurse should never leave the room of a client in distress (option 3). **Cognitive Level:** Application **Client Need:** Safe Effective Care Environment: Management of Care **Integrated Process:** Nursing Process: Implementation **Content Area:** Leadership/Management **Strategy:** Evaluate each of the options systematically. Option 1 seems plausible, but it does not obtain help from the charge nurse, who is needed in this situation. Options 2 and 3 allow the nurse to leave the room; rule these out. This client's condition is deteriorating and the assigned nurse should stay with the client; however, the nurse should call for help from the appropriate people. Use the ABCs of prioritization (airway, breathing, and circulation) and delegation principles to select the correct response. **References:** Finkelman, A. W. (2006). *Leadership and management in nursing*. Upper Saddle River, NJ: Pearson Education, pp. 224–233; Sullivan, E. J., & Decker, P. (2005). *Effective leadership and management in nursing* (6th ed.). Upper Saddle River, NJ: Pearson Education, pp. 143–152.

Posttest

1 **Answer: 1** The administration of IVP morphine for the client with pain is within the scope of practice for the RN, but not in the scope of practice for the LPN/LVN. The administration of oral medications for the client with CHF is within the scope of an LPN/LVN. The administration of vitamins for the client with wounds is in the scope of practice for the LPN/LVN; the client is stable and does not require immediate assessment. **Cognitive Level:** Application **Client Need:** Safe Effective Care Environment: Management of Care **Integrated Process:** Nursing Process: Implementation **Content Area:**

Leadership/Management **Strategy:** Think about scope of practice. Recall that the LPN/LVN should not administer IVP medications; however, the LPN/LVN may administer oral medications. This will enable you to eliminate options 2 and 3. Consider that option 4 is incorrect because it makes a very general statement *all*, and one medication is to be administered IVP. Therefore, the best option is 1. Use knowledge of delegation and the process of elimination to select the correct answer. **References:** Finkelman, A. W. (2006). *Leadership and management in nursing*. Upper Saddle River, NJ: Pearson Education, pp. 224–233; Sullivan, E. J., & Decker, P. (2005). *Effective leadership and management in nursing* (6th ed.). Upper Saddle River, NJ: Pearson Education, pp. 143–152.

2 **Answer: 3** A 76-year-old client with a chronic condition, type 2 diabetes, who was admitted three days ago should be stable, and the care of this client can be delegated to the LPN/LVN. A client with sickle cell anemia who requires pain medications every three hours needs frequent observations and assessments. Because the RN's scope of practice includes problem solving and critical thinking, this client should be assigned to an RN. The client who has a hemoglobin of 6.4 grams/dL may need a blood transfusion and may have unpredictable outcomes; therefore, an RN should be assigned to this client. The four-day postoperative client who will be discharged today is stable but requires teaching, which is within the scope of practice for the RN. **Cognitive Level:** Application **Client Need:** Safe Effective Care Environment: Management of Care **Integrated Process:** Nursing Process: Implementation **Content Area:** Leadership/Management **Strategy:** The core issue of the question is knowledge of scope of practice of both the RN and the LPN/LVN. Recall that assessment and teaching are within the RN's scope of practice to systemaically eliminate options 1, 2, and 4. **References:** Finkelman, A. W. (2006). *Leadership and management in nursing*. Upper Saddle River, NJ: Pearson Education, pp. 224–233; Sullivan, E. J., & Decker, P. (2005). *Effective leadership and management in nursing* (6th ed.). Upper Saddle River, NJ: Pearson Education, pp. 143–152.

3 **Answer: 1** In this scenario, various members of the nursing team are performing different elements of client care on the unit, a characteristic of task nursing. When primary nursing is utilized, the nurse assigned to the client performs most of the duties for assigned clients. In team nursing, a team of an RN and an LPN/LVN or CNA provides care to a group of assigned clients. Operational nursing is not a name for a type of care delivery system and is utilized solely as a distracter in the question.

Cognitive Level: Application **Client Need:** Safe Effective Care Environment: Management of Care **Integrated Process:** Nursing Process: Analysis **Content Area:** Leadership/Management **Strategy:** Recall information about the types of nursing care delivery systems. First, note that option 2 is not a formal nursing care delivery system. Then, note that the stem does not provide data to support primary or team nursing (options 3 and 4). Finally, identify that the stem includes specific tasks given to specific nurses to choose correctly. **References:** Finkelman, A. W. (2006). *Leadership and management in nursing.* Upper Saddle River, NJ: Pearson Education, pp. 224–233; Sullivan, E. J., & Decker, P. (2005). *Effective leadership and management in nursing* (6th ed.). Upper Saddle River, NJ: Pearson Education, pp. 143–152.

4 Answer: 2 The skilled RN should be assigned to the postoperative client who underwent hip replacement and the client who had an abdominal hysterectomy. Postoperative clients are potentially unstable clients because of the risk for hypovolemia and shock. The experienced nurse should receive the surgical clients. The RN on orientation should care for the clients with medical conditions such as DM. In this case, the LPNs should assume duties such as vital signs and assisting with ADLs.
Cognitive Level: Application **Client Need:** Safe Effective Care Environment: Management of Care **Integrated Process:** Nursing Process: Implementation **Content Area:** Leadership/Management **Strategy:** Option 1 is plausible, but not prudent depending on the level of skill and experience of the new RN orientee. The client in option 3 is not stable, making the LPN/LVN an unlikely provider of care for this client. The client in option 4 requires frequent assessments; rule it out. The best option is 2; this client requires frequent assessment, which is performed by the RN. **References:** Finkelman, A. W. (2006). *Leadership and management in nursing.* Upper Saddle River, NJ: Pearson Education, pp. 224–233; Sullivan, E. J., & Decker, P. (2005). *Effective leadership and management in nursing* (6th ed.). Upper Saddle River, NJ: Pearson Education, pp. 143–152.

5 Answer: 2 The charge nurse does not need to assume total care for these clients. In this case, the charge nurse needs to assist in the care of these clients. The charge nurse should administer the IV medications. The LPN can administer any oral medications and provide wound care. The CNA should not perform wound care because CNAs are not trained to observe wound characteristics.
Cognitive Level: Application **Client Need:** Safe Effective Care Environment: Management of Care **Integrated Process:** Nursing Process: Implementation **Content Area:** Leadership/Management **Strategy:** CNAs should assist

clients with activities of daily living. Intravenous push medications should be provided by the charge nurse. This rules out options 1, 3, and 4. Use knowledge of scope of practice and delegation to select the correct answer. **References:** Finkelman, A. W. (2006). *Leadership and management in nursing.* Upper Saddle River, NJ: Pearson Education, pp. 224–233; Sullivan, E. J., & Decker, P. (2005). *Effective leadership and management in nursing* (6th ed.). Upper Saddle River, NJ: Pearson Education, pp. 143–152.

6 Answer: 4 In team nursing a small group of nursing staff provide care to a small group of clients. In task nursing (option 1), each member of the nursing team has to provide specific care activities to clients on the unit. In primary nursing (option 2), the nurse assigned to the client assumes the majority of care for most of the clients. Paired nursing (option 3) is a false label and is a distracter.
Cognitive Level: Comprehension **Client Need:** Safe Effective Care Environment: Management of Care **Integrated Process:** Nursing Process: Analysis **Content Area:** Leadership/Management **Strategy:** Notice that the stem of the question provides characteristics of team nursing. Eliminate option 3 first because it is not a formal delivery system for nursing. Next, eliminate options 1 and 2 because the stem does not provide data to support task or primary nursing. Use knowledge of delivery care systems and delegation to make the selection. **References:** Finkelman, A. W. (2006). *Leadership and management in nursing.* Upper Saddle River, NJ: Pearson Education, pp. 224–233; Sullivan, E. J., & Decker, P. (2005). *Effective leadership and management in nursing* (6th ed.). Upper Saddle River, NJ: Pearson Education, pp. 143–152.

7 Answer: 2 The nurse should complete an incident report and document the fall in the client's medical record. The nurse should never place an incident report in the client's chart. The incident report is an internal risk management tool to monitor incidents within the facility. A copy of the incident report does not enter the nurse's record, nor does the client's caregiver receive a copy.
Cognitive Level: Application **Client Need:** Safe Effective Care Environment: Management of Care **Integrated Process:** Communication and Documentation **Content Area:** Leadership/Management **Strategy:** Eliminate option 1 first as being incorrect because incident reports are not filed in the client's medical record. Next, eliminate option 2 because incident reports are not filed in the nurse's record. Finally, eliminate option 4 because incident reports are not given to caregivers. The incident report is completed and given to the nurse manager and is then forwarded to the risk management department. The nurse documents the facts regarding the client's fall

in the client's medical record. **References:** Finkelman, A. W. (2006). *Leadership and management in nursing.* Upper Saddle River, NJ: Pearson Education, pp. 224–233; Sullivan, E. J., & Decker, P. (2005). *Effective leadership and management in nursing* (6th ed.). Upper Saddle River, NJ: Pearson Education, pp. 143–152.

8 Answer: 1 The float nurse should receive clients who are not compromised by chronic conditions exacerbated by acute conditions. The float nurse should not receive postoperative clients due to their high acuity. Generally, older adult clients may have fluctuations in status placing them at higher risk for complications, which is not an ideal situation for the float nurse. The float nurse's expertise is in obstetrics; the care of medical-surgical clients will be new to the nurse. The charge nurse should not overwhelm the float nurse. The best selection is option 1.

Cognitive Level: Application **Client Need:** Safe Effective Care Environment: Management of Care **Integrated Process:** Nursing Process: Evaluation **Content Area:** Leadership/Management **Strategy:** Option 2 is incorrect because the client with atrial fibrillation and the client with the colectomy are potentially more unstable. Options 3 and 4 are incorrect because those options contain clients whose condition may also fluctuate and become unstable. Option 1 is correct because those clients are more stable than the clients in the other options. Use knowledge of delegation and the process of elimination to select the correct answer. **References:** Finkelman, A. W. (2006). *Leadership and management in nursing.* Upper Saddle River, NJ: Pearson Education, pp. 224–233; Sullivan, E. J., & Decker, P. (2005). *Effective leadership and management in nursing* (6th ed.). Upper Saddle River, NJ: Pearson Education, pp. 143–152.

9 Answer: 3 The Health Information Portability and Accountability Act (HIPAA) has created regulations that do not permit healthcare workers to disclose information about clients unless the client has signed a release of information form. The nurse does not have a method

to verify the person's identity over the phone. The nurse should respond truthfully yet in a mild tone in an effort to make the son aware of confidentiality policies. **Cognitive Level:** Application **Client Need:** Safe Effective Care Environment: Management of Care **Integrated Process:** Nursing Process: Communication **Content Area:** Leadership/Management **Strategy:** Note that option 1 does not address the privacy issue to rule it out. Then note that option 2 is confrontational and eliminate that option also. Option 4 discloses information about the client, making it incorrect. Option 3 does address the major issue, client privacy. Use knowledge of communication and the process of elimination to select the correct response. **References:** Finkelman, A. W. (2006). *Leadership and management in nursing.* Upper Saddle River, NJ: Pearson Education, pp. 224–233; Sullivan, E. J., & Decker, P. (2005). *Effective leadership and management in nursing* (6th ed.). Upper Saddle River, NJ: Pearson Education, pp. 143–152.

10 Answer: 3 The best choice is to allow the LPN/LVN to change the client's dressing. The CNA may ambulate the client and provide morning hygiene care. The RN should perform all assessments and provide care to those clients who have unpredictable outcomes. **Cognitive Level:** Application **Client Need:** Safe Effective Care Environment: Management of Care **Integrated Process:** Nursing Process: Implementation **Content Area:** Leadership/Management **Strategy:** Eliminate options 1 and 2 first because they require assessment. Note then that option 4 should be delegated to a CNA. Option 3 considers the LPN's scope of practice and utilizes the LPN efficiently. Use knowledge of delegation and the process of elimination to select the correct answer. **References:** Finkelman, A. W. (2006). *Leadership and management in nursing.* Upper Saddle River, NJ: Pearson Education, pp. 224–233; Sullivan, E. J., & Decker, P. (2005). *Effective leadership and management in nursing* (6th ed.). Upper Saddle River, NJ: Pearson Education, pp. 143–152.

References

American Nurses Association (ANA). (2005). *Principles for delegation.* Silver Spring, MD: Author.

Anthony, M. K., Casy, D., Chau, T., & Brennan, P. F. (2000). Congruence between registered nurses and unlicensed assistive personnel perceptions of nursing practice. *Nursing Economics, 18,* 285–298.

Blais, K. K., Hayes, J. S., Kozier, B., & Erb, G. (2002). *Professional nursing practice: Concepts and perspectives* (pp. 75–76, 100). Upper Saddle River, NJ: Prentice Hall.

Curtis, E., & Nicholl, H. (2004). Delegation: A key function of nursing. *Nursing Management, 11*(4), 26–31.

Dessler, G. (2004). *Management: Principles and practices for tomorrow's leaders* (pp. 185–188). Upper Saddle River, NJ: Prentice Hall.

Finkelman, A. W. (2006). *Leadership and management in nursing.* Upper Saddle River, NJ: Pearson Education.

Grohar-Murray, W., & DiCroce, H. R. (2003). *Leadership and management in nursing* (pp. 172–182). Upper Saddle River, NJ: Prentice Hall.

Hansten R. I., & Washburn M. J. (2004). *Clinical delegation skills: A handbook for professional practice* (3rd ed.). Gaithersburg, MD: Aspen.

Heller, B. R., Oros, M.T., & Durney-Crowley, J. (n.d.). *The future of nursing education: Ten trends to watch*. National League for Nursing. Retrieved January 2, 2007, from www.nln.org/nlnjournal/infotrends.htm

Marquis, B. L., & Huston, C. J. (2003). *Leadership roles and management functions in nursing* (4th ed.). Philadelphia: Lippincott Williams & Wilkins.

McCloskey, J. C., & Grace, H. K. (Eds.). (2001). Should nurses use assistants? *Current issues in nursing* (4th ed.). St. Louis: Mosby-Year Book.

National Council of State Boards of Nursing & Contact Sites. (n.d.). Retrieved January 3, 2007, from www.ncsbn.org/public/regulation/boards_ofnursing_board.htm

National Council of State Boards of Nursing. (1995). *Delegation: Concepts and decision making process*. Position Paper. Retrieved January 3, 2007, from www.ncsbn.org/public/regulation/delegation_documents.htm

National Council of State Boards on Nursing. (n.d.). *Delegation of UAP issues: Delegation documents*. Retrieved January 3, 2007, from www.ncsbn.org/public/regulation/delegation_documents.html.

National Council of State Boards on Nursing. (1997). *Role development: Critical components of delegation curriculum outline*. Retrieved January 3, 2002, from www.ncsbn.org/public/res/uap/roledevelopment.pdf

Orne, R. M., Garland, D., O'Hara, M., Perfetto, L., & Stielau, J. (1998). Caught in the cross fire of change: Nurses' experience with unlicensed assistive personnel. *Applied Nursing Research, 11*(3), 101–110.

Poole, V. L., Davidhizar, R. E., & Giger, J. N. (1995). Delegating to transcultural team. *Nursing Management, 26*(8), 33–34. Retrieved January 9, 2007, from www.ncbi.n1m.nih.gov/entrez/query.fcgi?cmd=Retrieve&db=PubMed&listuids=7630597&dopt=Abstract

Sullivan, E. J., & Decker, P. J. (2005). *Effective leadership and management in nursing* (6th ed.). Upper Saddle River, NJ: Pearson Education.

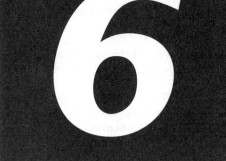

6 Improvement and Excellence in the Care Environment

 NCLEX-RN® Test Prep

Use the CD-ROM enclosed with this book to access additional practice opportunities.

Objectives

➤ Discuss the nurse leader's role in quality management within the healthcare delivery system.

➤ Differentiate between quality management and quality assurance.

➤ Identify the principles of quality management.

➤ Identify the factors required to build a culture of safety within the clinical practice setting.

➤ Discuss the role of risk management and risk reduction in healthcare.

➤ Describe sources for accreditation and regulation that influence quality measures in healthcare and their scope of responsibility.

Review at a Glance

benchmarking comparison of one's own performance or activity with level of performance or activity of another department or organization (best practices, processes, or systems); continuous measurement of a process, product, or service compared to those of the toughest competitor, to those considered industry leaders, or to similar activities in the organization in order to find and implement ways to improve it

clinical pathway treatment regime, agreed upon by consensus, that includes all the elements of care, regardless of the effect on client outcomes

continuous quality improvement comprehensive program designed to continually improve quality of client care; used interchangeably with total quality management, quality management, quality improvement, and performance management

failure mode, effect, and criticality analysis (FMECA) systematic way of examining a design prospectively for possible ways in which failure can occur; assumes that no matter how knowledgeable or careful people are, errors will occur in some situations and may even be likely to occur

Plan-Do-Study-Act (PDSA) cycle four-part method for discovering and correcting assignable causes to improve the quality of processes

process standards standards focused on actual delivery of care

quality assurance process that examines clinical aspects of health provider's care in response to an identified problem

quality management culture focused on customer satisfaction, innovation, and employee involvement in the quality improvement process; used interchangeably with total quality management, continuous quality improvement, quality improvement, and performance improvement

risk management clinical and administrative activities undertaken to identify, evaluate, and reduce the risk of injury to clients, staff, and visitors and the risk of loss to the organization itself

root-cause analysis process for identifying the basic or causal factor(s) that underlie variations in performance, including the occurrence or possible occurrence of a sentinel event

sentinel event unexpected occurrence involving death or serious physical or psychological injury, or the risk thereof; serious injury specifically includes loss of limb or function; "or the risk thereof" includes any process variation for which a recurrence would carry a significant chance of a serious adverse outcome; such events are called "sentinel" because they signal the need for immediate investigation and response

utilization review JCAHO-mandated review based on appropriate allocation of resources

PRETEST

1 After noting an increase in the number of medication errors on the night shift, the nurse manager wishes to reduce them. The manager decides to review the processes used on the unit and in the hospital from the time an order is written until the medication arrives on the unit. A nurse who is assisting the manager understands that what process is being used?

1. Quality assurance
2. Quality improvement
3. Process management
4. Evidence-based research

2 A nurse manager is analyzing the nurse/client ratio and the process of client care assignments on the nursing unit. A nurse working on the unit anticipates that which of the following is the best expected outcome for this task?

1. Identification of errors due to poor staffing
2. Assessment of client falls and incidents
3. Identification of a new process of client assignments
4. Identification of weak areas in client care assignments

3 A nurse leader plans to discharge a client and considers the reasons for the client's admission and types of treatment. Reasons for admission and types of treatments are data used in which of the following?

1. Risk management
2. Utilization review
3. Quality assurance
4. Benchmarks

4 The nurse attends a hospital inservice program on customer relations as part of a major hospital effort at improving the public image of the hospital. The nurse learns that which of the following is the best example of an external customer?

1. Client
2. Nurse in the emergency department
3. Physician
4. Phlebotomist

5 A nurse manager surveys clients about their perception of services while receiving care on the nursing unit. The nurse assisting with data collection understands that this activity represents which component of quality improvement?

1. Intermittent analysis
2. Process effectiveness
3. Error prevention
4. Customer satisfaction

6 A nurse who is the nursing unit representative to the hospital Nursing Practice Committee gathers information about the frequency and severity of client falls on the assigned nursing unit. The nurse explains to a new graduate nurse that this activity represents which step of the quality improvement process?

1. Priority setting
2. Data collection
3. Evaluation
4. Communication

7 A nurse manager plans to start data collection about venipuncture as it is performed on the nursing unit. Which tool should the manager use to facilitate this process?

1. Plan-Do-Study-Act (PDSA)
2. National Quality Forum (NQF)
3. Agency Healthcare Research & Quality (AHRQ)
4. Quality Plus Program

8 A nurse manager of an orthopedic nursing unit implements clinical pathways to facilitate decisions for nursing care of orthopedic clients. The nurse working on the unit is aware that a clinical pathway is an example of which of the following?

1. Data collection tool
2. Clinical outcome
3. Communication tool
4. Benchmarking tool

9 A nurse leader audits clients' charts to identify documentation errors. After analyzing the data gathered, which action should the nurse take to prevent documentation errors?

1. Educate nursing staff on documentation techniques.
2. Reinforce importance of proper documentation.
3. Identify nurses who made documentation errors.
4. Develop a documentation quick reference sheet for nurses.

10 Which of the following strategies should the nurse manager use in building a culture of safety on the nursing unit? Select all that apply.

1. Utilize highly specialized equipment.
2. Implement automated medication dispensing systems.
3. Create systems to monitor client safety.
4. Create a detailed system of checks and balances.
5. Provide inservices to teach use of new equipment.

➤ *See pages 126–129 for Answers and Rationales.*

I. UNDERSTANDING QUALITY IN HEALTHCARE

A. Key points

1. Rapid changes within healthcare have created a new climate focused on client outcomes, prevention of client care problems, and mitigation of adverse events
2. The Institute of Medicine (IOM) defines quality as the degree to which health services for individuals and populations increase likelihood of the desired health outcomes and are consistent with current professional knowledge
3. Healthcare organizations have begun to focus on the bottom line, requiring the staff to do "more" and "better" for "less"
4. Reliance on inspection and control using pre-established standards (traditional quality assurance model) are no longer enough or sufficient

5. Total quality improvement requires a vision of ongoing improvement combined with a well-developed structure to ensure implementation

6. Understanding quality means understanding that most problems lie within systems, not individuals; to improve quality, most improvements must be made within the system

7. Health professionals are required to possess specific knowledge tools and techniques to create new quality initiatives, including multidisciplinary teamwork, lifelong learning, and process improvement

8. The reason behind safety and quality management within healthcare organizations is to provide a systematic approach to prevent errors before they occur or identify and correct errors to decrease adverse events and maximize safety and quality client outcomes

9. Benchmarking is process of comparing one's own performance (best practices, processes, or systems) with best practices with others in the healthcare organization or industry

   a. Internal benchmarking occurs when similar processes within the same organization are compared

   b. Competitive benchmarking occurs when an organization's processes are compared with best practices within the industry

   c. Functional benchmarking occurs when an organization compares a specific function or process (such as scheduling) to others in the industry

10. **Continuous quality improvement** is a not separate management tool; it is a philosophy and process of need to shape healthcare delivery to assess, measure, and evaluate client care

11. Health delivery systems are creating environments in which quality and client safety are top priorities

II. TOTAL QUALITY MANAGEMENT

A. **Defined as a philosophy that ensures that a healthcare organization creates a culture committed to customer satisfaction, innovation, and total employee participation**

   1. It focuses on the client instead of the healthcare provider

   2. It addresses prevention instead of inspection

   3. It focuses on process instead of person

   4. It builds infrastructure that endorses quality

   5. It is an ongoing process focused on client safety, quality improvement, error prevention, and professional staff development in which a quality management philosophy is integrated into the healthcare organization

B. **Cultivating a workplace of mutual respect and support**

   1. Unhealthy work environments contribute to medical error, ineffective delivery of care, and conflict and stress among health professionals

   2. The American Association of Critical Care Nurses (AACN) developed *Standards for Establishing and Sustaining Healthy Work Environments* (2005); these are six standards that represent evidence-based and relationship-centered principles of professional performance:

      a. Skilled communication

      b. True collaboration

      c. Effective decision making

        d. Appropriate staffing

        e. Meaningful recognition

        f. Authentic leadership

  3. The American Association of Nurse Executives (AONE, 2007) developed the *AONE Guiding Principles Toolkit—The Role of the Nurse Executive in Patient Safety*, which provides information about strategies and approaches that will assist the nurse leader to improve the work environment including:

        a. Developing practice environments that prioritize client- and family-centered care, interdisciplinary collaboration, and a culture of safety, respect, and transparency

        b. Using client safety principles and practices

        c. Attaining and developing competencies that specifically address culture of safety skills, knowledge, and commitments, including mastering the following characteristics of leadership:

            1) Clinical practice knowledge

            2) Client care delivery models and work design knowledge

            3) Healthcare economics knowledge

            4) Healthcare policy knowledge

            5) Understanding of governance

            6) Understanding of evidence-based practice

            7) Outcome knowledge of and dedication to client safety

            8) Understanding of utilization/case management

            9) Knowledge of quality improvement

           10) Knowledge of risk management

C. Creating centers of nursing excellence through a magnet culture

  1. The Magnet Recognition Program was developed by the American Nurse Credentialing Center (ANCC) to recognize healthcare organizations that provide nursing excellence

  2. This program also provides a vehicle for disseminating successful nursing practices and strategies by recognizing quality client care, nursing excellence, and innovations in professional nursing practice

  3. The Magnet Recognition Program is based on quality indicators and standards of nursing practice as defined in the American Nurses Association's (ANA) *Scope and Standards for Nurse Administrators* (2004)

  4. The *Scope and Standards for Nurse Administrators* form the base upon which the Magnet designation work culture is built; this work culture includes nursing leadership that:

        a. Is visionary and enthusiastic

        b. Is supportive and knowledgeable

        c. Maintains high practice standards

        d. Holds positions of power and status within the organization

        e. Is visible to staff nurses

        f. Is actively involved in professional organizations

        g. Responds to nurses' needs

        h. Conducts open communication with staff nurses

D. Authentic leadership: nurse leaders must fully embrace the imperative of a healthy work environment, authentically live it, and engage others in its achievement

1. Nurse leaders demonstrate understanding of requirements and dynamics at the point of care and within this context successfully translate vision of healthy work environment

2. Nurse leaders excel at generating visible enthusiasm for achieving standards that create and sustain healthy work environments

3. Nurse leaders lead design of systems necessary to effectively implement and sustain standards for healthy work environments

4. Nurse leaders create and sustain a healthy work environment by providing necessary time and financial and human resources

5. The healthcare organization provides formal co-mentoring for all nurse leaders who actively engage in a co-mentoring program

6. The nurse leaders role model skilled communication, true collaboration, effective decision making, meaningful recognition, and authentic leadership

E. Nursing work environments and promoting client safety

1. Recognizing nurses' contribution to client safety and quality outcomes, the National Quality Forum (NQF) began the "Nursing Care Performance Measures" project in February 2003 to:

   a. Identify a framework for how to measure nursing care performance

   b. Endorse a set of voluntary consensus standards for evaluating the quality of nursing care

   c. Identify and prioritize unresolved issues regarding nursing care performance measurement and research needs

2. The Nursing Care Performance Measures project resulted in the Nursing Quality Forum endorsement of a set of nursing-sensitive consensus standards

   a. NQF endorsement of these measures marked a pivotal step in efforts to increase understanding of nurses' influence on inpatient hospital care and promote uniform metrics for use in internal quality improvement and public reporting activities

   b. NQF15, as the measure set has come to be called, includes measures that examine nursing contributions to hospital care from three perspectives:

      1) Client-centered outcome measures:

         a) Death among surgical inpatients with treatable serious complications (failure to rescue): percentage of major surgical inpatients who experience hospital-acquired complications and die

         b) Pressure ulcer prevalence: percentage of inpatients who have hospital-acquired pressure ulcers

         c) Falls prevalence: the number of inpatient falls per inpatient days

         d) Falls with injury: the number of inpatient falls with injuries per inpatient days

         c) Restraint prevalence: percentage of inpatients who have vest or limb restraints

         f) Urinary catheter-associated urinary tract infection for intensive care unit (ICU) clients: rate of urinary tract infections associated with use of urinary catheters for ICU clients

g) Central line catheter-associated bloodstream infection rate for ICU and high-risk nursery clients: rate of blood stream infections associated with use of central line catheters for ICU and high-risk nursery clients

h) Ventilator-associated pneumonia for ICU and high-risk nursery clients: rate of pneumonia associated with use of ventilators for ICU and high-risk nursery clients

2) Nursing-centered intervention measures:

a) Smoking cessation counseling for acute myocardial infarction

b) Smoking cessation counseling for heart failure

c) Smoking cessation counseling for pneumonia

d) Each measure above related to smoking cessation counseling evaluates the percentage of clients with a history of smoking within past year who received smoking cessation advice or counseling during hospitalization

3) System-centered measures:

a) Skill mix: percentage of registered nurses (RNs), licensed vocational/practical nurses (LPNs/LVNs), unlicensed assistive personnel (UAPs), and contracted nurses care hours to total nursing care hours

b) Nursing care hours per client day: the number of RNs per client day and number of nursing staff hours (RN, LPN/LVN, and UAP) per client day

c) Practice Environment Scale—Nursing Work Index: composite score and scores for five subscales: nurse participation in hospital affairs; nursing foundations for quality of care; nurse manager ability, leadership, and support of nurses; staffing and resource adequacy; and collegiality of nurse-physician relations

d) Voluntary turnover: number of voluntary uncontrolled separations during month by category (RNs, advanced practice nurses or APNs, LVN/LPNs, nursing assistants)

F. **Quality work environments seek to integrate following guiding principles:**

1. Put client care and safety first

2. Focus on reducing waste and improving clinical outcomes

3. Encourage reporting of errors and potential errors, thus significantly increasing and enabling better client care—key in promoting quality care

4. Cease focusing on blame (applies to hospital administrators)

5. Understand that poor work environments for nurses adversely impact client safety

6. Understand that decreased nurse staffing may adversely affect client outcomes and lead to increasing incidence of:

a. Urinary tract infections

b. Pneumonia

c. Shock

d. Upper gastrointestinal bleeding

e. Extended length of stay

G. **Healthy working environments have the following characteristics (see also Box 6-1):**

1. Ensure client safety

2. Enhance staff recruitment and retention

3. Maintain the organization's financial viability

Box 6-1	1. Create a client-centered environment; agree as a team that the client is the center of all unit activities and efforts.

Factors for Building a Quality Work Environment

1. Create a client-centered environment; agree as a team that the client is the center of all unit activities and efforts.

2. Team members are part of the solution, not the problem:

   a. Members are committed to the collective team and not just nursing personnel.

   b. Members contribute to a work ethic of respect and mutual trust.

   c. Members participate in team meetings through effective communication and constructive conflict resolution strategies.

   d. Members support a culture of client safety and quality.

   e. Members celebrate and reward best practices and benchmarking.

H. Principles of total quality management and quality improvement

1. **Quality management** is organized best within a flat, democratic organizational structure

2. Nurse leaders and staff are committed to quality improvement as a philosophy and a process

3. Quality management seeks to improve systems and processes while removing individual blame

4. Customers are respected, valued, and define quality

5. Total quality improvement processes focus upon achieving outcomes

6. Care decisions are always based upon data

I. Quality benefits and gains

1. A quality management program offers the healthcare organization substantial benefits and gains for clients and employees alike

2. Examples of such benefits and gain include the following:

   a. Greater efficiency

   b. Reduction in malpractice lawsuits due to "do it right first time philosophy"

   c. Increased staff morale and satisfaction due to individual/team contributions to improvement initiatives

J. Incorporation of quality management into healthcare settings

1. Non-healthcare corporations have integrated process improvement as a core business strategy or approach to quality management and continuous quality improvement

2. The DMAIC methodology (see below) can be adapted in healthcare to improve client safety and client satisfaction; a nurse leader using this process can foster accountability and teamwork by encouraging the team to:

   a. *Define* (project, goals, and customers/clients both internally and externally)

   b. *Measure* (processes to determine performance)

   c. *Analyze* (determine root cause(s) of defect)

   d. *Improve* (eliminate defect)

   e. *Control* (future process and performance)

3. Using DMAIC methodology has allowed corporations to develop a nearly error-free environment with improvement teams to minimize variation

4. Using and adapting quality improvement within the healthcare industry assures assessment of the following infrastructure:
   a. Structure—by assessing adequacy of staffing, effectiveness of documentation (computerized charting), and availability of medication delivery systems
   b. Process—by assessing timeliness of documentation and adherence to critical pathways
   c. Outcomes—by assessing client falls, client satisfaction, length of stay, and infection rates
5. Quality improvement outcomes:
   a. Describe the result of healthcare encounters
   b. Are specific and measurable
   c. Describe client's behavior
   d. Emerge from standard data systems or tools
   e. Are formulated upon ethical and legal standards of practice

Practice to Pass

Use the DMAIC methodology to describe a problem you have observed while caring for a client.

III. QUALITY IMPROVEMENT PROCESS

A. **Quality improvement:** an ongoing process of continuous improvement; involves four important components:
   1. Continual analysis
   2. Product evaluation
   3. Error prevention
   4. Customer satisfaction

B. **The quality improvement process involves a series of steps designed to plan, implement, and evaluate healthcare delivery; this process:**
   1. Assigns responsibility
   2. Delineates scope of practice
   3. Identifies important care priorities
   4. Establishes evaluation process
   5. Collects and organizes data
   6. Initiates evaluation
   7. Takes appropriate actions to improve care
   8. Assesses effectiveness of action
   9. Communicates results
   10. Identifies breakdowns in communication
   11. Documents client care and results of interventions

C. **Determining quality improvement (QI) based on client needs**
   1. The nurse leader has a responsibility to assess clinical care and determine ways to improve clinical care activities
   2. Information gathered directly from clients has the greatest effect in quality improvement efforts
   3. Client satisfaction surveys and client interviews about nursing care experiences can drive QI efforts
   4. Teamwork supports and sustains unit-based quality improvement processes by:
      a. Promoting open communication between nurses and other health professionals

b. Encouraging nurses to act as team

c. Ensuring other health professionals are included in unit-based quality improvement activities

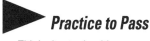 **D. Data collection and tools**

1. Doing quality improvement requires representation from all healthcare disciplines

2. QI team members are responsible for data collection to measure the current status of an activity, service, or procedure

a. Plan-Do-Study-Act cycle: Plan—develop plan to change; Do—implement change; Study—summarize results or lessons; Act—determine what changes are required

b. The **Plan-Do-Study-Act (PDSA) cycle** assists in the data collection process of quality improvement by asking three key questions:

1) What is change trying to accomplish?

2) How will change be assessed to determine if improvement occurred?

3) What change is needed that will result in improvement?

3. Tools for improvement can be divided into three categories, those used for:

a. Process description, such as flow charts and cause-and-effect diagrams

b. Data collection, such as data sheets and check sheets

c. Data analysis, such as bar and pie charts and the Pareto diagram

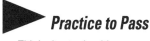 **E. Setting outcome measures**

1. Standards of practice and client-care outcomes evaluate the efforts of quality improvements by healthcare professionals

2. A variety of sources (see Box 6-2 for websites) assist professionals to determine acceptable standards of care and practice, including:

a. The American Nurses Association (ANA) Standards of Nursing Practice and state nurse practice acts provide standards and parameters for nursing practice

b. The National Quality Forum (NQF) develops sets of conditions that should never happen; the goal is to enable national quality measurement and reporting

c. The Centers for Medicare/Medicaid (CMS) develop and implement pay for performance initiatives to support QI in care of Medicare beneficiaries

d. The Agency for Healthcare Research & Quality (AHRQ) supports the National Guidelines Clearing House, National Quality Measures Clearing House, and quality tools inventory

Practice to Pass

Think about a healthcare team that you have been a member of. Explain how this team supports and sustains quality improvement efforts.

Box 6-2		
National Quality Organizations	American Nurses Association (ANA)	www.nursingworld.org
	The National Quality Forum (NQF)	www.qualityforum.org
	Centers for Medicare/Medicaid (CMS)	www.cms.hhs.gov
	Agency for Healthcare Research & Quality	www.ahcpr.gov/fund/funding.htm
	Joint Commission on Accreditation of Healthcare Organizations	www.jcaho.org
	Institute of Safe Medical Practices	www.ismp.org
	Institute of Healthcare Improvement	www.ihi.org
	Leapfrog Group	www.leapfroggroup.org/safety.htm

     e. The Joint Commission on Accreditation of Healthcare Organizations (JCAHO) supports the "**sentinel event**" program

     f. The National Committee on Quality Assurance measures the quality of the nation's managed care plans and the "Quality Plus" program for Web-enabled health plans

     g. The Leapfrog Group is coalition of purchasers providing specific strategies for metropolitan hospitals as well as development of a quality index of 27 safe practices

F. *Benchmarking*

  1. Definition: data-driven quality improvement program to identify quality and efficiency in healthcare delivery

  2. Compares best performance of one's own activity or results with level of activity or results of another department or organization; uses a variety of means to ensure an optimum level of client service, including use of report cards

     a. Report cards have been instituted within the healthcare delivery system to provide consumers with quality measures upon which to base decisions regarding care and to improve quality by encouraging competition among providers

     b. Quality reports allow for increasing accountability and funding tied to outcomes; tying participation in the report card to Medicare reimbursement will ensure hospitals and physicians stay engaged with performance improvement

     c. The Health report card for hospitals has been launched by the U.S. Centers for Medicare and Medicaid Services (CMS); the CMS public Website (www.hospitalcompare.hhs.gov) provides consumers with information on how often participating hospitals follow guidelines for clients with three specific conditions: heart attacks, heart failure, and pneumonia

     d. The Report card is a project of CMS and the Hospital Quality Alliance, a public-private collaboration of organizations that support the reporting of hospital quality of care; data is collected on all clients with the selected conditions regardless of age

     e. Reporting of hospital data quarterly to a state agency allows for greater transparency of hospital information

     f. Consumers can search for hospital information by state, county, city, zip code, or by hospital name, then choose the condition and treatment of interest; the system provides a bar chart comparing selected hospitals to the national and regional averages

G. Nursing standardized classifications systems

  1. Nurses can use information from standardized data to understand health problems across a variety of settings, populations, and care providers

  2. There are three leading nursing classification systems:

     a. The North American Nursing Diagnosis Association (NANDA) uses diagnosis labels as clinical judgments about actual or potential client health problems

     b. The Nursing Intervention Classification System (NIC) uses interventions representing both general and specialty nursing practice; each intervention provides a label, definition, and a set of activities for nurses to perform

     c. The Nursing Outcome Classification (NOC) contains outcomes for clients, including client behavior, perceptions, and statements sensitive to interventions

Box 6-3	1. Remember: quality management is a system. When something goes wrong, it is usually a flaw in the system.
Tools for Managing and Improving Quality	2. Become familiar with standards and outcome measures and use them to guide and improve your practice.
	3. Strive for perfection but be prepared to tolerate failure in order to encourage innovation.
	4. Be sure that performance appraisals and incident reports are not used for discipline but rather form the basis for improvements to the system and/or development of individuals.
	5. Remind yourself and your colleagues that a caring attitude is the best prevention for problems.

Source: Sullivan, E. J. & Decker, P. J. (2005). *Effective leadership and management in nursing* (6th ed.). Upper Saddle River, NJ: Pearson Education, p. 193. Reprinted by permission.

H. Quality follow-up and evaluation

1. The quality management process is cyclic and requires the following steps for monitoring and evaluation (see Box 6-3):

   a. Ongoing management of clinical and managerial performance

   b. Continuous feedback to ensure problems stay solved

   c. Setting standards of care

   d. Taking measures according to selected standards

   e. Evaluating care from multiple sources

   f. Recommending improvements

   g. Ensuring recommendations are implemented

2. Tracer methodology

   a. The Joint Commission's on-site survey process includes use of the tracer methodology

   b. This is an evaluation method in which surveyors select a client or resident and use that individual's record as a roadmap to move through an organization to assess and evaluate the organization's compliance with selected standards and the organization's systems of providing care and services

   c. Surveyors retrace specific care processes that an individual experienced by observing and talking to staff in areas where the individual received care; as surveyors follow the course of a client's or resident's treatment, they assess the healthcare organization's compliance with Joint Commission standards; they conduct this compliance assessment as they review the organization's systems for delivering safe, quality healthcare

   d. While conducting tracer activities, the surveyor may identify compliance issues in one or more elements of performance; surveyors will look for compliance trends that might point to potential system-level issues in the organization

   e. Tracer activity also provides several opportunities for surveyors to provide education to organization staff and leaders, as well as to share best practices from other similar healthcare organizations

   f. If problem trends are identified, surveyors issue the organization a Requirement for Improvement; the organization has 45 days from the end of the survey to submit Evidence of Standards Compliance and identify the Measures

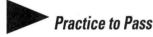

Practice to Pass

You are the nurse leader of a surgery unit. There as been a sudden rise in the number of surgical clients admitted to the unit. Clients, physicians, and other providers have started to complain about long delays for a surgical bed. How would you attempt to fix this problem? Describe how you would analyze the process.

of Success it will use to assess sustained compliance over time; four months after approval of the Evidence of Standards Compliance, the organization will submit data on its Measure of Success to demonstrate a track record

IV. PERIODIC INSPECTION

A. *Quality assurance* (QA)

1. Defined as a program to monitor healthcare
    a. Emerged in healthcare delivery in 1950s as an inspection approach to ensure that minimum standards of care are present within healthcare organizations
    b. QA focused on "doing it right," but often failed at preventing problems from occurring
2. Nurse leaders should communicate importance of ongoing QA activities and how unit-based monitoring improves overall quality program of organization through proactive prevention
3. Examines clinical aspects of healthcare provider's care, usually in response to identified issue or problem
4. Quality assurance tasks focus on **process standards**, which describe how health care should be provided, or what nursing actions are used to provide care
    a. Examples of process elements are staff satisfaction, pain management, client education, discharge planning, documentation, or adherence to practice standards
    b. Standards of practice focus on competency of practice for safe delivery of care to the public
    c. Standards of practice are determined by a professional organization such as the American Nurses Association
    d. Clinical practice guidelines are statements of practice expectations developed by health professionals to make decisions about care and guide clinical management; they are also a method to improve quality of care
    e. **Clinical pathway** is a systematic description or schematic representation of specific care decisions for nursing care for a client with a specific health problem
        1) Expected outcomes and care strategies outlined in the clinical pathway are developed by a collaborative team
        2) The pathway provides a daily outline of outcomes to be achieved for each client
        3) Alterations in expected outcomes are categorized as variances to be analyzed by the case manager
5. Chart review or chart auditing is a method used in QA
    a. Audits use either active (concurrent audit) or discharge chart records (retrospective audit)
    b. Audits are done to detect error and determine the responsible party
    c. Audits are done to improve client care at the unit level, such as to reinforce policies, procedures, or standards of documentation
        1) Charts are usually randomly selected for review by a health professional
        2) Charts may be audited both internally (performed by qualified professional from within the organization) and externally (performed by qualified professional outside the organization)

V. BUILDING A CULTURE OF SAFETY

A. Culture: a specific collection of values and norms shared by people and groups in an organization that control the way they interact with each other and with stakeholders outside the organization

1. Organizational culture comprises attitudes, experiences, beliefs, and values of the organization

2. Beliefs and ideas include what kinds of goals members of the organization should pursue and ideas about appropriate kinds or standards of behavior organizational members should use to achieve goals

3. From organizational values emerge organizational norms, guidelines, or expectations that prescribe appropriate behavior by employees in particular situations and control the behavior of organizational members toward one another

B. Culture can also be defined as observable:

1. Customs

2. Behavioral norms

3. Stories

4. Rites

5. Organizational values

C. Why measure or monitor culture?

1. One key reason is to achieve safest care possible

2. A fundamental predictor of success with a client is the current organizational culture

3. Building and sustaining excellence is born out of organizational culture

4. A culture of safety is a means to design systems geared toward preventing, detecting, and minimizing hazards and the likelihood of error rather than attaching blame to individuals

5. Nurse leaders play a vital role in creating a positive, fair, and balanced work environment that provides a culture of safety, support, and atmosphere of respect and tolerance; nurse leaders are accountable for ensuring client safety on their assigned units including:

   a. Delegating assignments and activities based on team members' clinical competencies and personal confidence

   b. Creating systems to monitor client safety

   c. Promoting confidence in the efficacy of preventive measures

   d. Implementing well-developed safety principles

   e. Providing safe working conditions

   f. Standardizing and simplifying equipment, supplies, and processes (such as electronic medical records, automated drug-ordering systems)

   g. Avoiding reliance on memory

   h. Collecting and sharing information about incidents, near misses, and the overall state of error prevention in the clinical environment

D. Transparency is a vital element in the culture of safety; it provides for meaningful orientation and professional development around client safety that:

1. Describes to staff what errors are to be reported

2. Encourages staff to report and supports those who report near misses and adverse events

3. Explains how staff will be treated when a report is made

4. Ensures expectations are clear about safety and the need for maintaining on-going feedback and transparency

5. Reduces fear, anxiety, and punishment when errors occur

E. **Clients as a safety check:** clients themselves can be major safety check; nurses have critical role ensuring that clients:

1. Know which medications they are taking

2. Know the appearance of their medications

3. Know side effects of medications

4. Are responsible for notifying their healthcare providers of medication discrepancies

F. **Standards for client safety**

1. Begin with fostering blameless culture built upon vigilance of learning, improvement, and resilience

2. Standards for client safety serve several functions:

   a. Systematic and transparent approach to safety and problem solving

   b. Establishment of minimum levels of performance

   c. Establishment of consistency or uniformity across disciplines and organizations

   d. Setting expectations

3. Standards can be used also in public regulatory processes:

   a. Licensure for health professionals

   b. Licensure for healthcare organizations (hospitals)

   c. Private voluntary processes (professional certification or organizational accreditation)

VI. RISK MANAGEMENT

A. **Seeks to analyze problems and minimize losses after an adverse event; such problems can be:**

1. The final result of a malpractice lawsuit

2. Absorbed costs due to extended length of stay for client

3. Negative public relations

4. Employee dissatisfaction

B. **Functions of risk management**

1. Identify and define circumstances of financial risk for an organization such as client falls, medication errors, or personnel injuries

2. Assess and determine frequency of occurrence of circumstances

3. Investigate and intervene in events involved in these circumstances

4. Identify areas of potential risk and seek to improve care

C. **Nurse leader responsibilities in risk management**

1. Nurse leader must ensure that individual nurses understand that they are viewed as risk managers

2. Responsibilities of the nurse leader include:

   a. Anticipate and seek sources of risk

      b. Identify and report unusual occurrences

      c. Develop a plan to avoid and manage risk

      d. Reduce fear of punishment for acknowledging, reporting, or discussing error

      e. Gather data that demonstrates success in avoiding and minimizing risk

      f. Evaluate and modify the risk reduction program

VII. RISK REDUCTION

A. Involves changing behavior, preventing risk when foreseeable, and focusing on clients with attention to outcomes

B. The nurse leader can engage staff actively in risk reduction activities to prevent adverse events and decrease negative outcomes; activities might include:

1. Ensuring accurate physical assessment upon admission and throughout hospitalization

2. Providing for early identification of problems

3. Correcting any physiologic abnormality

4. Adhering to best practice standards for high-risk/high volume practices (pressure ulcers, client falls, restraint use, and medication administration)

5. Conducting frequent safety rounds

6. Acknowledging staff's demonstration of safe practice and encouraging best practice standards

C. Reinforce adverse event reduction as a key risk management strategy

1. This strategy seeks to reduce client mortality and morbidity

2. It seeks to reduce number of the clients who experience adverse events and frequently die or suffer permanent disability

D. Use a risk-reduction program (*Failure Mode, Effects, and Criticality Analysis [FMECA]*) to identify and prioritize the high-risk processes to improve client safety

1. JCAHO's new client safety standard requires hospital leaders to implement a program to reduce the risk of sentinel events and medical/healthcare errors by conducting proactive risk assessment activities

2. Each year, hospitals are required to select at least one high-risk process for proactive risk assessment, based in part on information published by JCAHO, that identifies the most frequently occurring types of sentinel events and client safety risk factors; key steps and findings of a proactive risk assessment can be reported by using Failure Mode, Effects, and Criticality Analysis (FMECA)

3. For high-risk circumstances, nurse leaders can seek to manage adverse events by:

    a. Recognizing an event as a near miss or sentinel event; a near miss event often results in no harm but signals that an imminent problem or situation must be corrected

    b. Identify a sentinel event as a serious, unexpected occurrence, usually involving death or physical or psychological harm (see Box 6-4 for common sentinel events) when it has occurred

    c. Root-cause analysis: a retrospective review of an incident or event to identify sequences leading to the event for the purpose of identifying root causes

    d. A root-cause analysis can lead to specific risk-reduction strategies:

      1) In some circumstances, the risk-reduction plan is reported to JCAHO; all risks and/or adverse events are internally reported to the Risk Management Department on an incident report or other form

Box 6-4		
Common Sentinel Events	Client suicide	Client elopement (unauthorized departure)
	Operative/postoperative complications	Infection-related event
	Wrong-site surgery	Fire
	Medication error	Anesthesia-related event
	Delay in treatment	Maternal death
	Client falls	Ventilator death
	Death/injury of a client in restraints	Medical equipment related event
	Assault/rape/homicide	Infant abduction/wrong family
	Perinatal death/loss of function	Utility systems related event

Source: Joint Commission on Accreditation of Health Care Organizations. Retrieved December 20, 2007, from www.jcaho.org. © The Joint Commission, 2008. Reprinted with permission.

> ### Practice to Pass
>
> Identify an error that you have observed in the healthcare setting. Explain what you would do after observing the error and what events should follow. Explain what can be done to avoid a recurrence.

2) Incident reports are not kept with the client record but rather are filed separately with risk management after review by nurse manager or other department head; they are used as a method of communication to the organization that an incident caused harm or had potential to cause harm

3) Identified errors are viewed as opportunities for improvement; apology, honesty, and transparency characterize the relationship with clients who have been harmed or injured through error; and there is constant vigilance for emerging risks

VIII. UTILIZATION REVIEW

A. Defined as a process of assessing medical necessity, the appropriateness of healthcare services in a particular setting, and the efficiency of care

B. The focus of utilization review includes:

1. Reason for admission

2. Type and extent of treatment

3. Length of hospitalization

4. Discharge planning

5. Follow-up considerations

C. Utilization review is done by employees (often nurses) employed in a specific department known as Utilization Review or Case Management

D. Nurses play a key role in communicating with utilization review staff about individual clients and their health status to ensure they receive sufficient length of stay and services

IX. PROTECTING CLIENTS AND PROMOTING OPTIMAL OUTCOMES

A. Nurse leaders have a responsibility to ensure quality care; this requires a change in attitude that error is part of client care

B. A multidisciplinary approach to quality management and risk reduction leads to optimal client outcomes

C. **Diminished resources and poor communication place healthcare members at risk for unsafe practices**

D. **A culture of quality management and risk management ensures client safety and improves job satisfaction**

Case Study

During medication administration on the evening shift, you notice that a client on the day shift received 100 mg of meperidine (Demerol) intravenously instead of the ordered 50 mg by the intramuscular (IM) route. As the nurse manager, you represent the nursing unit on the hospital's Risk Management Committee. As part of this role, you are aware that risk management is directed at identifying, evaluating, and taking corrective action against potential risks that could threaten the well-being of the client, staff, or visitors.

1. What would your first action be?

2. Define what is meant by a reportable incident, a medical-legal incident, and a medication error.

3. Explain what documentation should appear in the client's chart.

4. Discuss the nurse manager's role in risk management.

5. Determine if an incident report is required for this incident. Why or why not?

For suggested responses, see pages 236–237.

POSTTEST

1 Which of the following safety measures on a unit should be included by a nurse manager on a plan to reduce errors and improve client safety? Select all that apply.

1. Use lock options on all IV pumps.
2. Implement targeted check and balance systems.
3. Utilize chart audits.
4. Attempt to identify critical errors.
5. Adopt the use of scanners for medication administration.

2 A nurse identifies a client at high risk for development of pressure ulcers and orders an air mattress for the client. This nurse is attempting to accomplish which of the following?

1. Risk management
2. Culture of safety
3. Quality assurance
4. Risk reduction

3 The nurse attends a hospital inservice program on customer relations as part of a major hospital effort at improving the public image of the hospital. The nurse learns that, in addition to clients, which of the following is an example of an internal customer?

1. Nurse working on the labor and delivery unit
2. Local chapter of the American Red Cross
3. Vascular surgeon
4. Blue Cross/Blue Shield insurance company

4 An accrediting body has guidelines that "healthcare facilities must run controls on blood glucose monitors once daily." The nursing representative to the hospital nurse practice committee explains to co-workers that this guideline is an example of which of the following?

1. Quality assurance
2. Risk management
3. Standards of care
4. Utilization review

5 The nurse manager who is conducting a staff development program on improving client care explains that which of the following best represents quality nursing care?

1. Clients with histories of pressure ulcers will receive an air mattress within 6 hours of admission.
2. Clients with heart failure will have a urinary drainage catheter inserted to measure output precisely.
3. A chemistry panel will be drawn daily on clients with peripheral edema.
4. All clients will be screened for methicillin-resistant *staphylococcus aureus* (MRSA).

6 A 27-year-old client is admitted with pneumonia and dies from a myocardial infarction within 24 hours of admission. The nurse manager works with staff to investigate this incident as which of the following?

1. Accident
2. Error
3. Sentinel event
4. Malpractice

7 A nurse leader reviews the client's chart for which of the following because they indicate effectiveness of treatment and care?

1. Indicators
2. Outcomes
3. Critical pathways
4. Standards

8 The nurse manager would recommend which of the following as the best measure to improve the culture of safety on a nursing unit?

1. Have certified nursing assistants monitor clients when nurses are busy with an emergency.
2. Have two nurses verify warfarin (Coumadin) doses.
3. Ask nurses to purchase back support devices to use for all lifting.
4. Assist with a plan to install automated medication dispensing stations on the unit.

9 A nurse manager reviews a chart for critical indicators of quality care to prepare a report for the Quality Improvement Department. The nurse explains to a new staff member that this activity represents which of the following?

1. External audit
2. Internal audit
3. Benchmarking
4. Control

10 The nurse manager who is attempting to increase client safety would work on which of the following within the nursing unit and as a representative on various hospital committees? Select all that apply.

1. Setting clear expectations
2. Developing an intricate approach to problem solving
3. Establishing consistent policies across disciplines
4. Developing maximum levels of expectations
5. Rewriting policies and procedures yearly

➤ *See pages 129–131 for Answers and Rationales.*

ANSWERS & RATIONALES

Pretest

1 **Answer: 2** Quality improvement is the ongoing effort of identifying potential errors in processes and systems and improving work and preventing errors. Quality assurance, on the other hand, is the identification of errors, but without the focus on prevention of errors. Evidence-based research is clinical research that is conducted with the intention of improving clinical practice by providing frameworks and guidelines for safe practice. Process management is not a formal method of performance improvement.
Cognitive Level: Comprehension **Client Need:** Safe Effective Care Environment: Management of Care **Integrated Process:** Nursing Process: Evaluation **Content Area:** Leadership/Management **Strategy:** First rule out process management because it is not a formal method of performance improvement. The definition of evidence-based research does not fit the stem; rule it out as well. Note that quality assurance and quality improvement

are different, and select option 2 because the manager is seeking to reduce errors, and this fits the definition of quality improvement. **References:** Finkelman, A. W. (2006). *Leadership and management in nursing.* Upper Saddle River, NJ: Pearson Education, pp. 482–516; Sullivan, E. J., & Decker, P. (2005). *Effective leadership and management in nursing* (6th ed.). Upper Saddle River, NJ: Pearson Education, pp. 182–192.

2 Answer: 4 The best expected outcome for this analysis is a compilation of data that helps to identify areas in need of improvement. This is a broad outcome that is consistent with the broad information in the question. The purpose of this task is to analyze the nurse/client ratio and client assignments, not client falls and incidents, as noted in option 2. Identification of errors due to poor staffing is also a narrower and more focused option, which is not consistent with wording of the question. Options 3 and 4 seem similar initially but the manager is accomplishing option 4, while option 3 may be an outcome if deficiencies are identified.
Cognitive Level: Application **Client Need:** Safe Effective Care Environment: Management of Care **Integrated Process:** Nursing Process: Assessment **Content Area:** Leadership/Management **Strategy:** The critical words in the stem of the question are *nurse/client ratios.* Based on these words, rule out options 2 and 3 because they do not specifically address the analysis of the nurse/client ratio. While identification of errors may seem plausible, it is not the best choice. The nurse manager is not looking for errors (quality assurance). Option 4 is correct because it addresses the main issue in the stem. Use nursing knowledge and the process of elimination to make the correct selection. **References:** Finkelman, A. W. (2006). *Leadership and management in nursing.* Upper Saddle River, NJ: Pearson Education, pp. 482–516; Sullivan, E. J., & Decker, P. (2005). *Effective leadership and management in nursing* (6th ed.). Upper Saddle River, NJ: Pearson Education, pp. 182–192.

3 Answer: 2 Utilization review is the process of assessing appropriateness of services provided to clients and consists of reasons for admission, type of treatment, length of hospital stay, discharge planning, and follow-up considerations. Benchmarks identify best practices and performances. Quality assurance is focused on getting the task done correctly. Risk management analyzes problems.
Cognitive Level: Comprehension **Client Need:** Safe Effective Care Environment: Management of Care **Integrated Process:** Nursing Process: Analysis **Content Area:** Leadership/Management **Strategy:** Choose the option that best fits the description in the stem. Focus on reasons for admission and types of treatment. By definition you can

rule out options 1, 3, and 4 because they do not analyze reasons for admission and types of treatments. The definition of utilization review fits the description in the stem. Use knowledge of quality improvement to select the correct answer. **References:** Finkelman, A. W. (2006). *Leadership and management in nursing.* Upper Saddle River, NJ: Pearson Education, pp. 482–516; Sullivan, E. J., & Decker, P. (2005). *Effective leadership and management in nursing* (6th ed.). Upper Saddle River, NJ: Pearson Education, pp. 182–192.

4 Answer: 3 External customers are individuals outside the healthcare system who receive products or services including physicians, community agencies, and families. An internal customer is an individual who receives products or services from the healthcare organization including clients, nurses, and other hospital departments.
Cognitive Level: Comprehension **Client Need:** Safe Effective Care Environment: Management of Care **Integrated Process:** Nursing Process: Analysis **Content Area:** Leadership/Management **Strategy:** Consider that an external customer is an individual outside the healthcare system who receives either products or services and then analyze which of the options fits this description. Eliminate option 1 first because a client is an internal customer. Next, eliminate the nurse in the emergency room (option 2) and the phlebotomist in the laboratory department (option 4), who are hospital employees and are therefore also internal customers. Using the process of elimination, the option that fits the description of an external customer is a healthcare provider such as a physician. **References:** Finkelman, A. W. (2006). *Leadership and management in nursing.* Upper Saddle River, NJ: Pearson Education, pp. 482–516; Sullivan, E. J., & Decker, P. (2005). *Effective leadership and management in nursing* (6th ed.). Upper Saddle River, NJ: Pearson Education, pp. 182–192.

5 Answer: 4 The nurse manager is collecting client data on satisfaction with services provided. Most surveys do not address error prevention. Intermittent analysis and process effectiveness are not components of quality improvement.
Cognitive Level: Comprehension **Client Need:** Safe Effective Care Environment: Management of Care **Integrated Process:** Nursing Process: Assessment **Content Area:** Leadership/Management **Strategy:** The critical words are *client satisfaction.* Choose the option that includes *customer satisfaction*—option 4. Note that the other options do not fit the stem. Use knowledge of quality improvement to select the correct answer. **References:** Finkelman, A. W. (2006). *Leadership and management in nursing.* Upper Saddle River, NJ: Pearson Education, pp. 482–516; Sullivan, E. J., & Decker, P. (2005). *Effective*

leadership and management in nursing (6th ed.). Upper Saddle River, NJ: Pearson Education, pp. 182–192.

6 **Answer: 2** The nurse is clearly in step five of the quality improvement process, which is data collection and organization. Priority identification is earlier in the process, and this question does not indicate priority. Evaluation occurs after data collection, and communication is last in the process.
Cognitive Level: Application **Client Need:** Safe Effective Care Environment: Management of Care **Integrated Process:** Nursing Process: Assessment **Content Area:** Leadership/Management **Strategy:** The critical words in the question are *collects information.* Choose an option that fits the stem. Note that the information in the stem does not provide data to support options 1, 3, or 4. **References:** Finkelman, A. W. (2006). *Leadership and management in nursing.* Upper Saddle River, NJ: Pearson Education, pp. 482–516; Sullivan, E. J., & Decker, P. (2005). *Effective leadership and management in nursing* (6th ed.). Upper Saddle River, NJ: Pearson Education, pp. 182–192.

7 **Answer: 1** The PDSA is a tool used for data collection. It measures the current status of procedures. This guideline provides quick and easy direction in data collection. The NQF and Quality Plus Program (options 2 and 4) provide resources to evaluate standards of care and practice. The AHRQ provides evaluation tools for inventory of standards of practice.
Cognitive Level: Application **Client Need:** Safe Effective Care Environment: Management of Care **Integrated Process:** Nursing Process: Assessment **Content Area:** Leadership/Management **Strategy:** Note that the question specifically asks for a tool. First rule out options 3 and 4 because they are not tools; they are resources that provide tools. The NQF is also a resource that provides tools. The only tool listed is in option 1. Use knowledge of quality improvement to select the correct answer. **References:** Finkelman, A. W. (2006). *Leadership and management in nursing.* Upper Saddle River, NJ: Pearson Education, pp. 482–516; Sullivan, E. J., & Decker, P. (2005). *Effective leadership and management in nursing* (6th ed.). Upper Saddle River, NJ: Pearson Education, pp. 182–192.

8 **Answer: 4** Benchmarks are part of quality improvement, but they are used to identify the best performance of the nurse's care. Communication does not apply to this scenario. Clinical pathways are not data collection tools nor are they clinical outcomes, but they are used to improve client outcomes.
Cognitive Level: Application **Client Need:** Safe Effective Care Environment: Management of Care **Integrated**

Process: Nursing Process: Evaluation **Content Area:** Leadership/Management **Strategy:** It helps to know the use of clinical pathways. Rule out option 1 because clinical pathways are not examples of data collection tools. Next, determine that clinical pathways do not fall under the genre of clinical outcomes or communication. This leaves clinical pathways as the item that is an example of a benchmark. **References:** Finkelman, A. W. (2006). *Leadership and management in nursing.* Upper Saddle River, NJ: Pearson Education, pp. 482–516; Sullivan, E. J., & Decker, P. (2005). *Effective leadership and management in nursing* (6th ed.). Upper Saddle River, NJ: Pearson Education, pp. 182–192.

9 **Answer: 1** A preventive measure to avoid documentation errors is comprehensive education on approved documentation techniques. A documentation quick reference sheet should not be used without proper education in documentation techniques. In fact, inappropriate use of these sheets could create errors. Reinforcing documentation techniques is effective, but the nurse must first know the proper documentation techniques for this strategy to be effective. Nurses should not be punished for making errors nor should they be singled out; this strategy is punitive and should be avoided.
Cognitive Level: Application **Client Need:** Safe Effective Care Environment: Management of Care **Integrated Process:** Nursing Process: Evaluation **Content Area:** Leadership/Management **Strategy:** The question asks for prevention of documentation errors. Option 3 is a poor method of resolution; rule it out. Options 2 and 4 are fragmented educative measures that may not prevent documentation errors. They are reactive measures to the documentation problem. Option 1 is correct because it is a proactive measure. Identify critical words in the question or stem to select the right answer. **References:** Finkelman, A. W. (2006). *Leadership and management in nursing.* Upper Saddle River, NJ: Pearson Education, pp. 482–516; Sullivan, E. J., & Decker, P. (2005). *Effective leadership and management in nursing* (6th ed.). Upper Saddle River, NJ: Pearson Education, pp. 182–192.

10 **Answers: 2, 3, 5** Equipment and processes should be simple to use with clear instructions. Errors are more likely to occur when equipment isn't user friendly and instructions are too detailed to understand. Unfortunately, many nurses and healthcare staff develop ways to work around elaborate check and balance systems; subsequently, this strategy may be more detrimental than the older system already in place.
Cognitive Level: Application **Client Need:** Safe Effective Care Environment: Management of Care **Integrated Process:** Nursing Process: Implementation **Content Area:**

Leadership/Management **Strategy:** Options 1 and 4 can be ruled out on the basis of the use of complicated systems. The other options focus on safety measures and staff education. Use communication concepts and the process of elimination to select the correct response. **References:** Finkelman, A. W. (2006). *Leadership and management in nursing.* Upper Saddle River, NJ: Pearson Education, pp. 482–516; Sullivan, E. J., & Decker, P. (2005). *Effective leadership and management in nursing* (6th ed.). Upper Saddle River, NJ: Pearson Education, pp. 182–192.

Posttest

1 Answers: 1, 2, 5 Safety measures on any medical unit should include lock options on IV pumps to prevent clients or staff from changing the program. Check and balance systems allow staff to verify the right care is given to the right client at the right time. Scanners for medication administration are components of a system that assures the nurse is giving the correct medication to the right client. Chart audits and error identification are not safety measures.
Cognitive Level: Analysis **Client Need:** Safe Effective Care Environment: Management of Care **Integrated Process:** Nursing Process: Implementation **Content Area:** Leadership/Management **Strategy:** Identify the critical words in the question—*safety measures.* Note that chart audits and error identification are not safety measures; rule them out. Identify that options 1, 2, and 5 are all safety measures and are therefore correct. **References:** Finkelman, A. W. (2006). *Leadership and management in nursing.* Upper Saddle River, NJ: Pearson Education, pp. 482–516; Sullivan, E. J., & Decker, P. (2005). *Effective leadership and management in nursing* (6th ed.). Upper Saddle River, NJ: Pearson Education, pp. 182–192.

2 Answer: 4 In risk reduction, the nurse identifies that the client may develop poor outcomes and takes measures to prevent negative client outcomes. Risk management analyzes problems. Quality assurance is focused on getting the task done correctly. Providing a culture of safety is a strategy in which the organization designs systems to prevent and detect errors.
Cognitive Level: Application **Client Need:** Safe Effective Care Environment: Management of Care **Integrated Process:** Nursing Process: Implementation **Content Area:** Leadership/Management **Strategy:** Identify the critical words *high risk* in the stem and match them with the option that fits the stem. Options 1 and 4 both contain the word *risk* so rule out options 2 and 3. Next, evaluate the action of the nurse, *identifies and orders.* In other words, the nurse reduces the client's chances of con-

tracting a pressure ulcer. Option 4 is the best option because it is risk reduction. Use knowledge of quality improvement to select the correct answer. **References:** Finkelman, A. W. (2006). *Leadership and management in nursing.* Upper Saddle River, NJ: Pearson Education, pp. 482–516; Sullivan, E. J., & Decker, P. (2005). *Effective leadership and management in nursing* (6th ed.). Upper Saddle River, NJ: Pearson Education, pp. 182–192.

3 Answer: 1 An internal customer is an individual/entity who receives products or services from the healthcare organization. This includes clients, nurses, and other hospital departments. External customers are individuals outside the healthcare system who receive products and services including physicians, community agencies, and families.
Cognitive Level: Comprehension **Client Need:** Safe Effective Care Environment: Management of Care **Integrated Process:** Nursing Process: Analysis **Content Area:** Leadership/Management **Strategy:** Consider that an internal customer receives products or services from the healthcare organization and analyze which of the options fits this description. Eliminate options 2 and 4 (American Red Cross and Blue Cross/Blue Shield) first as entities that are external to the hospital. Next, eliminate option 3 because the vascular surgeon is an external customer, although he or she provides services at the hospital. Using the process of elimination, the nurse on the obstetric unit is considered an internal customer. Use nursing knowledge and the process of elimination to make the correct selection. **References:** Finkelman, A. W. (2006). *Leadership and management in nursing.* Upper Saddle River, NJ: Pearson Education, pp. 482–516; Sullivan, E. J., & Decker, P. (2005). *Effective leadership and management in nursing* (6th ed.). Upper Saddle River, NJ: Pearson Education, pp. 182–192.

4 Answer: 3 Standards of care are levels of quality that are considered safe, acceptable practice. Quality assurance is focused on getting the task done correctly. Risk management analyzes problems. Utilization review is the process of assessing appropriateness of services provided to clients and consists of reasons for admission, type of treatment, length of hospital stay, discharge planning, and follow-up considerations.
Cognitive Level: Application **Client Need:** Safe Effective Care Environment: Management of Care **Integrated Process:** Nursing Process: Evaluation **Content Area:** Leadership/Management **Strategy:** Look at each option. The stem is stated as a *standard.* Option 3 includes the term *standard.* This option is very specific. The other options do not apply to this case. Use knowledge of quality improvement to select correctly. **References:**

Finkelman, A. W. (2006). *Leadership and management in nursing*. Upper Saddle River, NJ: Pearson Education, pp. 482–516; Sullivan, E. J., & Decker, P. (2005). *Effective leadership and management in nursing* (6th ed.). Upper Saddle River, NJ: Pearson Education, pp. 182–192.

⑤ Answer: 1 Two options are correct, but option 1 is a more specific expression of quality. Option 4 is just a screening; it does not provide a specific strategy. If option 4 included "contact precautions will be initiated," this option would be more viable. All clients with heart failure do not need urinary drainage catheters; these place clients at risk for infection. Chemistry panels may not be warranted daily on clients with edema. **Cognitive Level:** Analysis **Client Need:** Safe Effective Care Environment: Management of Care **Integrated Process:** Nursing Process: Implementation **Content Area:** Leadership/Management **Strategy:** Option 4 contains a very general term, *all*; rule it out. Option 2 can be ruled out based on the increased infection rate that occurs with urinary drainage catheters. Option 3 can be ruled out because clients with peripheral edema may not need daily chemistry panels. Option 1 is an aggressive measure to prevent skin breakdown in high-risk clients. Use nursing knowledge and the process of elimination to make the correct selection. **References:** Finkelman, A. W. (2006). *Leadership and management in nursing*. Upper Saddle River, NJ: Pearson Education, pp. 482–516; Sullivan, E. J., & Decker, P. (2005). *Effective leadership and management in nursing* (6th ed.). Upper Saddle River, NJ: Pearson Education, pp. 182–192.

⑥ Answer: 3 A sentinel event is a very serious, unexpected incident that leads to death or major injury. The cause of the event is usually determined in debriefing. Often, an accident or error in care or treatment may contribute to the sentinel event. Malpractice is a tort that may be pursued in a court of law. **Cognitive Level:** Comprehension **Client Need:** Safe Effective Care Environment: Management of Care **Integrated Process:** Nursing Process: Assessment **Content Area:** Leadership/Management **Strategy:** While all options seem plausible, sentinel event is the global answer. Options 1 and 2 are causes of death. Option 4 is a legal term. Use knowledge of quality improvement to select correctly. **References:** Finkelman, A. W. (2006). *Leadership and management in nursing*. Upper Saddle River, NJ: Pearson Education, pp. 482–516; Sullivan, E. J., & Decker, P. (2005). *Effective leadership and management in nursing* (6th ed.). Upper Saddle River, NJ: Pearson Education, pp. 182–192.

⑦ Answer: 2 Client outcomes are key indicators of the effectiveness of treatment and care received during hospitalization. Option 1 does not fit; the term indicate is used in the sentence. Critical pathways are not indicators of effective treatment, but they are guidelines to deliver effective, safe treatment. Standards are not considered a concept in performance improvement. **Cognitive Level:** Knowledge **Client Need:** Safe Effective Care Environment: Management of Care **Integrated Process:** Nursing Process: Evaluation **Content Area:** Leadership/Management **Strategy:** The question is looking for a term that speaks to *effectiveness of treatment and care*. Use nursing knowledge and the process of elimination to make the correct selection. **References:** Finkelman, A. W. (2006). *Leadership and management in nursing*. Upper Saddle River, NJ: Pearson Education, pp. 482–516; Sullivan, E. J., & Decker, P. (2005). *Effective leadership and management in nursing* (6th ed.). Upper Saddle River, NJ: Pearson Education, pp. 182–192.

⑧ Answer: 4 Automated medication dispensing stations provide safety features that help prevent medication errors. Two nurses are not needed to verify warfarin doses or orders unless there is a discrepancy, and, if so, the prescribing physician should verify the order. The healthcare facility should provide back support devices for the staff to prevent back injuries. Some clients may be monitored by nursing assistants during an emergency, but some who require assessment should still be monitored by a registered nurse. **Cognitive Level:** Application **Client Need:** Safe Effective Care Environment: Management of Care **Integrated Process:** Nursing Process: Evaluation **Content Area:** Leadership/Management **Strategy:** Identify the critical words in the question, which include *best measure* and *culture of safety*. Anticipate that the correct answer is one that will affect a large number of clients and focus on reduction of common errors in healthcare to choose correctly. **References:** Finkelman, A. W. (2006). *Leadership and management in nursing*. Upper Saddle River, NJ: Pearson Education, pp. 482–516; Sullivan, E. J., & Decker, P. (2005). *Effective leadership and management in nursing* (6th ed.). Upper Saddle River, NJ: Pearson Education, pp. 182–192.

⑨ Answer: 2 Chart reviews for quality indicators are part of quality assurance and are referred to as internal audits since the nurse employed by the agency is performing the chart review. If an outside agency or consultant conducts the chart review, this is considered an external audit. Benchmarking is the comparison of a unit's performance against another unit's performance or standard of care/practice. Control is a function of management. **Cognitive Level:** Comprehension **Client Need:** Safe Effective Care Environment: Management of Care **Integrated Process:** Nursing Process: Implementation **Content Area:**

Leadership/Management **Strategy:** The critical information in the stem is that the nurse is conducting a chart review. Note that the nurse is one who works in the hospital and note the similarity with the term *internal audit*. Apply knowledge of quality assurance to select the correct answer. **References:** Finkelman, A. W. (2006). *Leadership and management in nursing.* Upper Saddle River, NJ: Pearson Education, pp. 482–516; Sullivan, E. J., & Decker, P. (2005). *Effective leadership and management in nursing* (6th ed.). Upper Saddle River, NJ: Pearson Education, pp. 182–192.

10 Answers: 1, 3 Standards for client safety include identifying clear, concise expectations and establishing uniform policies across disciplines. To ensure client safety there must be a systematic approach to problem solving and minimum levels of performance must be established. Policies and procedures are rewritten based on evidence-based research and changes in standards of care and are rewritten as needed, not yearly.
Cognitive Level: Analysis **Client Need:** Safe Effective Care Environment: Management of Care **Integrated Process:** Nursing Process: Evaluation **Content Area:** Leadership/Management **Strategy:** Identify critical words in the question or stem to select the right answer. Note that the focus is on the nursing unit and across the hospital to help you choose correctly. **References:** Finkelman, A. W. (2006). *Leadership and management in nursing.* Upper Saddle River, NJ: Pearson Education, pp. 482–516; Sullivan, E. J., & Decker, P. (2005). *Effective leadership and management in nursing* (6th ed.). Upper Saddle River, NJ: Pearson Education, pp. 182–192.

References

American Association of Critical Care Nurses. (2005). *AACN standards for establishing and sustaining healthy work environments.* Retrieved May 15, 2008, from http://www.aacn.org/aacn/pubpolcy.nsf/Files/HWEStandards/$file/HWEStandards.pdf

American Nurses Association. (2004). *Scope and standards for nurse administrators* (2nd ed.). Silver Spring, MD: Author.

American Nurses Credentialing Center (ANCC) (2007). *What is the Magnet Recognition Program?* Retrieved November 25, 2007, from www.nursecredentialing.org/magnet/index.html

American Organization of Nurse Executives. (2007). *Role of the nurse executive in patient safety. Guiding principles toolkit.* Retrieved May 15, 2008, from http://www.aone.org/aone/pdf/Role%20of%the%20Nurse%20Executive%20in%20Patient%20Safety%20Toolkit_July 2007.pdf

Cook, A. F., Hoas, H., Guttmannova, K., & Joyner, J. C. (2004). An error by any other name. *American Journal of Nursing, 104*(6), 32–34.

Finkelman, A. W. (2006). *Leadership and management in nursing.* Upper Saddle River, NJ: Pearson Education.

Gantz, N. R., Sorenson, L., & Howard, R. L. (2003). A collaborative perspective on nursing leadership in quality improvement: The foundation for outcomes management and patient/staff safety in health care environment. *Nursing Administration Quarterly, 27*(4), 324–329.

Hudon, S. (2003). Leapfrog standards: Implications for nursing practice. *Nursing Economics, 21*(5), 233–236.

Hughes, R. G. (2004). First, do no harm: Avoiding the near misses taking into account one ever-present factor: Human fallibility. *American Journal of Nursing, 104*(5), 81–84.

Improving the Quality of Health Care for Mental and Substance-Use Conditions: Quality Chasm Series, www.nap.edu/catalog/11470.html

Institute of Medicine. (2001). *Crossing the quality chasm: A new health system for the 21st century—summary.* Washington, DC: National Academy Press, 2–4. Available from www.nap.edu/books/0309072808/html.

Institute of Medicine (IOM). (2000). *To err is human: Building a safer health care system.* Washington, DC: National Academy Press.

Institute of Medicine (IOM). (2004). *Keeping patients safe: Transforming the work environment of nurses.* Washington, DC: National Academy Press.

Joint Commission on Accreditation of Healthcare Organizations. This Month for State Hospitals Associations. Retrieved December 2, 2007, from www.jcaho.org.

Joint Commission on the Accreditation of Healthcare Organizations. (2001). Joint Commission Public Policy Initiative. *Health care at the crossroads: Strategies for addressing the evolving nursing crisis.* Chicago, IL: Author.

Joint Commission on the Accreditation of Healthcare Organizations. (2003a). 2003 JCAHO national patient safety goals: Practical strategies and helpful solutions for meeting these goals. *Joint Commission Perspectives on Patient Safety, 3*(1).

Joint Commission on the Accreditation of Healthcare Organizations. (2003b). JCAHO national patient safety goals approved. *Joint Commission Perspectives, 23*(9), 1, 3.

Kohn, K. T., Donaldson, M. S., & Corrigan, J. M. (2000). *To err is human: Building a safer health system.* Washington, DC: National Academy Press.

Lin, L., & Liang, B. (2007). Addressing the nursing work environment to promote patient safety. *Nursing Forum, 42*(1), 20–30.

Massachusetts Coalition for the Prevention of Medical Error. (2006). *When things go wrong. Responding to adverse events.* Retrieved August 7, 2007 from www.macoalition.org.

Morath, J., & Leary, M. (2004). Creating safe spaces in organizations to talk about safety. *Nursing Economics, 22*(6), 344–351, 354.

Reeves, K. (2007). New evidence report on nursing staffing and quality of patient care. *MEDSURG Nursing, 16*(2), 73–78.

Schloman, B. (2005, May 9). Information Resources Column: Health care report cards: Pass or fail? *Online Journal of Issues in Nursing*. Retrieved November 25, 2007, from http://nursingworld.org/ojin/infocol/info_17.htm

Smith, A. (2007). Nursing-sensitive care measures: A platform for value and vision. *Nursing Economic$, 25*(1), 43–46.

Sullivan, E. J., & Decker, P. J. (2005). *Effective leadership and management in nursing* (6th ed.). Upper Saddle River, NJ: Pearson Education.

Sutcliffe, K. M., & Weick, K. E. (2001). *Managing the unexpected*. San Francisco, CA: Jossey-Bass.

Swan, B. A., Lang, N. M., & McGinley, A. M. (2004). Access to quality health care: Links between evidence, nursing language, and informatics. *Nursing Economics, 22*(6), 325–331.

Woodward, S. (2004). Achieving a safer health service. Part 3: Investigating root cause and formulating solutions. *Professional Nurse, 19*(7), 390–394.

Yoder-Wise, P. (2007). *Leading and managing in nursing* (4th ed.). St. Louis, MO: Mosby, Inc.

Online Resources

Joint Commission for Accreditation of Healthcare Organizations at www.jcaho.org

Institute for Healthcare Improvement at www.ihi.org

Institute of Medicine at www4.nationalacademies.org

National Council for Quality Assurance at www.ncqa.org/Programs/HEDIS/index.htm

PDCA cycle at http://hci.com.au/hcisite2/toolkit/pdcacycl.htm

Teamwork Through Effective Communication, Collaboration, and Conflict Management

7

Chapter Outline

Dimensions of Teamwork
Managing Cultural Diversity
Working in Interdisciplinary Teams
Communication
Conflict Management

Objectives

➤ Describe the difference between a team and a group team.
➤ Identify the characteristics of an effective team.
➤ Describe ways to promote and build an interdisciplinary team.
➤ Discuss ways to manage cultural diversity with the team.
➤ Detail current trends in society that impact communication.
➤ Explain how the barriers to communication impede team performance.
➤ Define the term *conflict*.
➤ Discuss the positive and negative aspects of conflict.
➤ Describe the conflict process and approaches to resolve conflict.

> **NCLEX-RN® Test Prep**
>
> Use the CD-ROM enclosed with this book to access additional practice opportunities.

Review at a Glance

avoiding unassertive, uncooperative approach to conflict in which avoider neither pursues his or her own needs, goals, and concerns nor helps others

coaching strategy used to help others learn, think critically, and grow through communication about performance

collaboration conflict management style in which both sides work together to achieve agreement; process in which two or more individuals work together, jointly influencing one another

communication exchange of information and transmission of meaning; exchange of ideas or feelings such that sender and receiver perceive common meaning

competition approach to conflict management and negotiating that presumes win-lose situation

compromise settling conflict through mutual concessions

conflict perceived difference among people

cooperation act of working together with others for common purpose, respecting opinions of others and being willing to examine alternative points of view and change personal beliefs and perspectives

coordination process of achieving unity of action among interdependent activities

feedback a form of communication; a message that receiver returns to sender in response to sender's message

group two or more persons interacting in such a way that each person influences and is influenced by the other

group norms informal rules that groups adopt to regulate and regularize group members' behavior

interpersonal occuring between or among individuals

intrapersonal occuring within an individual

message a component of communication, includes verbal and nonverbal behaviors and total impact conveyed by these behaviors

receiver a component of communication; refers to person who receives message

sender a component of communication; refers to individual who is sending message

team group of people committed to a common purpose, set of performance goals, and approach for which team members hold each other mutually accountable

PRETEST

1 A nurse manager who is working on developing unit staff regarding teamwork explains in a staff meeting that which characteristics are noted in an effective team? Select all that apply.

1. Trustworthiness
2. Respect for each other
3. Open communication
4. Tolerance of each others flaws
5. Eagerness to get the job done

2 Which strategy should the nurse leader use to foster a climate of collaboration on the nursing unit?

1. Place emphasis on tasks to be accomplished during each shift.
2. Display an open attitude toward new ideas and suggestions.
3. Focus on high-quality care and benchmarking results.
4. Use firm communication about items of importance to the nurse leader.

3 The nurse leader in a healthcare facility works with other organizational leaders to review and possibly revise the organization's mission statement. The nurse leader requests input from staff on the nursing unit, explaining that the mission statement should do which of the following?

1. Provide direction and keep the group focused
2. Foster open communication between members
3. Increase amount and diversity of problem solving
4. Promote team building and personal bonding

4 A new nurse who wishes to eventually become a team leader would focus on developing which of the following characteristics? Select all that apply.

1. Commitment to action
2. Passion for learning
3. Delegation of planning
4. Ability to determine rules
5. Eagerness to succeed

5 A nurse leader collaborates with team members to establish new goals. Which of the following is the best action for the nurse leader to take to foster success in this project?

1. Establish "buy-in" from other team members.
2. Only supervise when necessary.
3. Analyze the structure of the organization.
4. Reorganize the group.

6 The nurse leader needs to develop a plan with the nursing staff about how to best reduce the number of client falls on the unit. Several nurses have ideas about the best actions to take. Which approach should the nurse take to achieve consensus with the team?

1. Change the rules for decision making according to how the conversation progresses.
2. Pay special attention to the details of what is being discussed.
3. Use firm words when communicating with each staff member.
4. Encourage continued discussion and point out areas of agreement.

7 A certified nursing assistant (CNA) reports clients' complaints to the nurse manager. The manager understands that this represents which type of organizational communication?

1. Upward communication
2. Downward communication
3. Lateral communication
4. Horizontal communication

8 A nursing team implements an agreed-upon plan of action, and most goals are achieved. The nurse leader concludes that this team is in which phase of team development?

1. Forming
2. Performing
3. Storming
4. Norming

9 A nurse team member consistently refuses to follow up on assignments and questions the purpose of the team. Which strategy represents the best action the team leader should use to coach the team member?

1. Allow the member to write an action plan.
2. Ask the nurse to listen attentively.
3. Focus on the problem and behavior.
4. Listen to the team member's excuses.

10 The nurse who is the chairperson of an agency committee recognizes that the committee is collaborating after noting which of the following behaviors in the group?

1. A compromise occurs between two of the committee members.
2. One member stands firm by a preset goal.
3. There is effective negotiation among the committee members.
4. All members uphold goals created by the administration.

➤ *See pages 151–154 for Answers and Rationales.*

I. DIMENSIONS OF TEAMWORK

A. *Team*

1. Defined as a group of people with complementary skills who are committed to a purpose, goal, and approach for which they hold themselves accountable

2. A team performs work that otherwise could not be accomplished easily, effectively, or efficiently by an individual alone

B. Teamwork and the nurse leader

1. To provide safe and high-quality care, healthcare professionals must successfully work together

2. Teamwork is a solution no nurse leader can do without

3. Teams succeed when the nurse leader understands the essentials of teamwork, including:

   a. Honesty and trustworthiness

   b. Respect and tolerance for diversity of opinions

   c. Use of direct, open, and free communication of ideas, thoughts, and feelings

   d. The ability of the team leader to be both leader and coach

   e. Use of successful teambuilding strategies (develop a winning strategy)

4. When teams do not succeed, the problem often lies with leadership, focus, or capability

C. Benefits of effective teamwork: effective teamwork sustains and builds the performance of the team by:

1. Increasing the number and diversity of creative problem-solving solutions possible

2. Allowing team members to grow and develop in their roles and responsibilities

3. Enhancing the ability of team members to become more efficient in use of available resources

4. Fostering a work environment that is more enjoyable, thus increasing personal satisfaction of the team

D. Characteristics of a high performance team

1. Team leaders set the stage and expectations for team building and are responsible for the team's growth, development, and success

2. The team leader seeks to build characteristics that produce a high performance team, including:

   a. A clear mission statement with direction and that motivates the team

   b. Clearly identifiable goals

   c. Mastery of fundamentals—clear roles, competency in skills, constant training, and development of standards of performance

   d. Clear lines of communication—relationships are built on openness and trustworthiness; upward, downward, and lateral communication are promoted

   e. Trust and intimacy—the glue that holds a team together

   f. Attention to team building effectiveness and continuous improvement—setting standards, measuring progress, and fixing problems rather than blaming (collaborative problem solving)

   g. Mutual support and balance of task and social responsibility—work hard, play hard, and support each other; know how to have fun together

   h. Selection of members for skill and for skill potential and development

   i. Creation of vision

   j. Keeping team on track toward implementing and sharing and achieving visions

   k. Finding solutions and creating results

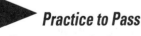
Practice to Pass

How can a nurse leader go about building a high performance team?

E. The team-building process is one that empowers and sustains the work environment through the efforts of all its members; process includes:

1. **Coordination**: getting the right people to work together; to keep the team achieving goals the nurse leaders must:

   a. Commit to action—look for individuals with the passion to succeed

   b. Possess a thirst for learning

   c. Do background preparation for the group's charge/task

   d. Have a passion for success

   e. Have love of laughter

2. **Collaboration:** getting the right people to generate ideas for solving problems, making decisions, and keeping team members oriented toward goal achievement; nurse leaders must take the time to:

   a. Build structures of support and integrity

   b. Maintain interpersonal relationships

   c. Establish "buy-in" on change

   d. Create a climate of safety for clients and team members

   e. Ask questions and challenge the status quo

   f. Actively listen and encourage dialogue

   g. Paraphrase and clarify when confusion and chaos emerge

   h. Summarize and provide ongoing feedback

   i. Enforce ground rules, regulations, and organizational policies

   j. Frequently evaluate team members' performance

3. Consensus: getting the right people to agree and commit to action; to keep the team achieving, nurse leaders must:

   a. Have patience

   b. Have an eye for detail

   c. Be an effective decision maker

   d. Be insightful in managing chaos

   e. Be diplomatic and fair

   f. Set priorities

   g. Have a bias toward action

F. Group dynamics

1. All teams are groups

2. **Group:** two or more individuals who are interacting in such a way that each individual influences and is influenced by the other

G. *Group norms*

1. Groups norms are informal rules of behavior that are shared, accepted by, and enforced by group members

2. May have some influence on how group members perform within the group

H. Phases of team development

1. Forming: teams work out their specific role responsibilities, build friendships/relationships, and work through issues related to team's purpose, structure, and leadership

2. Storming: a period of confusion; team members begin to raise questions about leadership and what is the structure and purpose of the team

3. Norming: team members now agree on matters of purpose, structure, and leadership; prepared to perform their tasks or assigned activities with cooperation, mutual support, and agreement

4. Performing: period of productivity, achievement, and pride as team members work together to achieve goals and get the job done

5. Adjoining: some members may leave the team and others may join; team members face mixed emotions of both separation and satisfaction over a job well done

I. **Team-building challenges**

1. Teams occasionally lose footing because most problems require more than a simple goal or single set of solutions to solve them; when team building begins to break down, it is sometimes easier to switch people in the group rather than try to change individuals

2. When team members cannot be removed from the team, the nurse leader must use effective **coaching** skills, including:

   a. Stating the problem in behavioral terms

   b. Focusing on the problem, not the person

   c. Connecting the problem to functioning of the organization and to person's self-interest

   d. Bringing reasons for the problem into the open

   e. Asking team members for suggestions and discussing ideas on how solve problem

   f. Listening openly

   g. Agreeing on steps and solutions to the problem

   h. Committing steps to writing (putting words down on paper)

   i. Planning and recording a specific follow-up date

3. Hidden agendas: member's unspoken objectives that interfere with commitment or enthusiasm; often impede teamwork

II. MANAGING CULTURAL DIVERSITY

A. Healthcare organizations have an obligation to manage a highly skilled and diverse workforce; the nurse leader plays a key role in helping the organization understand cultural differences among team members, other healthcare professionals, and clients

B. Diversity in nursing includes age, gender, and ethnicity

C. Contemporary nursing practice includes four generations of professionals working in teams; can lead to generational differences in priorities, expectations, and motivations

D. Workforce diversity requires enthusiasm for shared values and tolerance of dissimilar preferences; team members must learn to value everyone's differences and recognize their similarities

E. Team members need to pay close attention to both verbal and nonverbal communications for cultural cues

F. When doubt emerges, team members will need to ask for clarification; the nurse leader cannot assume they understand the differences

G. **Team members must learn to alter assumptions about others based on their membership in certain groups; they must assist those not of majority cultural group to be successful by including them in informal networking and the organization's culture as a starting point**

III. WORKING IN INTERDISCIPLINARY TEAMS

A. **One of five core competencies of that all clinicians should possess, regardless of their discipline, to meet needs of 21st century health system (as reported in the Institute of Medicine report, *Health Professions Education: A Bridge to Quality*) is working effectively in interdisciplinary teams**

B. **This includes knowing how to effectively cooperate, collaborate, communicate, and integrate care to ensure that care is continuous and reliable**

C. **Collaboration is described as a face to-face interchange; contributions from each team member are valued and used in problem solving, integration of ideas, and formulation of a new plan or change initiative**

D. **Collaboration is recognition that this type of interaction can improve the solution of mutually acknowledged clinical or client problems**

1. Interaction is characterized by activities directed toward an agreed-upon goal by two or more persons among whom exists a norm of equity and mutual recognition of the complementarity of their knowledge and ability

2. To collaborate is to:
   a. Work together, especially in joint intellectual efforts
   b. Work reasonably well with others outside one's discipline
   c. Coordinate and share vital information and resources

3. For collaboration to be truly effective, the following essential factors must be present:
   a. Effective and efficient communication
   b. High-level performance and competence
   c. Accountability
   d. Trust
   e. Administrative support

4. Equity implies that although there may not be constant equality in decision making in any particular activity, dominance in decision making does tend to even out over time

5. Fostering a climate for collaboration among team members calls for the following:
   a. Openness and trust among interested parties
   b. Emphasis on reward for quality work, not simply for quantity and speed of task accomplishment
   c. Shared organizational resources and support that consider experience in collaborative activities as positive attributes of professional interaction

6. Critical attributes of collaboration include:
   a. Sharing in planning
   b. Making decisions
   c. Solving problems
   d. Setting goals

      e. Assuming responsibility

      f. Working together

      g. Coordinating

      h. Communicating

  7. Principles of collaboration include learning how to:

      a. Compliment before criticizing

      b. Deal with the outside world by being careful to use "we" instead of "I"

      c. Ask for a partner's opinion and be clear about what is wanted at the time of asking

      d. Beware of unsolicited commentary

      e. Speak up if it is felt that something is not working

      f. Keep each other informed on daily basis

      g. Yield to the passionate side when two are debating without a compelling argument on either side and one feels much more passionate about the matter

      h. Avoid raising an issue again once that issue is decided

      i. Ask to postpone discussion when an agreement cannot be reached on something of significance and fatigue sets in

      j. Accept a capable person's responsibility for a phase or portion of the project

  8. Barriers to effective collaboration can emerge in any work environment:

      a. Nurses may feel threatened by increased responsibility and accountability crucial to collaboration

      b. Those with low-status collaboration may defer to those with high status collaboration; this may lead to conflict between the desire to be accepted and the duty to advocate for the client

Practice to Pass

What behaviors can you use to increase your effectiveness with collaboration within the clinical setting?

IV. COMMUNICATION

  A. Defined as:

    1. Exchange of information or opinions

    2. Interactive process that is a means to an end

    3. Influenced by the context in which it occurs

  B. Effective *communication* is key to building quality teams; a nurse leader who builds a caring and supportive workplace does so through effective communication (see Box 7-1); people will not care how much knowledge is possessed until they know they are cared for

  C. Factors aiding effective communication

    1. Feedback: give back information to allow the communicator to determine whether the purpose of the communication has been achieved

    2. Appropriateness: replies by the nurse leader to staff or client must fit the circumstances, match the message, and be of an amount that is neither great nor small

    3. Efficiency: use simple, clear words that are timed and paced for the nursing staff or client

    4. Flexibility: send messages on and about the immediate situation rather than on preconceived expectations

    5. Listening: involves focus on nursing staff or client needs rather than just the task at hand; make eye contact

Box 7-1	1. Identify and use the appropriate method (in person, phone, voice mail, e-mail, letter) for your communications.
Tools for Communicating Effectively	2. Evaluate your communication skills in various situations. Think of ways to improve.
	3. Practice using the skills described in specific situations, such as with your supervisor, with the medical staff, or with difficult people.
	4. Become sensitive to others' responses, both verbal and nonverbal, and craft your messages appropriately.
	5. Gather feedback and continue to assess the effectiveness of your communications.
	6. Strive to improve your communication skills.

Source: Sullivan, E. J. & Decker, P. J. (2005). *Effective leadership and management in nursing* (6th ed.). Upper Saddle River, NJ: Pearson Prentice Hall, p. 131. Reprinted by permission.

6. Astuteness in communication: communication skills can be learned and developed over time; nurse leaders must work on improving their communication skills

7. Being helpful and nonjudgmental; demonstrate and provide:

   a. Empathy: awareness of and sensitivity to feelings of another person

   b. Open-ended questions: requires giving more than a yes or no answer

   c. Giving information: provide information to clients and, with client's permission, to their significant others

   d. Reflection: a method of encouraging staff or clients to think through problems for themselves

   e. Silence: allow periods of reflection

   f. Congruence: matching the verbal and nonverbal elements of messages sent to others

8. See also Box 7-2 for discussion of how nurse leaders can foster effective communication

D. Benefits of effective communication:

   1. It leads to greater influence and collective power

   2. Team members become more productive with higher performance

Box 7-2	Effective communication fosters a caring workplace.
The Nurse Leader's Role in Fostering Effective Communication	➤ Be mindful of the words you use and the actions you take.
	➤ Capture the attention of your team.
	➤ Present an impeccable image and take the time to evaluate your communication patterns:
	▪ Engage in frank, open, two-way communication.
	▪ Take time to listen and listen carefully.
	▪ Teach yourself to concentrate.
	▪ Do not interrupt.
	▪ Listen to what a person is saying not how he or she is saying it.
	▪ Suspend judgment; be sensitive to others.
	▪ Listen between the lines.
	▪ Listen with your eyes!

   3. There is a higher level of competency in skills and abilities

   4. It provides for wholeness and balance of self and others

   5. It accomplishes a great deal when done well

   6. There is clarity and accuracy in communication patterns with others

E. **Challenges and trends in society that impact communication**

   1. Increasing social diversity

   2. Changing/differing beliefs

   3. An aging population

   4. A shift to computerized communication

F. **Patterns of communication emerge from the direction of the communication**

   1. Downward flow of communication from top executive or administrators often involves:

      a. Directives, policies, procedures, and regulations

      b. Specific instructions

      c. Employer expectations

      d. Performance feedback

   2. Upward flow of communication from subordinates or team members often involves:

      a. Reporting of employee attitudes and feelings

      b. Suggestions for improvements and new ideas

      c. Requests for resources

      d. Sharing of employee grievances

   3. Horizontal flow of communication often involves:

      a. A peer to peer exchange

      b. Coordination between units and services

      c. Socialization

      d. Information sharing

      e. Problem solving

      f. Conflict management and resolution

      g. Client and family dialogues

G. **Types of communication**

   1. Interpersonal communication: the process of exchanging information and meaning either between two people or in a small group of people

   2. Organizational communication: a process whereby the nurse leader uses established communication systems to receive and relay information to individuals within the organization and to relevant individuals and groups outside the organization

H. **Elements of the communication process**

   1. **Sender**: "who" in communication, i.e., person who initiates the communication

   2. **Receiver**: person who takes in the message and analyzes it

   3. **Message**: "what" in communication; consists of verbal and/or nonverbal stimuli taken in by the receiver

4. Encoding: how we translate the message into verbal or nonverbal symbols that will communicate the intended meaning to the receiver

    a. The nurse leader must decide the appropriate degree of intensity of a message

    b. Know that words mean different things to different people

    c. Encode in the simplest terms; if terms are complex, the message should be expressed in several ways or broken down into simple bits (sound bites)

    d. Language used should reflect values, culture, and personality of the receiver

5. Transmitting the message: is how the sender gets information to the receiver (direct verbal, telephone, email, internet, cell phone, or television)

6. Decoding: the mechanism for translating message into a form that the receiver can use (in humans beings, it is the sensory receptor mechanisms)

7. Action: behavior taken by the receiver as result of the message sent, received, and perceived

    a. Communication is not considered successful until the message received has been understood and acted on appropriately

    b. The receiver can ignore, store, or respond by saying one thing and doing another or can respond according to the sender's wishes

8. Feedback: a new message generated by the receiver in response to the original message from the sender

    a. Sender and receiver exchange information and clarify messages

    b. Accurate feedback is best achieved with face-to-face communication

I. Levels of communication

1. Public: communication with a group of people with a common interest; the communicator acts primarily as the sender of information; feedback typically is limited

2. Intrapersonal: internal communication within an individual; used to process observations, analyze situations, resolve doubts, or reaffirm beliefs

3. Interpersonal: communication between individuals, person to person, or in small groups

J. Communication skills include the following:

1. Attending: active listening

2. Responding: verbal and nonverbal acknowledgment of the sender's message

3. Clarifying: communicating as specifically as possible to help the message become clear

4. Confronting: working jointly with others to resolve a problem or conflict

K. Channels of communication have the following components:

1. Visual (seeing): is nonverbal and includes facial expressions, posture, gait, body movements, position, gestures.

2. Auditory (hearing): is verbal (spoken)

3. Kinesthetic (touching): is also nonverbal

4. Electronic: uses electronic media that don't have characteristics of other modes

L. Barriers to effective communication

1. Physical barriers

    a. Space

    b. Distance

Practice to Pass

What can you do as a healthcare provider when encountering a team member, another health professional, or a client whose nonverbal behavior fails to match his or her verbal messages?

      c. Temperature

      d. Ventilation

      e. Structure

      f. Equipment

      g. Distracting noises

    2. Social and psychological barriers

      a. Arise from judgments, emotions, and social values

      b. Communication cannot be separated from personality and social implications because personal emotions at the time affect the communication process

    3. Semantic barriers (interpretation of meanings)

      a. Interpretation of message through signs and symbols

      b. It is important to encode and decode accurately

      c. Remember that difficulties may arise in verbal and listening processes

M. Factors influencing communication: to enhance communication within the work environment, recognize how the following factors may enhance communication:

    1. Gender: men and women may process information differently

    2. Culture: different cultures may have different beliefs, practices, and assumptions; cross-cultural communication involves:

      a. Respect

      b. Empathy

      c. Tolerance for nonjudgmental attitudes toward people with different behaviors, values, and attitudes

    3. Culturally competent communication occurs when a person from one culture understands the message sent from a person of another culture

N. Organizational challenges to effective communication: no single organization can overcome all challenges to effective communication; however, knowing how to deal with such challenges can improve communication channels

    1. Organizational culture and climate:

      a. Accessibility of information (Who has access to information?)

      b. Communication channels (What are the modes of communication?)

      c. Organizational structures

      d. Clarity of message (How clear/effective are the messages?)

      e. Flow control and information load (What rules affect organizational communication?)

      f. Communicator effectiveness (Does one receive enough/too much information?)

    2. Organizational stress: every organization experiences a certain level of stress during its daily operations; health organizations in particular are known to have increased levels of stress because of:

      a. High levels of tension due to increased workloads

      b. High levels of criticism from internal and external customers

      c. Anger and bad feelings among employees

   d. Low morale in team members

   e. High use of sick time

   f. High number of medical errors

   3. Overcoming organizational stress: to address the issues surrounding organizational stress, the nurse leader can:

   a. Find out what is wrong with communication patterns and work to fix them

   b. Know issues causing low morale of the team

   c. Find out what motivates the team and make an effort to support it

O. Ways to enhance workplace communication

   1. Nurse leaders have an obligation to enhance communication in the workplace; they act as role models and demonstrate effective strategies to enhance daily communications by:

   a. Observing professional courtesies

   b. Being prepared to state concerns clearly and accurately

   c. Providing supportive evidence and anticipating resistance to change and requests

   d. Learning to separate out needs from desires

   e. Stating a willingness to cooperate in finding solutions and then matching behaviors to words; being in the pursuit of solutions

   2. Co-workers also have an obligation to communicate clearly and effectively with one another

   a. Report client information accurately, informatively, and succinctly

   b. Change of shift reports should include:

   1) Name, age, room number of client, medical diagnoses, major procedures or surgery with date

   2) Name of physician or group of physicians

   3) Significant nursing diagnoses and progress toward goals during shift

   4) Significant assessment findings during shift

   5) Any pertinent diagnostic test or laboratory results during the shift

   6) Specific treatments to be completed by the incoming nurse

   7) IV rate and credits (amount remaining)

   c. Delegate clearly and concisely

   d. Offer positive feedback continually

   3. Physicians/other healthcare professionals are vital to clients' and families' health and well-being; thus, clear and open communication is beneficial to all who are involved in healthcare delivery; communication requires:

   a. Striving for collaboration and keeping client care as the goal central to the discussion

   b. Allowing for open and direct telephone reporting to healthcare providers about changes in client's condition

   c. Presenting information in a straightforward manner

   d. Being sure to have the client's chart on hand and providing the healthcare provider with:

   1) Client's name and diagnosis

   2) Stated symptoms

3) Changes in nursing assessments

4) Vital signs compared with baseline

5) Laboratory test results compared with baseline

6) Nursing interventions initiated and client response

e. Remaining calm and objective even if healthcare provider is not helpful

f. Following institution's procedure for getting the client treated and then documenting actions taken

4. Because clients and families need support and freedom to communicate their concerns about their healthcare and conditions, the healthcare team needs to incorporate diverse communication strategies, including:

a. Using touch as way to communicate caring and concern; occasionally, language barriers will limit communication to the nonverbal mode

b. Being open and honest while respecting clients and families

c. Honoring and protect clients' privacy with both actions and words

d. Assessing client's baseline understanding before providing extensive information about nursing care

e. Using plain language, not nursing jargon, vague terms, or words that may have different meanings to client

f. Encouraging the client to ask questions

g. Confirming that the client understands either by repeating back or using return demonstration

V. CONFLICT MANAGEMENT

A. The nurse leader must learn to confront conflict for what it is—a difference in perception or opinion

B. *Conflict*

1. A consequence of real or perceived differences in mutually exclusive goals, values, ideas, attitudes, beliefs, feelings, or actions

2. A perceived struggle between two or more interdependent individuals

3. Disagreement about something of importance to each person involved

4. Not necessarily bad

5. A natural, inevitable condition in organizations and often a prerequisite to change in people and organizations

C. Role and responsibility of nurse leaders during conflict (see also Box 7-3 and 7-4)

1. Model conflict resolution behaviors

2. Lessen perceptual differences of involved parties

3. Assist involved parties to identify resolution techniques

4. Create an environment conducive to conflict resolution; if conflict cannot be resolved, minimize or lessen the perceptions of the conflicting parties

D. Barriers that create conflicts include the following:

1. Preconceived expectations

2. Prejudices

3. Cherished beliefs

Box 7-3	
Role of the Nurse Leader in Managing Conflict	➤ Survey the landscape. ➤ Identify the nature of the challenge. ➤ Monitor the tension. ➤ Decide on a mechanism for resolution. ➤ Consider the level of participation. ➤ Protect minority opinion or voices. ➤ Focus on achievement and outcomes. ➤ Encourage humanism. ➤ Promote self-actualization. ➤ Promote full participation in new and different ways.

    4. Need to control

    5. Lack of clarity of the goal

    6. Role misconceptions

E. Types of conflict

    1. Content conflict or value conflict involves the beliefs and values of the individuals involved; different beliefs and/or values that prevent resolution of conflict situation include:

        a. Different criteria for evaluating ideas or behaviors

        b. Exclusive goals

        c. Different ways of life, philosophy, or religion

    2. Procedural conflict or interest conflict occurs when individuals have the same goal but differ in how they want to reach these goals:

        a. Perceived or actual competition over substance

        b. Procedural interests

        c. Psychological interests

    3. Substantive conflict or data conflict causes individuals to differ about what the goals are in a particular situation and can include:

        a. Lack of information

        b. Misinformation

Box 7-4	
How to Lead and Manage Difficult People	There will be times when difficult people will challenge the nurse leader's abilities and leadership. When this occurs: ➤ Keep focused. ➤ Ask them to join you. ➤ Encourage and engage them to work as team players. ➤ Remain calm. ➤ Lower your voice. ➤ Determine whether it is the person or the situation that is difficult. ➤ Avoid internalizing or taking the behavior personally.

  c. Different views on relevance

  d. Different interpretations

  e. Different assessment

 4. Relationship conflict causes issues of self-esteem; individuals do not feel that others are dealing with them in a respectful way; this can be triggered by:

  a. Issues of control—individuals are primarily concerned with who is controlling the situation

  b. Issues of affiliation—individuals do not feel they are getting their need for warmth and affection met by other person(s)

 5. Other causes of conflict involve strong emotions, misperceptions or stereotypes, and poor communication:

  a. Intrapersonal—within one individual

  b. Interpersonal—between two or more individuals

  c. Intragroup—between two or more groups

F. Sources of conflict may arise from a variety of sources, including:

 1. Allocation/availability of resources

 2. Personality differences

 3. Differences in values

 4. Internal/external pressures

 5. Cultural differences

 6. Competition

 7. Differences in goals

 8. Issues of personal/professional control

G. The process of conflict involves:

 1. Antecedent conditions

  a. Incompatible goals

  b. Structural conflicts

  c. Competition for resources

  d. Values and beliefs

 2. Perceived or felt conflict

 3. Manifest behavior

 4. Outcomes

  a. Suppression or resolution

  b. Resolution aftermath

H. Basic methods for resolving conflict (see Box 7-5):

 1. **Avoiding**/withdrawing: failing to acknowledge that conflict exists

 2. Accommodation: abandoning one's own needs and submitting to satisfy the needs of others, but often at own expense; willing to lose and let other side win; cooperative and assertive

 3. **Competition**: trying to defeat the other person or pursue own goals; wanting to win and make other side lose; competitor is assertive and does not want to cooperate

 4. **Cooperation** or **compromise:** exchanging equivalent values or agreeing not to get in each other's way; willing to accept loss of own needs in order to achieve a solution; mildly cooperative and assertive

Box 7-5	1. Evaluate conflict situations to decide if and when to intervene.
Tools for Handling Conflict	2. Understand the antecedent conditions for the conflict and the positions of those involved.
	3. Enlist others to help solve conflicts.
	4. Select a conflict management strategy appropriate to the situation.
	5. Practice the conflict management strategies discussed in the chapter and evaluate the outcomes.

Source: Sullivan, E. J. & Decker, P. J. (2005). *Effective leadership and management in nursing* (6th ed.). Upper Saddle River, NJ: Pearson Prentice Hall, p. 141. Reprinted by permission.

5. Collaboration: focusing on action in the interest of future relationships; attempting to define and satisfy needs of all at the table; the goal is for everyone to win; both assertive and cooperative

I. Key prerequisites to collaboration

1. Ability to listen, comprehend, and trust
2. Ability to interpret client needs to others

J. Steps to successful collaboration include:

1. Establishing a common vision: what similar aspirations/goals do both parties have; establish commonalties that a solution is possible and provide a sense of direction
2. Creating a situation of balanced power; trust others and have willingness to work together; know own expertise, limits, and discipline boundaries
3. What is best use of all resources in the interest of the common goal?
4. Engaging in relational thinking: how can the parties see themselves in relation to "three fields of influence" (ourselves, others, and overall system of which we are a part) in conflict
5. Importance of listening: partners in conflict also require compassion, best demonstrated through listening with genuine interest to another person; understand and appreciate what others do
6. Negotiation: a key response in which both parties are willing to give and take on issues; the nurse leader can use any of following strategies to successfully negotiate conflict:

   a. Clarify a common purpose
   b. Keep the discussion relevant
   c. Get agreement on terminology
   d. Avoid abstract principals; use facts
   e. Look for potential tradeoffs
   f. Use active listening
   g. Avoid debating tactics; use persuasion
   h. Look for solutions that satisfy real interests

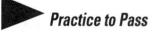

Practice to Pass

Think about a conflict situation that you have witnessed in the clinical setting. Describe the conflict process. Discuss effective tools for handling conflict.

K. Constructive functions of conflict: conflict is neither good nor bad; however, knowing how to constructively manage the functions of conflict will always enhance the workplace environment

1. Interpersonal challenges may result in improved coping skills
2. May release tension in a relationship

▶ *Practice to Pass*

Even though many conflicts cannot be fully resolved, explain why negotiation may be a reasonable strategy to use when parties are willing to discuss an issue. Describe the skills the nurse leader can use to successfully negotiate conflict.

3. Sometimes promotes intimacy
4. Changes or clarifies goals
5. Provides a cooling-off period
6. Uses intermediaries
7. May divide resources among parties

L. Not all conflicts can be solved or are worth fighting
1. Some differences are irreconcilable
2. Agreement may not be worth the effort needed to reach it
3. There may be no good solution

Case Study

On the morning of surgery to remove infected tissue from an abdominal surgical procedure, a female client tells the staff nurse that she is furious with her doctor. She demands to know how she got this abdominal infection in the first place.

1. Discuss which responses would indicate that the staff nurse is a holistic communicator.

2. Describe communication facilitators that would be useful for the nurse to use when communicating with this client.

3. Identify and describe communication barriers that are present in this situation when the nurse is communicating with this client.

4. Explain how the client might feel about undergoing an additional surgery.

5. Using simple, clear words explain how the staff nurse could show sensitivity to the client during this interaction.

For suggested answers, see page 237.

POSTTEST

1 A nurse leader attempts effective collaboration with charge nurses. Which components of effective leadership should the leader use? Select all that apply.

1. Downward communication
2. Trust
3. Administrative support
4. Accountability
5. Dominant decision making

2 The nurse leader who is trying to build an effective work team tries to motivate staff nurses by explaining that which of the following are benefits of a productive team? Select all that apply.

1. Diverse solutions to problems
2. Personal satisfaction
3. Solitary work
4. Efficiency of services
5. Use of resources

3 A nurse leader reviews the work of the team. The nurse leader interprets that which attribute of the group is consistent with effective collaboration?

1. Independent work
2. Setting goals
3. Decision making
4. Delegating responses

4 Which of the following strategies would be best for the nurse leader to use when communicating with team members at the beginning of a team project?

1. Give clear directions about the nature and scope of the project.
2. Start with constructive criticism.
3. State that something isn't working and needs to be fixed.
4. Take ownership of the project.

5 A nurse communicates changes in practice to the certified nursing assistant (CNA). The nurse is aware that the direction of this communication is considered to be:

1. Upward flow.
2. Downward flow.
3. Lateral flow.
4. Horizontal flow.

6 Team members working on a quality improvement project for the nursing unit debate among themselves about the direction of the team. The nurse leader of the team interprets that this behavior indicates which phase of team development?

1. Norming
2. Forming
3. Storming
4. Performing

7 A staff nurse who volunteers to record minutes for a staff meeting uses the agency intranet to inform the nursing staff of outcomes from a staff meeting. The nurse reading this communication understands that the nurse who recorded the minutes has used the computer to facilitate which type of communication?

1. Upward communication
2. Downward communication
3. Distant communication
4. Horizontal communication

8 A nurse leader attempts to resolve conflict between two nurses. Which communication skill should the leader use first?

1. Clarification
2. Confrontation
3. Nonverbal acknowledgement
4. Active listening

9 A charge nurse explains a new procedure to a staff nurse; however, the staff nurse is upset about working understaffed. The charge nurse recognizes that which barrier to communication is influencing this dialogue?

1. Distracting noise
2. Emotions
3. Structure
4. Space

10 The nurse leader is starting to work on a team project with members of a diverse agency workforce. The nurse is aware that which of the following will primarily influence communication among group members because they have different beliefs, practices, and assumptions?

1. Gender
2. Culture
3. Time orientation
4. Ethnicity

➤ *See pages 154–156 for Answers and Rationales.*

ANSWERS & RATIONALES

Pretest

1 **Answers: 1, 2, 3, 5** Characteristics of a productive team are trustworthiness among each other, respect for each other, and open communication. Effective teams are eager to get the job done. Although everyone has flaws, tolerance of these is not an accepted characteristic when defining effective teams.

Cognitive Level: Comprehension **Client Need:** Safe Effective Care Environment: Management of Care **Integrated Process:** Nursing Process: Implementation **Content Area:** Leadership/Management **Strategy:** Select options that signify positive attributes in a team. Rule out options that are negative attributes of a team. Options 1, 2, 3, and 5 are positive attributes, making them correct answers. Option 4 is a more negative attribute. **References:**

POSTTEST

ANSWERS & RATIONALES

Finkelman, A. W. (2006). *Leadership and management in nursing*. Upper Saddle River, NJ: Pearson Education, pp. 70–84, 200–221, 535–536; Sullivan, E. J., & Decker, P. (2005). *Effective leadership and management in nursing* (6th ed.). Upper Saddle River, NJ: Pearson Education, pp. 133–139, 155–166.

2 **Answer: 2** The best strategy the nurse can use to foster collaboration is developing openness toward ideas and suggestions of the nursing staff. Emphasis on tasks (option 1) and firm communication (option 4) are not effective in collaboration. Focusing on quality care is an appropriate strategy for a nurse leader, but this question focuses on collaboration as a process. Quality care might be an outcome of high-level collaboration among staff. **Cognitive Level:** Analysis **Client Need:** Safe Effective Care Environment: Management of Care **Integrated Process:** Nursing Process: Planning **Content Area:** Leadership/Management **Strategy:** Look for the option that focuses on collaboration—option 2. Emphasis on tasks, resistance, and firm communication are not measures that foster collaboration. These strategies function as barriers to collaboration. Use collaboration principles to select the correct response. **References:** Finkelman, A. W. (2006). *Leadership and management in nursing*. Upper Saddle River, NJ: Pearson Education, pp. 70–84, 200–221, 535–536; Sullivan, E. J., & Decker, P. (2005). *Effective leadership and management in nursing* (6th Ed.). Upper Saddle River, NJ: Pearson Education, pp. 133–139, 155–166.

3 **Answer: 1** The mission statement is a broad statement that describes the purpose of the organization to internal and external constituents and provides the team with guidance and focus. Fostering communication (option 2), increasing problem solving (option 3), and team building/personal bonding (option 4) are too specific for a mission statement. **Cognitive Level:** Comprehension **Client Need:** Safe Effective Care Environment: Management of Care **Integrated Process:** Communication and Documentation **Content Area:** Leadership/Management **Strategy:** Identify the option that includes the purpose of the mission, option 1. The other options focus on topics that fail to include the purpose of the mission. Use knowledge of team building to select the correct response. **References:** Finkelman, A. W. (2006). *Leadership and management in nursing*. Upper Saddle River, NJ: Pearson Education, pp. 70–84, 200–221, 535–536; Sullivan, E. J., & Decker, P. (2005). *Effective leadership and management in nursing* (6th ed.). Upper Saddle River, NJ: Pearson Education, pp. 133–139, 155–166.

4 **Answers: 1, 2, 5** Team leaders are committed to action with a passion for learning, and they are eager to suc-

ceed. They do not delegate planning (option 3) but are active participants in planning. They do not develop the rules singly (option 4) but share in establishing the rules of the group. **Cognitive Level:** Comprehension **Client Need:** Safe Effective Care Environment: Management of Care **Integrated Process:** Nursing Process: Planning **Content Area:** Leadership/Management **Strategy:** Choose options that are specific characteristics of leaders. This includes options 1, 2, and 5. Note that options 3 and 4 focus on the functions of leaders (not innate characteristics) so these must be eliminated. Use knowledge of team building to select the correct response. **References:** Finkelman, A. W. (2006). *Leadership and management in nursing*. Upper Saddle River, NJ: Pearson Education, pp. 70–84, 200–221, 535–536; Sullivan, E. J., & Decker, P. (2005). *Effective leadership and management in nursing* (6th ed.). Upper Saddle River, NJ: Pearson Education, pp. 133–139, 155–166.

5 **Answer: 1** Whenever planning new ideas, it is beneficial to get support from other members of the team because this action may decrease resistance. Supervising only when necessary (option 2) may not be appropriate in the goal setting process. Analyzing the organizational structure (option 3) is not within the scope of a single team. Reorganizing the group (option 4) does not address the issue of goal setting directly and may or may not be necessary. **Cognitive Level:** Application **Client Need:** Safe Effective Care Environment: Management of Care **Integrated Process:** Nursing Process: Planning **Content Area:** Leadership/Management **Strategy:** Rule out option 2 based on the term *only*, which is so exclusive. Note the critical word *best* in the question, which indicates that more than one option may be plausible but that one is better than the others. Note that the options for analyzing the organizational structure (option 3) and group reorganization (option 4) may or may not be instrumental in establishing new goals, but they are not the priority actions. Ascertaining buy-in from other members of the team is a priority action, making option 1 the correct choice. Use collaboration principles to select the correct response. **References:** Finkelman, A. W. (2006). *Leadership and management in nursing*. Upper Saddle River, NJ: Pearson Education, pp. 70–84, 200–221, 535–536; Sullivan, E. J., & Decker, P. (2005). *Effective leadership and management in nursing* (6th ed.). Upper Saddle River, NJ: Pearson Education, pp. 133–139, 155–166.

6 **Answer: 4** It's always best to include group members in decision making; this action increases adherence to rules and support for new ideas. Continuing to engage in dialogue and pointing out areas of agreement helps keep

the group energized and focused. Changing rules during the discussion (option 1) is inconsistent and can cause confusion and resentment within the team. The issue of fairness is also a concern. Focusing on details (option 2) can distract the group from the main discussion; details can be discussed once a course of action is established. Diplomacy (not firm words as in option 3) is the best way to communicate with a group of individuals.
Cognitive Level: Application **Client Need:** Safe Effective Care Environment: Management of Care **Integrated Process:** Communication and Documentation **Content Area:** Leadership/Management **Strategy:** Choose an option that includes consensus-building measures. Note that options 1 and 3 are not consensus-building strategies and that option 2 does not apply to this question. Use collaboration principles to select the correct response. **References:** Finkelman, A. W. (2006). *Leadership and management in nursing.* Upper Saddle River, NJ: Pearson Education, pp. 70–84, 200–221, 535–536; Sullivan, E. J., & Decker, P. (2005). *Effective leadership and management in nursing* (6th ed.). Upper Saddle River, NJ: Pearson Education, pp. 133–139, 155–166.

7 **Answer: 1** The assistant is communicating client concerns to the nurse manager, which flows up the chain of command. Downward flow starts with communication from someone in leadership to those in subordinate positions. Lateral or horizontal flow is communication on the same level such as communication from the nursing department to the lab department.
Cognitive Level: Comprehension **Client Need:** Safe Effective Care Environment: Management of Care **Integrated Process:** Communication and Documentation **Content Area:** Leadership/Management **Strategy:** Eliminate options 3 and 4 because they are the same. Choose option 1 over option 2 because the CNA works under the direction of the nurse manager. Use communication concepts and the process of elimination to select the correct response. **References:** Finkelman, A. W. (2006). *Leadership and management in nursing.* Upper Saddle River, NJ: Pearson Education, pp. 70–84, 200–221, 535–536; Sullivan, E. J., & Decker, P. (2005). *Effective leadership and management in nursing* (6th ed.). Upper Saddle River, NJ: Pearson Education, pp. 133–139, 155–166.

8 **Answer: 2** The "performing" stage of team development (option 2) is characterized by carrying out the action plan. The members are focusing on getting the tasks done to achieve the goals of the team. In the "storming" phase (option 3), members may lose confidence in the leader, team direction, and purpose of the group. The "norming" phase (option 4) is characterized by agreement of rules, direction, and a plan. The "forming" phase (option 1) is represented by familiarization of

group members and identification of the group's goals and mission.
Cognitive Level: Application **Client Need:** Safe Effective Care Environment: Management of Care **Integrated Process:** Nursing Process: Assessment **Content Area:** Leadership/Management **Strategy:** Look for the critical word *implementation.* This word implies that the team is working on specific strategies to achieve goals. Identify best practice options to select the correct response. **References:** Finkelman, A. W. (2006). *Leadership and management in nursing.* Upper Saddle River, NJ: Pearson Education, pp. 70–84, 200–221, 535–536; Sullivan, E. J., & Decker, P. (2005). *Effective leadership and management in nursing* (6th ed.). Upper Saddle River, NJ: Pearson Education, pp. 133–139, 155–166.

9 **Answer: 3** When attempting to handle difficult behavior demonstrated by staff, employees, or team members, it is always best to focus on the problem and the negative behavior. This dialogue should include the goals of the group and expectations. Writing an action plan may be implemented, but it is not the focus of the meeting. The team leader should listen to the nurse, but this is not the best strategy to move toward improvement.
Cognitive Level: Application **Client Need:** Safe Effective Care Environment: Management of Care **Integrated Process:** Nursing Process: Planning **Content Area:** Leadership/Management **Strategy:** Identify an option that focuses on the team member's behavior, which is option 3. Consider that option 1 is necessary, but it is not the best action. Options 2 and 4 are also plausible, but are not the most important item in moving toward effective change. Identify critical words in the question or stem to select the right answer. **References:** Finkelman, A. W. (2006). *Leadership and management in nursing.* Upper Saddle River, NJ: Pearson Education, pp. 70–84, 200–221, 535–536; Sullivan, E. J., & Decker, P. (2005). *Effective leadership and management in nursing* (6th ed.). Upper Saddle River, NJ: Pearson Education, pp. 133–139, 155–166.

10 **Answer: 3** Option 3 represents the best characteristic of collaboration because everyone on the team has a voice that is heard and considered. Compromise (option 1) does not necessarily yield effective results for some parties. Option 2 yields results for one party, but perhaps not for all. Option 4 illustrates a shared vision but not necessarily collaboration.
Cognitive Level: Application **Client Need:** Safe Effective Care Environment: Management of Care **Integrated Process:** Nursing Process: Assessment **Content Area:** Leadership/Management **Strategy:** Focus on the option that includes characteristics of collaboration—negotiation. A compromise is not a characteristic of

collaboration. Options 2 and 4 are not characteristics of collaboration, and option 2 is a biased approach to problem solving. Use communication concepts and the process of elimination to select the correct response. **References:** Finkelman, A. W. (2006). *Leadership and management in nursing.* Upper Saddle River, NJ: Pearson Education, pp. 70–84, 200–221, 535–536; Sullivan, E. J., & Decker, P. (2005). *Effective leadership and management in nursing* (6th ed.). Upper Saddle River, NJ: Pearson Education, pp. 133–139, 155–166.

Posttest

1 **Answers: 1, 2, 3, 4** Effective collaboration includes communication, trust among staff, support from administration, and accountability of leadership and staff. Dominant decision making is not effective in collaboration.
Cognitive Level: Application **Client Need:** Safe Effective Care Environment: Management of Care **Integrated Process:** Nursing Process: Implementation **Content Area:** Leadership/Management **Strategy:** Select the options that focus on positive aspects of collaboration. This includes all options except dominant decision making, which is not synonymous with collaboration. Use communication concepts and the process of elimination to select the correct response. **References:** Finkelman, A. W. (2006). *Leadership and management in nursing.* Upper Saddle River, NJ: Pearson Education, pp. 70–84, 200–221, 535–536; Sullivan, E. J., & Decker, P. (2005). *Effective leadership and management in nursing* (6th ed.). Upper Saddle River, NJ: Pearson Education, pp. 133–139, 155–166.

2 **Answers: 1, 2, 4** Benefits of a productive team include diverse solutions to problems, personal satisfaction, and efficiency of services. Teams work in groups; team members do not work in a solitary fashion.
Cognitive Level: Comprehension **Client Need:** Safe Effective Care Environment: Management of Care **Integrated Process:** Nursing Process: Implementation **Content Area:** Leadership/Management **Strategy:** Eliminate option 5 first because use of resources is not related to the question being asked. Next, eliminate solitary work because it is not a benefit of a productive team. Recall that the benefits of a team include diverse solutions problems to personal satisfaction, and efficiency of services. Use knowledge of team building to select the correct response. **References:** Finkelman, A. W. (2006). *Leadership and management in nursing.* Upper Saddle River, NJ: Pearson Education, pp. 70–84, 200–221, 535–536; Sullivan, E. J., & Decker, P. (2005). *Effective leadership and management in nursing* (6th ed.). Upper Saddle River, NJ: Pearson Education, pp. 133–139, 155–166.

3 **Answer: 2** Goal setting is consistent with effective collaboration. Doing independent work (option 1), engag-

ing in decision making (option 3), and delegating responses (option 4) are not hallmarks of collaboration.
Cognitive Level: Application **Client Need:** Safe Effective Care Environment: Management of Care **Integrated Process:** Nursing Process: Evaluation **Content Area:** Leadership/Management **Strategy:** Choose an option that represents collaboration. Rule out option 1—independent work is not a characteristic of collaboration. Options 3 and 4 are indirectly linked to collaboration. Option 2 represents collaboration because it shows the team has worked to create a plan. Use collaboration principles to select the correct response. **References:** Finkelman, A. W. (2006). *Leadership and management in nursing.* Upper Saddle River, NJ: Pearson Education, pp. 70–84, 200–221, 535–536; Sullivan, E. J., & Decker, P. (2005). *Effective leadership and management in nursing* (6th Ed.). Upper Saddle River, NJ: Pearson Education, pp. 133–139, 155–166.

4 **Answer: 1** Leaders should be very clear and concise when providing directions and goals at the beginning of a project so that members have a clear vision about what is to be accomplished and the processes that will be used in the group. Criticism (option 2) should be sandwiched in the dialogue and never presented first. Focusing on problem solving (option 3) does not address collaboration. Ownership of the project (option 4) does not directly address collaboration.
Cognitive Level: Application **Client Need:** Safe Effective Care Environment: Management of Care **Integrated Process:** Communication and Documentation **Content Area:** Leadership/Management **Strategy:** First, rule out option 2 because it is too harsh. Next, eliminate option 4, since the team needs to feel ownership of the project for best results. Option 3 is mildly plausible; however, when working with the team it is important to lead with clarity, direction, and purpose. Use principles of communication and collaboration to select the correct response. **References:** Finkelman, A. W. (2006). *Leadership and management in nursing.* Upper Saddle River, NJ: Pearson Education, pp. 70–84, 200–221, 535–536; Sullivan, E. J., & Decker, P. (2005). *Effective leadership and management in nursing* (6th ed.). Upper Saddle River, NJ: Pearson Education, pp. 133–139, 155–166.

5 **Answer: 2** Downward flow starts with communication from someone in leadership to those in subordinate positions. Upward flow is characterized by communication coming from those in lower positions to those in higher positions. Lateral or horizontal flow is communication on the same level such as communication from the nursing department to the lab department.
Cognitive Level: Comprehension **Client Need:** Safe Effective Care Environment: Management of Care **Integrated Process:** Communication and Documentation **Content**

Area: Leadership/Management **Strategy:** Eliminate options 3 and 4 because they are the same. Choose option 2 over option 1 because the CNA works under the direction of the nurse. Use communication concepts and the process of elimination to select the correct response. **References:** Finkelman, A. W. (2006). *Leadership and management in nursing.* Upper Saddle River, NJ: Pearson Education, pp. 200–221, 70–84, 535–536; Sullivan, E. J., & Decker, P. (2005). *Effective leadership and management in nursing* (6th ed.). Upper Saddle River, NJ: Pearson Education, pp. 133–139, 155–166.

6 **Answer: 3** In the "storming" phase, members may lose confidence in the leader, team direction, and purpose of the group. The "norming" phase is characterized by agreement of rules, direction, and a plan. The "forming" phase is represented by familiarization of group members and identification of the group's goals and mission. The "performing" stage of team development is characterized by carrying out the action plan.
Cognitive Level: Application **Client Need:** Safe Effective Care Environment: Management of Care **Integrated Process:** Nursing Process: Planning **Content Area:** Leadership/Management **Strategy:** Consider the definitions of the various terms used in the options. The debate among team members is best interpreted as "storming." The other options do not apply. Use knowledge of team building to select the correct response. **References:** Finkelman, A. W. (2006). *Leadership and management in nursing.* Upper Saddle River, NJ: Pearson Education, pp. 70–84, 200–221, 535–536; Sullivan, E. J., & Decker, P. (2005). *Effective leadership and management in nursing* (6th ed.). Upper Saddle River, NJ: Pearson Education, pp. 133–139, 155–166.

7 **Answer: 4** The clinical coordinator is communicating with others on the same level of the organizational chain, so this is consistent with horizontal communication. Downward flow starts with communication from someone in leadership to those in subordinate positions. Upward flow is characterized by communication coming from those in lower positions to those in higher positions. Distant communication is not a term used to describe communication.
Cognitive Level: Comprehension **Client Need:** Safe Effective Care Environment: Management of Care **Integrated Process:** Communication and Documentation **Content Area:** Leadership/Management **Strategy:** First note that the nurse who is sending the communication is at the same level in the organization as the recipients of the information. Correlate this with the word *horizontal* in the correct option. Use communication concepts and the process of elimination to select the correct response. **References:** Finkelman, A. W. (2006). *Leadership and management in nursing.* Upper Saddle River, NJ: Pear-

son Education, pp. 70–84, 200–221, 535–536; Sullivan, E. J., & Decker, P. (2005). *Effective leadership and management in nursing* (6th ed.). Upper Saddle River, NJ: Pearson Education, pp. 133–139, 155–166.

8 **Answer: 4** The first action by the leader is active listening. The leader needs to listen to both nurses separately then together (meeting). During the meeting, the nurse leader should clarify issues that are ambiguous. Acknowledgment should occur during the meeting to indicate all parties are listening.
Cognitive Level: Application **Client Need:** Safe Effective Care Environment: Management of Care **Integrated Process:** Nursing Process: Planning **Content Area:** Leadership/Management **Strategy:** The critical word in the question is *first.* This tells you that there may be more than one plausible option, but that one is better than the others. Option 3 is a passive-aggressive skill; rule it out. Option 2 is unprofessional, so eliminate that next. Of the remaining two, consider that it is always best to start with listening. Clarification is a correct type of action, but the leader must listen first and clarify second. Use communication concepts and the process of elimination to select the correct response. **References:** Finkelman, A. W. (2006). *Leadership and management in nursing.* Upper Saddle River, NJ: Pearson Education, pp. 70–84, 200–221, 535–536; Sullivan, E. J., & Decker, P. (2005). *Effective leadership and management in nursing* (6th ed.). Upper Saddle River, NJ: Pearson Education, pp. 133–139, 155–166.

9 **Answer: 2** The only option that fits this scenario is emotions. The nurse is upset about the shortage of staff, and this prevents the nurse from focusing on the information the charge nurse attempts to convey. There is no information in the question that makes reference to distracting noise (option 1), structure (option 3), or space (option 4).
Cognitive Level: Comprehension **Client Need:** Safe Effective Care Environment: Management of Care **Integrated Process:** Nursing Process: Evaluation **Content Area:** Leadership/Management **Strategy:** Noise is not present in the scenario so rule it out. Structure and space are not addressed in the scenario so rule them out next. The nurse's emotions are quite clear. Use communication concepts and the process of elimination to select the correct response. **References:** Finkelman, A. W. (2006). *Leadership and management in nursing.* Upper Saddle River, NJ: Pearson Education, pp. 70–84, 200–221, 535–536; Sullivan, E. J., & Decker, P. (2005). *Effective leadership and management in nursing* (6th ed.). Upper Saddle River, NJ: Pearson Education, pp. 133–139, 155–166.

10 **Answer: 2** Culture plays a very vital role in communication. Gender and ethnicity may have some influence in

communication styles, but culture has a direct impact on the fashion in which people communicate with others. Time orientation does not have a role in communication although it is part of culture.
Cognitive Level: Comprehension **Client Need:** Safe Effective Care Environment: Management of Care **Integrated Process:** Nursing Process: Planning **Content Area:** Leadership/Management **Strategy:** Choose the option that is used to describe beliefs, practices, and assumptions. Gender, time orientation, and ethnicity do not describe different beliefs, practices, and assumptions; however, culture does. Use communication concepts and the process of elimination to select the correct response. **References:** Finkelman, A. W. (2006). *Leadership and management in nursing.* Upper Saddle River, NJ: Pearson Education, pp. 70–84, 200–221, 535–536; Sullivan, E. J., & Decker, P. (2005). *Effective leadership and management in nursing* (6th ed.). Upper Saddle River, NJ: Pearson Education, pp. 133–139, 155–166.

References

Amos, M., Hu, J., & Herrick, C. (2005). The impact of team building on communication and job satisfaction. *Journal for Nurses in Staff Development, 21*(1), 10–16.

Artford, P. (2005). Nurse-physician communication: An organizational accountability. *Nursing Economics, 23*(2), 72–77.

Bacal, R. (2004). Organizational conflict: The good, the bad, and the ugly. *The Journal for Quality & Participation, 27*(2), 21–22.

Baldoni, J. (2004). Powerful leadership communication. *Leader to Leader, 32,* 20–24.

Barker, A. M., Sullivan, D. T., & Emery, M. J. (2006). *Leadership competencies for clinical managers.* Sudbury, MA: Jones and Bartlett Publishers.

Conerly, K., & Tripathi, A. (2004). What is your conflict style? *The Journal for Quality & Participation, 27*(2), 16–20.

Dessle, G. (2004). *Management: Principles and practices for tomorrow's leaders.* Upper Saddle River, NJ: Pearson Education.

Giger, J. N., Davidhizar, R., Purnell, L., Harden, J. T., Phillips, J., & Strickland, O. (2007). Developing cultural competency to eliminate health disparities in ethnic minorities and other vulnerable populations. American Academy of Nursing Expert Panel Reports. *Journal of Transcultural Nursing, 18*(2), 100–101.

Porter-O'Grady, T. (2005). Managing conflict in the workplace. *Imprint, 50*(4), 66–68.

Sullivan, E. J., & Decker, P. J. (2005). *Effective leadership and management in nursing* (6th ed.). Upper Saddle River, NJ: Pearson Education.

Yoder-Wise, P. S. (2007). *Leading and managing in nursing* (4th ed.). St. Louis, MO: Mosby.

Ensuring a Quality Nurse Workforce

8

Objectives

➤ Identify ways to ensure a quality nurse workforce through staff development.

➤ Define the term *competency*.

➤ Explain the nurse's role as client advocate.

➤ Define the term *performance appraisal*.

➤ Describe criteria used to evaluate nursing staff.

➤ Explain the different methods used to evaluate performance.

➤ Identify skills and strategies to resolve personnel problems and challenges.

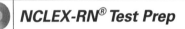

NCLEX-RN® Test Prep

Use the CD-ROM enclosed with this book to access additional practice opportunities.

Review at a Glance

absenteeism rate at which a staff member misses work on an unplanned basis

advocacy proactively speaking for another to ensure his or her needs or wishes are met

coaching strategy used by a nurse leader to assist others to learn, critically think, and develop through ongoing communication about job performance

competencies cluster of attributes consisting of knowledge, skills, attitudes, abilities, behaviors, and other characteristics

continuing education programs planned and organized to expand upon nurses' educational and experiential needs; professional learning experiences to augment the knowledge, skills, and attitudes of nursing staff

critical incident a brief example of good or bad performance that is used to support performance appraisals and development needs of staff

in-service training activity directed at assisting nursing staff in performing their assigned functions

orientation formal process of familiarizing nursing staff with an organization, including learning about the organization

performance appraisal evaluation process in which a nurse leader evaluates a staff member's work performance

standard a unit of measurement that serves as a reference point for evaluating results

PRETEST

1 The nurse educator on a nursing unit develops staff development programs to accomplish which of the following goals? Select all that apply.

1. Enhance social support and employee relations
2. Acquire new skills
3. Change undesired staff behavior
4. Investigate sources of errors
5. Increase professional competence

2 The nurse educator explains to a group of new nurse orientees to expect which of the following benefits from staff development programs?

1. Acquisition of technical skills
2. Personal development
3. Forum to share their views on client care issues
4. Opportunity to develop networks

3 Which strategy should a nurse leader use to build a culture for staff development?

1. Expect all staff to attend each activity.
2. Aggressively pursue funding from administration.
3. Add development activities based on managers' preferences.
4. Schedule staff development activities at a variety of times.

4 A nurse is hired and scheduled for orientation. The nurse anticipates learning about which of the following during orientation? Select all that apply.

1. Unwritten agency rules
2. Policies
3. Benefits
4. Procedures
5. Role expectations

5 A facility purchases new intravenous (IV) pumps. Which strategy should the nurse leader use to educate the current staff about the new pumps?

1. Web-enhanced instruction
2. In-service
3. Orientation
4. User manual

6 To be eligible for renewal of a nursing license, the nurse expects to complete a predetermined number of hours of which of the following to ensure practice competency?

1. Refresher courses
2. Virtual instruction
3. Continuing education
4. Orientation

7 A nurse who aspires to be a nurse manager understands that which of the following will be one of the competencies that will be needed in the new role?

1. Ability to demonstrate virtual instruction technology to staff
2. Visioning and strategic planning for the nursing unit
3. Use of technological devices
4. Proficiency in the use of nursing process

8 A staff nurse who has been in practice for one year is about to have the first annual employment evaluation. The nurse should be prepared to show evidence of proficiency in which of the following?

1. Nursing process
2. Financial management
3. Human resource benefits management
4. Visioning for the unit

9 A unit manager rates a staff member the same on all dimensions of the performance evaluation. The chief nurse officer counsels the manager about which type of appraisal error?

1. Ambiguous
2. Recency
3. Leniency
4. Halo

10 A nurse with fifteen years experience recognizes early signs of urosepsis in an older adult admitted with pneumonia and notifies the primary care provider of the physical assessment findings. This represents which stage of Benner's model?

1. Proficient practitioner
2. Advanced practitioner
3. Expert practitioner
4. Competent practitioner

➤ *See pages 172–174 for Answers and Rationales.*

I. STAFF DEVELOPMENT

A. Goals of staff development
1. Enable staff members to learn under conditions that foster changing behaviors, attitudes, and opinions that support nursing care and improved quality performance
2. Create a professional practice environment that encourages professional and personal growth and development
3. Provide staff with a development program that seeks to motivate the adult learner to consider learning as a natural part of living

B. Role of staff development: staff education, training, and development are essential to the recruitment and retention of staff because:
1. Staff development plays a significant role in the quality rating of an organization
2. It is an essential strategy for maintaining the competency of the nurse workforce
3. It provides for learning opportunities and assists the individual staff member to mature in his or her role
4. It provides for the needed technical skill (what has to be done) and human skill (how is it done) that are critical to the ongoing development of professional staff

C. Building a culture for staff development
1. The nurse leader is an educator and facilitator of staff learning
2. By seeking to improve the quality of staff members' performance the nurse leader ensures improvement in the quality and safety of care given to clients; this ensures that a culture for staff development emerges when:
   a. Supported and encouraged by the executive management and leadership team
   b. Incorporated and valued into the infrastructure of the organization
   c. Planned, purposeful, budgeted, and approved by nursing service
   d. Built on confidence in others

D. Components of staff development

1. **Orientation:** a formal process of familiarizing nursing staff to the organization, including learning about the organization; this orientation process is essential if newly hired personnel are to perform within the following core elements of the organization:

   a. Philosophy
   b. Goals
   c. Policies
   d. Procedures
   e. Personnel benefits
   f. Role expectations
   g. Physical facilities

2. **In-service training**

   a. Known as a key activity directed at assisting nursing staff in performing and maintaining their assigned activities and functions
   b. Provides for refining and developing new skills related to job performance in relation to new products or technology for healthcare delivery

3. **Continuing education** (CE)

   a. The nurse leader plays a key role in motivating and developing staff for peak job performance (see Box 8–1)
   b. CE programs are planned and organized to meet the educational needs and expand upon the experiential base of the nurse; they are professional learning experiences to augment the knowledge, skills, and attitudes of nursing staff
   c. CE programs often include state-board-approved continuing education programs needed for state license renewal and offerings in new approaches in care delivery and/or enhanced practice, education, administration, and research

II. PROFESSIONAL COMPETENCY

A. The National Council of State Board of Nursing (NCSBN) explains that *competency* is the application of knowledge and the interpersonal, decision-making, and psychomotor skills expected for the nurse's practice role, within the context of public health, welfare, and safety; having the knowledge, skills, and attitudes to be professionally competent means that an individual is able to do the job and do it well

Box 8-1
Tools for Motivating and Developing Staff

1. Become familiar with various theories of motivation and use the information to help you understand others' motivations.
2. Recognize that an employee's job performance includes both ability to do the job and motivation.
3. Identify staff and department educational needs and communicate those to the appropriate decision makers.
4. Participate in in-service and/or staff development activities as appropriate.
5. Evaluate staff members' abilities to transfer learning to the job.
6. Become sensitive to the needs of a multicultural staff and design programs and activities to meet those needs.

Source: Sullivan, E. J. & Decker, P. J. (2005). *Effective leadership and management in nursing* (6th ed.). Upper Saddle River, NJ: Pearson Prentice Hall, p. 275. Reprinted by permission.

B. Staff competency is a shared responsibility and must have the ongoing support of the nurse leader

1. The nurse leader and other nurses have a responsibility to ensure safe practice through state licensure requirements, continuing education, ongoing self-evaluation, and the organization's annual performance appraisal process

2. Regulatory boards (state boards of nursing) establish the state nurse practice act, determine the scope of practice, and monitor licensure to protect the public

3. Professional organizations provide standards of practice used by healthcare organizations, regulatory boards, and professional nurses to guide professional practice decisions

C. Nurse leader *competencies* are skills, attitudes, and behaviors that ensure the practice environment meets the requirements and standards of nursing care, including:

1. Customer needs and expectations

2. Visioning and strategic planning

3. Managing care across the continuum of healthcare delivery settings

4. Improving quality and performance

5. Human resource management

6. Financial outcomes management

D. Staff nurse competencies include managing:

1. Nursing process

2. Daily job performance activities and tasks

3. Safety measures

4. Continuing education requirements

5. Initiatives for increasing quality and performance

6. Satisfactory client care results

7. Adherence to policies and procedures

8. Absence of incidents, errors, and accidents

9. Personal behavior so that it is honest and trustworthy

10. Professional performance that is ethical and moral

III. BENNER'S MODEL OF NURSING PRACTICE

A. Benner's model includes five stages in nursing care delivery that range from novice to expert; stages measure three key aspects of the nurse's skill performance:

1. Reliance on abstract principles as well as the use of past concrete experiences

2. Nurse's perception of the demand of the situation in which parts of the situation are viewed in relation to the whole, and where only certain parts are important to the situation

3. Nurse as a detached observer versus an involved participant engaged in the situation

B. Stages of nursing expertise

1. Stage 1—Novice:

   a. No experience (nursing student)

   b. Performance is limited

Practice to Pass

Locate a job description for a registered nurse (RN) position on your assigned unit or organization during a clinical experience. Analyze the job description for specific categories and behaviors. What competencies do you already have? Explain how you will develop and master the ones you do not have. Identify the common competencies needed by all registered nurses.

        c. Inflexible

        d. Governed by context-free rules and regulations

   2. Stage II—Advanced Beginner:

        a. Demonstrates marginal accepted performance

        b. Recognizes meaningful aspects of real situations

        c. Has experienced enough real situations to make a judgment

   3. Stage III—Competent Practitioner:

        a. Has two or three years experience in a similar job situation

        b. Demonstrates organizational and planning abilities

        c. Differentiates more important from less important aspects of care

        d. Coordinates multiple complex care demands

   4. Stage IV—Proficient Practitioner:

        a. Has three to five years experience with a similar client population

        b. Perceives situations as a whole rather than in parts

        c. Uses maxims as guides for what to consider in a situation

        d. Has a holistic understanding of the client

        e. Focuses on long-term goals

   5. Stage V—Expert Practitioner

        a. Performance is fluid

        b. Is flexible

        c. Is highly proficient

        d. No longer requires rules, guidelines, or maxims to connect an understanding to the current situation

        e. Demonstrates highly skilled intuitive and analytic ability in new situations

        f. Takes action because "it feels right"

C. As professional nurses mature in their roles from novice to expert, they do so across seven domains of nursing practice, which are:

   1. Helping role

   2. Teaching-coaching role

   3. Diagnostic and client monitoring function

   4. Effective management of rapidly changing situations

   5. Administration and monitoring of therapeutic interventions and regimens

   6. Monitoring of healthcare practices and ensuring quality of client care

   7. Organizational and work role competencies

IV. *ADVOCACY*

A. Definition:

   1. Proactively speaking for another to ensure his or her needs/wishes are fulfilled

   2. Nurse leaders have an obligation to be advocates for their clients and staff members by ensuring their health and well-being are protected; advocacy within the organization may occur in multiple ways, including:

        a. Preparing and developing a staffing plan and annual budget that supports funds for staff training and development

  b. Requesting and gaining support from executive leadership for safety and quality initiatives to improve client care

  c. Seeking and obtaining support for an appropriate staff nurse to patient ratio and an appropriate mix of staff

B. Nurse as client advocate

 1. All professional nurses are client advocates regardless of their title or position; nurses are expected to act as client advocates by providing information that is useful to the client and supports his or her decisions; advocacy is accepting the responsibility to:

  a. Promote and protect the client's human and legal rights

  b. Ensure the client's needs are addressed and met

  c. Protect and prevent clients from sustaining injury from adverse events

  d. Educate client and families about the healthcare delivery system

 2. Being and becoming a client advocate; nurses are obligated to:

  a. Be aware of and knowledgeable about the cultural differences of the clients they care for

  b. Respect cultural beliefs of clients and other healthcare professionals

  c. Provide a professional medical interpreter for clients who do not speak or understand English

  d. Stay informed about federal regulations and accreditation standards pertaining to clients' rights

 3. Consultation as a method of advocacy

  a. The nurse leader and the team collect data from a variety of sources: primary (client) and secondary (family, support persons, health professionals, and records)

  b. Consultation with individuals who can contribute to the client's database is helpful in achieving the most complete and accurate information about a client

  c. Supplemental information from secondary sources (any source other than the client) can help verify information, provide information for a client who is unable do so on his or her own, and convey information about the client's status prior to admission

 4. Referrals are a route to advocacy: using referrals to gain needed or additional services for clients is another route to client advocacy; referrals:

  a. Help the nurse to assist the client to obtain the necessary resources to support his or her healthcare needs

  b. Involve knowledge about community resources and how to obtain them

  c. Present a clear picture of the client and his or her healthcare needs

Practice to Pass

Describe the nurse as a client advocate. Explain why this is a key nursing role and responsibility.

V. PERFORMANCE APPRAISAL

A. The nurse leader has a key role in ensuring the quality and successful work performance of others; *performance appraisal* is defined as an evaluation process in which the nurse leader evaluates the staff against predetermined standards; nurse leader's role responsibilities include:

 1. Assisting staff in job performance

 2. Maintaining high standards of client care

3. Providing a quality and safe work environment

4. Attaining work satisfaction for self and others

B. Performance appraisal process

1. The nurse leader has within the scope of his or her managerial responsibility the key function of control for those managed on a daily basis

2. The control or feedback mechanism includes conducting probationary or annual performance appraisals

3. The appraisal process:

    a. Is a dynamic and ongoing process of interaction

    b. Is used to justify merit increases, provide feedback, and identify candidates for promotion

    c. Ensures the organization meets legal requirements for standardized procedures, forms, job analysis, and evaluator's ability

4. Critical elements of a performance appraisal process include:

    a. Ability to motivate staff to perform tasks and accomplish the organizational mission and objectives

    b. Continuous feedback throughout the period of evaluation (day-to-day **coaching** and counseling)

    c. Written documentation notes about a staff member's behavior (good or bad)

    d. An annual formal interview

    e. Follow-up interviews between nurse leader and staff member as needed to give feedback, make decisions, and comply with fair employment practice law

    f. Enforcing policy and procedural updates and violations

    g. Providing ongoing discipline if needed

5. See Box 8-2 for tips to managers for maximizing the performance appraisal process

C. Performance expectations

1. Nurse leaders must ensure that staff members know in advance what performance and expectations are desired in regard to client care and professional behavior

2. Using a standard to measure performance allows the nurse leader to adequately evaluate nursing productivity against core measures

    a. A **standard** is defined as a unit of measurement that provides a reference point for evaluating results

    b. Job standards or professional standards include such elements as established criteria, planning goals, physical or quantitative measurements of units of service

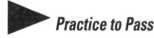

Practice to Pass

Discuss the reason why performance appraisal is considered an important process in guiding and directing nursing staff in their professional development and performance.

Box 8-2

Getting the Most Out of the Performance Appraisal Process

1. Create opportunities to reward staff performance verbally and in writing.

2. Motivate staff by setting high expectations and establishing goals that promote professional development.

3. Share the organization's and unit's visions and goals frequently with staff.

4. Describe each staff member's role and responsibility to the overall success of the unit and organization.

5. Establish unit and staff goals for professional development.

      c. Performance standards are associated with job tasks and need to be accomplished to achieve the job objectives

      d. American Nurses Association (ANA) Standards of Clinical Nursing Practice may be used as performance standards to evaluate clinical nurse practice

D. Performance evaluation methods

  1. Each organization formulates an approach to the evaluation process using evaluation method based on either *absolute judgment* or *comparative judgment*

      a. Absolute judgment uses an internal standard that allows the staff member to exceed or barely meet the standard of acceptable performance

      b. Comparative judgment rates or compares each staff member with another's performance

  2. See Figure 8-1 for a decision tree for evaluating staff performance

  3. Types of rating or evaluation tools: traditional rating scales evaluate a staff member for an entire evaluation period (usually 12 months but is often shorter for a probationary period); tool includes:

      a. General performance

      b. Equally weighted components

      c. Absolute judgment standards

      d. Judgments based on the nurse leader's idea of satisfactory performance

      e. Essay evaluation describing a staff member's performance through a detailed written narrative

      f. Forced distribution evaluation allowing for a staff member's performance to be rated in a fixed method or grading along a curve

      g. Behavior-oriented rating scales, which focus on a staff member's specific behavior and uses **critical incidents** grouped into various performance dimensions

      h. A focus on results, which promotes setting objectives that the staff member is expected to accomplish over a period of time

E. Preventing appraisal rating issues

  1. Nurse managers must be prepared to manage difficult and challenging appraisal issues as they emerge during the performance process

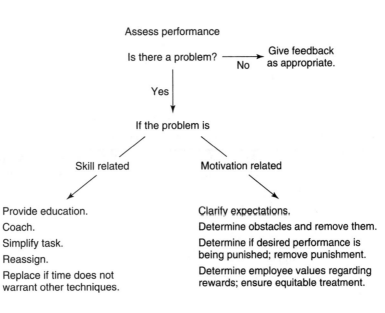

Figure 8-1

Decision tree for evaluating performance.

Source: Sullivan, E. J. & Decker P. J. (2005). *Effective leadership and management in nursing* (6th ed.). Upper Saddle River, NJ: Pearson Prentice Hall, p. 289. Reprinted by permission.

2. To safeguard against errors, the nurse leader can learn techniques to accurately carry out performance appraisal, including:

   a. Being an excellent appraiser—if don't know what to do, get help

   b. Being of the right mindset and free of distractions

   c. Setting the time to complete the process accurately and correctly

   d. Postponing the appraisal interview, if necessary

   e. Changing an inaccurate rating, if needed

   f. Using an appraisal evaluation system or tool that is error free

3. Nurse leaders can decrease potential appraisal problems by understanding how errors emerge:

   a. A leniency error occurs when the nurse leader overrates the staff member's performance (may rate all members of the team above average)

   b. A recency error occurs when the nurse leader rates the staff member's performance upon recent events rather than over the entire evaluation period

   c. A halo error occurs when the nurse leader fails to distinguish a staff member's performance on various dimensions of the rating scale and reflects identical or similar ratings on all dimensions

   d. Ambiguous evaluation standards occur when the nurse leader allows different meanings for words provided on the rating scale form, such as outstanding, above average, or below average

   e. Problems with written comments occur when the nurse leader either uses too few words or words that are meaningless to describe the true nature of a staff member's performance

F. **Performance appraisal interview:** the nurse leader:

   1. Schedules the interview by notifying the staff member in advance of the date, time, and place of appraisal interview

   2. Selects a quiet and relaxed atmosphere

   3. Sets the stage for the actual interview (arranges the table and chairs; has notes and the appraisal form ready)

   4. Remains calm, open, and receptive toward goal setting and problem-solving during the interview

   5. Prepares to accept staff member's thoughts, opinions, and concerns regarding the performance appraisal and process

   6. Describes and defines both positive and negative performance; is accurate and specific in the details

   7. Provides for an opportunity to develop a mutually acceptable action plan

   8. Discusses the need for a follow-up meeting if appropriate

G. **Helping staff members to improve performance**

   1. Nurse leaders have the responsibility to ensure that staff members carry out their delegated duties and assignments with full confidence and competence (see Box 8-3)

   2. Occasionally staff need appropriate and immediate feedback on their performance; day-to-day coaching offers an approach or intervention to deal with performance issues as they arise rather then waiting for a near miss or error to happen; intervention includes:

      a. Stating targeted performance in behavioral terms

Box 8-3	**1.** Set goals that are specific and relevant to the job position.
Criteria for Improving Performance	**2.** Make goals measurable.
	3. Maintain realistic and attainable goals.
	4. Focus performance on results not activities.
	5. Ensure performance contributes to the overall unit's goals and objectives.

  b. Connecting the problem to consequences

  c. Avoiding jumping to conclusions

  d. Asking the staff member for suggestions and discussing how to solve the problem

  e. Documenting required behavioral steps as indicated

  f. Arranging for a follow-up meeting to evaluate performance and progress toward agreed-upon targets

VI. DISCIPLINE

A. Sometimes discipline becomes necessary when staff members fail to meet job expectations

B. The nurse leader is obligated to investigate the incident carefully; the purpose is to teach new skills and encourage the staff member to improve performance or behave appropriately in the future

C. When an infraction occurs, the nurse leader:

 1. Should maintain close contact with the Human Resources Department for advice and assistance

 2. Understand the rules and regulations regarding discipline

 3. Clearly communicate the need for disciplinary action to the staff member

D. Dealing with policy or procedure incidents: when an incident occurs, the nurse leader must act immediately to address the infraction; the process includes:

 1. Determining whether the staff member is aware of current policy/procedure

 2. Describing the action/behavior violated

 3. Soliciting the staff member's reason for the action/behavior

 4. Providing for progressive discipline

 5. Allowing for consistent and ongoing evaluation of performance with feedback and sanctions if necessary

E. Steps in progressive discipline (see also Box 8-4)

 1. Each and every healthcare organization establishes a policy on progressive discipline

 2. Nurse leaders must be familiar with the procedural steps and know when and how to apply them; this includes knowing the terms, causes, and violations that warrant the discipline process to be implemented

 3. The progressive discipline process involves:

  a. Counseling

  b. A reprimand, either verbally or in writing

Box 8-4	1. To prepare and conduct a coaching session:
Tools for Coaching, Disciplining, and Terminating Staff	

1. To prepare and conduct a coaching session:
   a. Note the behavior and why it is unacceptable.
   b. Explore reasons for the behavior with the employee.
   c. Ask the employee for suggestions to solve the problem.
   d. Arrange for follow-up.
2. To conduct a discipline session:
   a. Be certain you are calm before beginning.
   b. Assure privacy before beginning.
   c. Apply rules consistently.
   d. Get both sides of a story.
   e. Keep the focus on the problem, not the person.
   f. Arrange for follow-up.
   g. Inform the human resources department and administration.
3. To prepare to terminate a staff member:
   a. Inform the human resources department and administration beforehand.
   b. State the offending behavior and the reason for termination.
   c. Explain the termination process.
   d. Remain calm.
   e. Arrange for employee to be escorted out.
   f. Report back to the human resources department and administration.

Source: Sullivan, E. J. & Decker, P. J. (2005). *Effective leadership and management in nursing* (6th ed.). Upper Saddle River, NJ: Pearson Prentice Hall, p. 289. Reprinted by permission.

▶ *Practice to Pass*

Discuss ways in which the nurse leader can help nursing staff to improve their performance over time.

   c. Suspension
   d. A set of agreed-upon terms to return to work
   e. Termination, if necessary

VII. OTHER WORKFORCE ISSUES IMPACTING QUALITY CARE: ABSENTEEISM AND TURNOVER

A. *Absenteeism:* the absentee rate is known as the time in which staff miss work on an unplanned basis; unscheduled absences often result in:
   1. Disruptions in work assignments for co-workers
   2. Rushed and sometimes poor quality client care
   3. Increased costs related to overtime or use of agency personnel
   4. Working shorthanded
B. **Employee attendance barriers**
   1. There are times when employees face unique challenges to their ability to attend to work; however, any absence that is unplanned and occurs on an ongoing basis may turn into a barrier

2. The nurse leader must address attendance barriers as they arise before they turn into a chronic problem

3. Attendance barriers often include:

   a. The job itself, including performance issues

   b. Organizational practices or policies that are not enforced

   c. An absence culture where absenteeism is not addressed

   d. Supervision that is inconsistent or lacking

   e. Labor market forces

   f. Personal characteristics where attendance is not valued

C. **Increase the desire and motivation to attend work by ensuring:**

   1. The job itself remains interesting, challenging, and fulfilling

   2. Organizational policies and procedures reward those who come to work

   3. A culture of "what does it mean to be absent?" is understood

   4. Staff member's attitudes, values, and goals are understood and match job expectations and job responsibilities

   5. That job-related stressors are attended to

   6. That advancement opportunities are encouraged and promoted

   7. That the issue of absenteeism is addressed sooner rather than later

Practice to Pass

Describe at least two ways that a nurse leader can solve the issue of absenteeism on the nursing unit.

D. **Managing an absentee employee:** nurse leaders must recognize that managing an absentee employee requires:

   1. Knowing the organizational policies on absenteeism

   2. Identifying the absence patterns or cycles of absenteeism

   3. Examining the motivation of individual staff member

E. **Turnover and its impact**

   1. High turnover rates for the health organization are costly; the nurse leader must attend to the reasons for turnover and seek to reduce the causes

   2. One method used to uncover such reasons is through a termination interview:

      a. Ask staff why they have chosen to leave voluntarily

      b. If the nurse leader has had an open and professional relationship with the staff member, he or she is more likely to undercover the true reasons for the termination

   3. Frequent causes of termination include:

      a. Inadequate compensation (wages)

      b. Inadequate benefits

      c. Scheduling conflicts or issues

      d. Lack of promotion or advancement opportunities

      e. Inadequate staff-nurse leader communication and staff-to-staff communication

      f. Unsafe working conditions

      g. Inadequate or lack of nursing leadership support or supervision

      h. Personal reasons unrelated to work: spouse transferred, to be married, illness or death in family, personal illness, personal injury, pregnancy

F. **Reducing unit turnover:** to address the issue of turnover and reduce a nursing unit's turnover rate, the nurse leader must first understand why it exists; since the best

Box 8-5	1. Recognize when turnover is voluntary or involuntary and when it is functional or dysfunctional.
Tools for Reducing Turnover, Retaining Staff	2. Assess the reasons for voluntary, dysfunctional turnover.
	3. Plan strategies individually and collectively to address voluntary, dysfunctional turnover, realizing the problem may be systemwide and beyond your control.

Source: Sullivan, E. J. & Decker, P. J. (2005). *Effective leadership and management in nursing* (6th ed.). Upper Saddle River, NJ: Pearson Prentice Hall, p. 310. Reprinted by permission.

approach to reducing turnover is to prevent it from occurring, nurse leaders can use the following strategies (see Box 8-5):

1. Build a culture of client safety and clinical excellence through appropriate staffing levels and effective hiring procedures
2. Provide for career advancement opportunities
3. Encourage effective communication and problem solving
4. Manage conflict as it arises
5. Provide for ongoing staff development and training
6. Promote trust, commitment, and meaningful work
7. Allow staff to have control over their practice environment
8. Foster teambuilding and relationships among the staff

G. **Creating a nurturing and supportive workplace**

1. The nurse leader is responsible for detecting, preventing, and correcting problems that negatively affect client care, staff morale, and welfare
2. The unit climate and culture is the responsibility of the nurse leader
3. A nurturing and supportive work environment results in lower turnover rates

Case Study

As the nurse manager of a 12-bed intensive care unit (ICU), you notice that a staff nurse is not using appropriate hand hygiene between clients when giving morning care.

1. What is the first step that you should take in confronting the staff nurse about a policy violation?

2. How would you assist the staff nurse to realize the unwanted behavior has consequences for client?

3. Identify and discuss the most important guideline in disciplining this employee.

4. Discuss why the goal of the nurse manager is to encourage the correct behavior.

5. Describe the key skills, behaviors, and communication approaches to supervising and disciplining this staff member.

For suggested answers, see pages 237–238.

POSTTEST

1 The newly hired nurse manager assesses that one of the staff nurses on the nursing unit is an expert practitioner after observing the nurse's expertise in which of the following areas?

1. Competency in the helping role
2. Work role competencies
3. Ability to monitor interventions
4. Ability to make medical diagnoses

2 A nurse manager overhears a nurse state during interdisciplinary rounds, "After learning he has an inoperable brain tumor, the client wishes to terminate dialysis for his renal failure. Since he has no family, I think we should consider his wishes." The nurse manager concludes that the nurse is functioning in which role at this time?

1. Clinical practitioner
2. Case manager
3. Client advocate
4. Staff educator

3 Which strategy would be best for the nurse to use to be an effective client advocate?

1. Maintain knowledge of standards and regulations about client rights.
2. Listen to the healthcare experiences of clients from different cultures.
3. Learn to speak different languages to facilitate communication.
4. Openly discuss cultural differences with clients and the staff.

4 The nurse leader who is a unit manager would take which action with a staff nurse who has one year of experience to best assist this nurse with performance improvement?

1. Review the original orientation documentation for any gaps.
2. Document and review with the nurse any errors or client complaints.
3. Review the original job description and point out areas of strength and weakness.
4. Collaboratively develop behavioral objectives with target dates for reevaluation.

5 A nurse leader needs to notify staff registered nurses (RNs) about a change in the staff RN position description. Which method should the nurse leader use to communicate the change?

1. Announce the change in a staff meeting.
2. Post a notice on the bulletin board in the nurses' lounge.
3. Speak to each nurse individually.
4. Provide notification and a copy of the changes in writing.

6 The nurse leader evaluates the staff nurse's performance by narrating a detailed description of the nurse's performance after making a decision to use which of the following types of performance evaluation tool?

1. Essay evaluation
2. Traditional rating scale
3. Forced distribution
4. Behavior orientation scale

7 Which strategy should the nurse leader use to facilitate the performance appraisal conference?

1. Refrain from adding comments to the evaluation form.
2. Include personal feelings in the comments section of the tool for clarity.
3. Begin the evaluation interview with an open-ended question.
4. Interview other staff about the employee's performance before meeting with the employee.

8 A nurse manager overrates a staff nurse on the performance evaluation. The chief nurse officer counsels the manager about which type of performance evaluation error?

1. Ambiguous
2. Recency
3. Leniency
4. Halo

9 The nurse is assigned to work for the shift with a nursing student. In planning to work with this student, the nurse who uses Benner's model of nursing practice anticipates that the student is at which stage of practice?

1. Pre-novice
2. Novice
3. Beginner
4. Advanced beginner

10 A novice nurse leader prepares to conduct a performance appraisal interview. How should this leader prepare? Select all that apply.

1. Remain calm and receptive toward goal setting.
2. Be prepared to reject the staff's comments.
3. Define positive and negative performance.
4. Allow the staff to select the time and place of the evaluation.
5. Set the stage for the interview.

➤ *See pages 174–176 for Answers and Rationales.*

ANSWERS & RATIONALES

Pretest

1 **Answers: 2, 5** The major goals of staff development include creating an environment that supports learning. Staff development also creates opportunities to learn new skills to improve competence. Although staff development programs may provide socialization opportunities, they are primarily learning opportunities. Option 3 in essence is correct, but the word "undesired behavior" implies the goal is to make staff change negative behavior, and this is not the goal of staff development. Investigation of errors is not a function of staff development. **Cognitive Level:** Comprehension **Client Need:** Safe Effective Care Environment: Management of Care **Integrated Process:** Nursing Process: Planning **Content Area:** Leadership/Management **Strategy:** Choose options that focus on learning. Options 2 and 5 include learning opportunities. Option 1 is incorrect because it implies the purpose of staff development is to increase socialization. Options 3 and 4 are incorrect because they presuppose staff members are inept. Identify best practice options to select the correct response. **Reference:** Finkelman, A. W. (2006). *Leadership and management in nursing.* Upper Saddle River, NJ: Pearson Education, pp. 397–399.

2 **Answer: 1** Staff development gives nurses opportunities to improve technical skills such as venipunctures and central venous access line care. Staff development is not a time for personal development (option 2). Staff development does not provide an outlet for nurses to discuss

their concerns about client care issues (option 3). In-house staff development does not provide for as much opportunity for networking as programs conducted outside the employee's organization, but this would be a secondary gain rather than a primary purpose. **Cognitive Level:** Application **Client Need:** Safe Effective Care Environment: Management of Care **Integrated Process:** Nursing Process: Planning **Content Area:** Leadership/Management **Strategy:** Eliminate distracters that do not focus on education. Option 3 is incorrect because it focuses on forums, which is not the purpose of staff development. While networking is a by-product of staff development, it is not the purpose of staff development. The purpose of staff development is to provide knowledge or information needed for development of necessary skills. Identify best practices in staff development to select the correct answer. **Reference:** Finkelman, A. W. (2006). *Leadership and management in nursing.* Upper Saddle River, NJ: Pearson Education, pp. 399–400.

3 **Answer: 4** The best strategy is to develop a list of planned events for staff, setup the activities with the individuals in charge of providing the education, and schedule the activities at various times convenient for all shifts to get better compliance from the staff. Not all staff may need to attend each activity (option 1). Option 2 uses the term *aggressively*, which gives a negative connotation, and option 3 may or may not meet the actual needs of staff. Instead, programs should be planned according to needs assessment results determined by unit staff, manager, or the staff development department. **Cognitive Level:** Application **Client Need:** Safe Effective Care Environment: Management of Care **Integrated Process:** Nursing Process: Implementation **Content Area:** Leadership/Management **Strategy:** Eliminate option 1 based on the use of a very general term, *all.* Option 2 is incorrect because aggressiveness is not a useful strategy. To eliminate option 3, consider that managers may not always be in the best position to be aware of the total staff development needs of the aggregate nurses in a healthcare institution. Use nursing knowledge and the process of elimination to make the correct selection. **Reference:** Finkelman, A. W. (2006). *Leadership and management in nursing.* Upper Saddle River, NJ: Pearson Education, pp. 389–392.

4 Answers: 2, 3, 4, 5 Orientation should provide information about current policies, procedures, role expectations, and employee benefits. Rules should be written, and if there are unwritten expectations regarding behavior, these are not learned at orientation. **Cognitive Level:** Application **Client Need:** Safe Effective Care Environment: Management of Care **Integrated Process:** Nursing Process: Planning **Content Area:** Leadership/Management **Strategy:** Evaluate each option and consider whether it is part of a formal orientation program for a healthcare facility. Consider that unwritten rules are ascertained over time from other members of the staff and that the other options are part of orientation. **Reference:** Finkelman, A. W. (2006). *Leadership and management in nursing.* Upper Saddle River, NJ: Pearson Education, pp. 355–356, 399–400.

5 Answer: 2 The most effective strategy is an in-service, which gives the nurses an opportunity to handle the pumps and ask questions. During orientation, nurses are educated on the use of the pumps, but this question asks specifically about educating the current staff about the new pumps. Web-enhanced instruction and user manuals are helpful for ancillary information but a hands-on approach works best for learning to operate equipment. **Cognitive Level:** Application **Client Need:** Safe Effective Care Environment: Management of Care **Integrated Process:** Nursing Process: Planning **Content Area:** Leadership/Management **Strategy:** Option 1 is a newer form of education; however, for the use of an IV pump it is not the ideal form of education. Orientation should be used in conjunction with other forms of education. A manual is used as a reference. An in-service includes an orientation and directions; it is more comprehensive than the other options. Identify best practices in staff development to select the correct answer. **Reference:** Finkelman, A. W. (2006). *Leadership and management*

in nursing. Upper Saddle River, NJ: Pearson Education, p. 399.

6 Answer: 3 Many states require practicing nurses to fulfill a predetermined number of continuing education hours to ensure safe practice and current knowledge of standards of care. Refresher courses are a specific type of continuing education intended for nurses who have not been in practice for some years. Virtual instruction is a newer method of delivery of information. Orientation assists a nurse to learn about the requirements and role for a specific nursing position. **Cognitive Level:** Comprehension **Client Need:** Safe Effective Care Environment: Management of Care **Integrated Process:** Nursing Process: Analysis **Content Area:** Leadership/Management **Strategy:** The question specifically asks about methods for obtaining the number of hours for verification of practice competency. Virtual instruction is a delivery method for education, but this option does not answer the question. Orientation is related to a specific nursing position. Recall that refresher courses fall under the genre of continuing education to eliminate this option. Then recall that option 3, continuing education, is the term used to ensure practice competency. **Reference:** Finkelman, A. W. (2006). *Leadership and management in nursing.* Upper Saddle River, NJ: Pearson Education, pp. 392–393.

7 Answer: 2 The leader should show proficiency in providing and articulating the vision of the unit and/or facility and the strategic plan. While the leader should know the nursing process and technological devices, these areas are needed most by staff nurses. The leader needs to demonstrate capability in managerial attributes and characteristics, not instructional technology. **Cognitive Level:** Application **Client Need:** Safe Effective Care Environment: Management of Care **Integrated Process:** Nursing Process: Planning **Content Area:** Leadership/Management **Strategy:** Analyze each option and eliminate first those options that apply to staff nurses. Consider that staff nurses are required to show competence in technological devices or the nursing process to eliminate options 3 and 4. Next, determine that staff development personnel should be proficient in delivery methods for education to eliminate option 1. Alternatively, realize that leaders must be able to share the vision of the organization and provide or develop a strategic plan. Identify best practice options to select the correct response. **Reference:** Sullivan, E. J., & Decker, P. (2005). *Effective leadership and management in nursing* (6th Ed.). Upper Saddle River, NJ: Pearson Education, pp. 26–27.

8 Answer: 1 Bedside nurses should be knowledgeable in using the nursing process to problem solve and note subtle changes in clients' conditions. The staff nurse does not need to show competency in financial management, but the nurse manager should have this capability. Nurses are provided with benefits, but the management of benefits that are under employee control is a personal matter and is not considered on an employment evaluation. The bedside nurse does not need to provide a vision; the nurse needs to understand the vision for the unit.

Cognitive Level: Comprehension **Client Need:** Safe Effective Care Environment: Management of Care **Integrated Process:** Nursing Process: Evaluation **Content Area:** Leadership/Management **Strategy:** Evaluate the competency identified in each option and determine the agency position to which it applies. Eliminate options 2 and 4 first, which are necessary for a nurse leader. Next, eliminate option 3, which is not evaluated in yearly performance assessments. Identify best practices in staff development to select the correct answer. **Reference:** Finkelman, A. W. (2006). *Leadership and management in nursing.* Upper Saddle River, NJ: Pearson Education, pp. 404–405.

9 **Answer: 4** A halo error occurs because of an appraiser's inability to recognize the differences among ratings in various areas. This information is not transcribed onto the evaluation, making the employee appear the same in every category with no variations of higher and lower ratings. Ambiguous errors denote vague evaluations. Recency errors occur when the employer evaluates the employee based on the most recent occurrence. Leniency implies the employer overrates the employee.

Cognitive Level: Comprehension **Client Need:** Safe Effective Care Environment: Management of Care **Integrated Process:** Nursing Process: Evaluation **Content Area:** Leadership/Management **Strategy:** Identify critical words in the question or stem such as *same* and *halo* to select the right answer. Look for an option that includes a lack of variation, option 4. **Reference:** Sullivan, E. J., & Decker, P. (2005). *Effective leadership and management in nursing* (6th ed.). Upper Saddle River, NJ: Pearson Education, pp. 279–284.

10 **Answer: 3** The nurse's years of nursing service have added intuitive insight into the care of clients. This expert nurse is able to recognize and adjust when the client's condition changes, demonstrates highly skilled intuitive and analytic ability in new situations, and takes action because "it feels right." The term *advanced practitioner* (option 2) is not part of Benner's model. A competent practitioner (option 4) demonstrates organizational and planning abilities and can differentiate more important from less important aspects of care. This level usually takes at least three years to achieve. The proficient practitioner (option 1) generally has

three to five years experience working with a client population that has similar characteristics, perceives situations as a whole rather than in parts, and uses maxims as guides for what to consider in a situation.

Cognitive Level: Application **Client Need:** Safe Effective Care Environment: Management of Care **Integrated Process:** Nursing Process: Analysis **Content Area:** Leadership/Management **Strategy:** Specific knowledge of the various stages of Benner's model is needed to answer the question. Consider the definitions at each level and choose the one that best matches the scenario in the stem of the question. **Reference:** Blais, K. K., Hayes, J. S., & Kozier, B. (2005). *Professional nursing practice: Concepts and perspectives* (5th ed.). Upper Saddle River, NJ: Pearson Education, pp. 21–22, 104–105.

Posttest

1 **Answer: 2** The expert practitioner is Benner's highest ranking practitioner who has matured into an individual who is intimate with work role competencies. Abilities in the helping role (option 1) and monitoring interventions (option 3) are characteristic of practitioners at lower levels in Benner's model. Determining medical diagnoses (option 4) is within the scope of medical practice, not nursing.

Cognitive Level: Application **Client Need:** Safe Effective Care Environment: Management of Care **Integrated Process:** Nursing Process: Evaluation **Content Area:** Leadership/Management **Strategy:** Identify critical words in the question such as *expert* and *expertise* to select the right answer. Recall that the helping role is the domain of the novice nurse. Next, recall that the advanced beginner focuses on observation of interventions and the proficient nurse is better able to hone in on problems. **Reference:** Blais, K. K., Hayes, J. S., & Kozier, B. (2005). *Professional nursing practice: Concepts and perspectives* (5th ed.). Upper Saddle River, NJ: Pearson Education, pp. 21–22, 104–105.

2 **Answer: 3** A nurse is a client's advocate when acting on the client's behalf to further the wishes of the client. This supports the ethical principle of autonomy for the client. The clinical practitioner role involves a wide range of assessments, care activities, and teaching that the nurse would engage in. The case manager would be involved in coordinating care across healthcare settings. A staff educator would provide new clinical information to staff, orientation to new hires, or provide in-services on new products and equipment.

Cognitive Level: Application **Client Need:** Safe Effective Care Environment: Management of Care **Integrated Process:** Nursing Process: Evaluation **Content Area:** Leadership/Management **Strategy:** Consider the content of the nurse's communication and note that the nurse is trying to further the client's wishes. Compare this interpretation to each of the options and use the process of elimination to make the correct selection, keeping in mind the various roles of the nurse. **Reference:** Finkelman, A. W. (2006). *Leadership and management in nursing.* Upper Saddle River, NJ: Pearson Education, pp. 329–330.

3 **Answer: 1** The nurse should accumulate a working knowledge of regulations and standards about client rights that should be applied to practice. The strategies outlined in options 2, 3, and 4 may be helpful in delivering culturally competent care.
Cognitive Level: Application **Client Need:** Safe Effective Care Environment: Management of Care **Integrated Process:** Nursing Process: Planning **Content Area:** Leadership/Management **Strategy:** The critical words in the question are *client advocate.* With this in mind, consider that the correct option is one that focuses on client rights. Note that the incorrect options focus on culturally sensitive or competent care to choose correctly. **Reference:** Finkelman, A. W. (2006). *Leadership and management in nursing.* Upper Saddle River, NJ: Pearson Education, pp. 329–330.

4 **Answer: 4** A nurse leader's role in performance improvement includes helping staff members improve overall job performance. This is accomplished best by assisting the staff member to identify areas of unsatisfactory performance and develop a plan for improvement. Reviewing the original job description to point out areas of weakness (option 3) is only a starting point but is not the best answer. Gaps in orientation (option 1) should be identified and corrected before orientation is completed. Performance improvement is not focused on merely identifying negative behavior (options 2 and 3).
Cognitive Level: Application **Client Need:** Safe Effective Care Environment: Management of Care **Integrated Process:** Communication and Documentation **Content Area:** Leadership/Management **Strategy:** Choose an option that addresses staff improvement. First, eliminate option 1 because of the timeframe. Next, eliminate options 2 and 3 because they are similar in that they identify negative aspects of performance but do not carry it a step further to improvement. Identify best practices in staff development to select the correct answer. **Reference:** Finkelman, A. W. (2006). *Leadership and management in nursing.* Upper Saddle River, NJ: Pearson Education, pp. 391–392.

5 **Answer: 4** If changes are made in a position description, the staff needs to be notified in writing. The position description contains performance standards against which an employee's job performance will be evaluated. Announcing the change at a staff meeting (option 1) and posting a notice (option 2) does not guarantee that

every nurse will be aware of the change. Speaking to each nurse individually (option 3) is not time efficient and does not provide documentation of notification.
Cognitive Level: Application **Client Need:** Safe Effective Care Environment: Management of Care **Integrated Process:** Communication and Documentation **Content Area:** Leadership/Management **Strategy:** The core issue of the question is knowledge of how to properly communicate important changes related to the work role. Consider that there needs to be evidence of notification to eliminate each of the incorrect options systematically. **Reference:** Finkelman, A. W. (2006). *Leadership and management in nursing.* Upper Saddle River, NJ: Pearson Education, p. 358.

6 **Answer: 1** A written narrative about a staff member's work performance characterizes the essay evaluation. It should include the entire evaluation period and describe both positive and negative behavior. Scales (options 2 and 4) are not narratives. A forced distribution (option 3) is also a rating system.
Cognitive Level: Application **Client Need:** Safe Effective Care Environment: Management of Care **Integrated Process:** Nursing Process: Evaluation **Content Area:** Leadership/Management **Strategy:** Note the connection between the word *narrative* in the question and the word *essay* in the correct option. Look for an option that includes a written, narrative form of evaluation. Essay evaluation includes a narration of the employee's performance. Scales do not include narration and recall forced distribution is a rating system. **Reference:** Sullivan, E. J., & Decker, P. (2005). *Effective leadership and management in nursing* (6th ed.). Upper Saddle River, NJ: Pearson Education, p. 281.

7 **Answer: 3** The performance appraisal interview is best started with an open-ended question, which draws the employee into conversation and thus into the process. Comments should be added to the evaluation form (option 1) for detail and clarity. Personal feelings (option 2) have no part in the process; rather, facts and behaviors should be included. Interviewing other staff (option 4) might be helpful in some instances, but inaccurate information could also be obtained, thus invalidating the accuracy of the data.
Cognitive Level: Application **Client Need:** Safe Effective Care Environment: Management of Care **Integrated Process:** Communication and Documentation **Content Area:** Leadership/Management **Strategy:** Focus on the critical word *facilitate* in the question. This tells you that the correct option is one that will ensure that the performance evaluation interview is completely accurately and maintains good relations between the nurse leader and employee. Use general nursing knowledge and the process of elimination to make a selection. **References:**

Sullivan, E. J., & Decker, P. (2005). *Effective leadership and management in nursing* (6th ed.). Upper Saddle River, NJ: Pearson Education, pp. 288–289; Finkelman, A. W. (2006). *Leadership and management in nursing.* Upper Saddle River, NJ: Pearson Education, p. 362.

8 **Answer: 3** An overrated appraisal of an employee characterizes leniency errors. This type of error can occur more frequently when the appraiser does not include the entire evaluation period. The term *ambiguous* means open to interpretation or unclear. *Recency* refers to an event that happened in the recent past. A halo error occurs when one aspect of the employee's performance affects the entire performance evaluation. **Cognitive Level:** Comprehension **Client Need:** Safe Effective Care Environment: Management of Care **Integrated Process:** Nursing Process: Evaluation **Content Area:** Leadership/Management **Strategy:** Identify the critical word *overrate* in the question to select the right answer. The option that fits with an overrater is leniency. The stem of the question does not include data to support the other options. **Reference:** Sullivan, E. J., & Decker, P. (2005). *Effective leadership and management in nursing* (6th ed.). Upper Saddle River, NJ: Pearson Education, pp. 281–284.

9 **Answer: 2** The nursing student is a novice with limited "hands-on" experience and critical thinking skills as applied to client care situations. The advanced beginner is different from the novice by way of more experienced decision making and acquisition of skills. The pre-novice and beginner are not part of Benner's model. **Cognitive Level:** Application **Client Need:** Safe Effective Care Environment: Management of Care **Integrated**

Process: Nursing Process: Evaluation **Content Area:** Leadership/Management **Strategy:** Specific knowledge of Benner's stages of development is needed to answer the question. Recall the definitions of each stage and use the process of elimination to select the correct answer. **Reference:** Finkelman, A. W. (2006). *Leadership and management in nursing.* Upper Saddle River, NJ: Pearson Education, pp. 382–400.

10 **Answers: 1, 3, 5** The appraiser should maintain calmness and reception toward goal setting. The appraiser should define both negative and positive behaviors, set the stage for the interview, and practice if necessary. The manager should not allow the employee to select the time and place. The employee may delay this interview for fear it may not go well. The appraiser should be open to comments from the employee. **Cognitive Level:** Application **Client Need:** Safe Effective Care Environment: Management of Care **Integrated Process:** Nursing Process: Evaluation **Content Area:** Leadership/Management **Strategy:** Choose options that are true and show the outcome of the appraisal interview in a positive light. Rule out option 2; it is a fallacy. Option 4 does not give clear and precise direction to the employee. The other options are true statements. **Reference:** Sullivan, E. J., & Decker, P. (2005). *Effective leadership and management in nursing* (6th ed.). Upper Saddle River, NJ: Pearson Education, pp. 288–290; Finkelman, A. W. (2006). *Leadership and management in nursing.* Upper Saddle River, NJ: Pearson Education, pp. 361–364.

References

Barker, A. M., Sullivan, D. T., & Emery, M. J. (2006). *Leadership competencies for clinical managers.* Sudbury, MA: Jones and Bartlett Publishers.

Benner, P. A. (1984). *Novice to expert.* Menlo Park, CA: Addison-Wesley.

Blais, K. K., Hayes, J. S., & Kozier, B. (2005). *Professional nursing practice: Concepts and perspectives* (5th ed.). Upper Saddle River, NJ: Pearson Education.

Creasia, J. L., & Parker, B. J. (2007). *Conceptual foundations: The bridge to professional nursing practice.* St. Louis, MO: Mosby.

Dessler, G. (2004). *Management: Principles and practices for tomorrow's leaders* (3rd ed.). Upper Saddle River, NJ: Prentice Hall.

Feuer, L. (2003). The management challenge: Making the best of your next performance appraisal. *Case Manager, 14*(15), 22–24.

Finkelman, A. W. (2006). *Leadership and management in nursing.* Upper Saddle River, NJ: Pearson Education.

Gelinas, L., & Bohen, C. (2002). Designing work for optimal care promotes patient safety and staff satisfaction. *Clinical Systems Management, 4*(7), 13–15.

Kerfoot, K. (2004). Building confident organizations by filling buckets, building infrastructures, and shining the flashlight. *Nursing Economic$, 22*(6), 333–335.

Roussel, L. (2006). *Management and leadership for nurse adminstrators* (4th ed.). Sudbury, MA: Jones and Bartlett Publishers.

Sullivan, E. J., & Decker, P. J. (2005). *Effective leadership and management in nursing* (6th ed.). Upper Saddle River, NJ: Pearson Education.

Yoder-Wise, P. S. (2007). *Leading and managing in nursing* (4th ed.). St. Louis, MO: Mosby.

Resource Management in Healthcare: Organizing and Managing Human/Fiscal Responsibilities

9

Chapter Outline

Resource Management
Healthcare Finance
Healthcare Funding
Types of Budgets
Budget Process
Cost Categories

Resource Allocation
Staffing
Scheduling
Nursing Informatics
Health Insurance Portability and Accountability
  Act (HIPAA)

Objectives

➤ Explain the role of the nurse leader in resource management.
➤ Explain how healthcare is financed and funded.
➤ Describe the budgeting process.
➤ Explain the various types of budgets.
➤ Identify cost categories.
➤ Describe how staffing requirements are determined.
➤ Explain the factors to consider when scheduling staff.
➤ Define nursing informatics.
➤ Describe the nurse's role in complying with the Health Insurance Portability and Accountability Act.

NCLEX-RN® Test Prep

Use the CD-ROM enclosed with this book to access additional practice opportunities.

Review at a Glance

average daily census average number of clients cared for per day of reporting period

benefit paid time vacation, holidays, and sick days for which there is no work output

budget detailed fiscal plan for carrying out organizational mission and goals

budget process planning and controlling future operations by comparing actual results with planned expectations

capital expenditure budget equipment and renovations needed by an organization to meet long-term goals

cash budget covers monthly receipts and expenses of a department and/or organization

computerized patient record (CPR) electronic version of the client's medical record

diagnostic related groups (DRGs) a prospective payment system used by Medicare to determine payment rates for hospital services, which are categorized into 495 case types

direct costs expenses that directly affect client care

electronic medical record (EMR) a computer-based client record that features electronic data processes

electronic medication administration record an electronic format of centralized information pertaining to client medication administration

fixed costs expenses that remain same for a budget period regardless of activity level of the organization

full-time equivalent (FTE) a position that can be equated to 40 hours of work per week for 52 weeks a year, or 2,080 hours per year

Health Insurance Portability and Accountability Act (HIPAA) a federal law that mandates a centralized database and assurance of public confidentiality about a client's healthcare

health management information system the hardware and software necessary to process data into information for multiple uses

indirect costs expenditures that do not affect client care directly

informatics use of knowledge technology

information competencies integration of knowledge, skills, and attitudes in performance of various nursing activities that involve data

information technology use of computer hardware and software to process data into information to solve problems

managed care a healthcare system that combines financing and delivery of health services into single entity

nonproductive hours benefitted time, either vacation or sick time

nursing informatics specialty that integrates nursing, computer science, and information technology to manage and communicate data, information, and knowledge in nursing

operating budget organization's statement of expected revenue and expenses for the upcoming year

personnel budget allocates budget expenses related to nursing personnel

prospective payment system (PPS) pay scale to compensate hospitals and other providers for Medicare or other government funded healthcare services; Medicare pays a fixed amount for covered client's procedure or service regardless of actual amount incurred by provider; system is designed to encourage providers to deliver services in a cost-effective manner

scheduling ongoing responsibility of assigning nursing personnel to specified time and location of duties

staffing placement of qualified human resources into budgeted positions for care delivery

telehealth telecommunications and information technologies for healthcare to clients at distance and transmission of information provided for care; uses two-way interactive video-conferencing, high-speed phone lines, fiber-optic cable, and/or satellite transmission

third-party payers financial intermediaries, such as insurance companies, that pay providers for services and collect premiums

variable costs expenses that depend on and change in direct proportion to client volume and acuity

PRETEST

1 Which resource is best used to foster an atmosphere of professional growth in staff?

1. Electronic medical record
2. Information technology
3. Resource management
4. Resource allocation

2 A nurse manager would draw on knowledge in which of the following areas to balance human and fiscal resources in fulfilling role responsibilities? Select all that apply.

1. Healthcare financing
2. Government resources
3. Consumer demographics
4. Nursing process
5. Adaptive equipment

3 Healthcare demand determines which services and/or products customers want and will pay for. Which of the following is the healthcare industry's ability to produce or provide the services and products?

1. Insurance
2. Reimbursement
3. Efficiency
4. Supply

4 Which of the following is an example of a third-party payer?

1. Centers for Medicare and Medicaid Services (CMS)
2. Cigna Insurance Company
3. Medicaid
4. Medicare

5 The nurse leader expects that under the managed care system:

1. Some clients "fall through the cracks" created by the system.
2. Clients may not receive the necessary care to prevent the onset of illnesses.
3. Healthcare providers must document reasons for extended length of stay.
4. Healthcare providers might not be able to order the necessary treatments for clients.

6 The nurse leader is aware that which of the following are internal factors that impact staffing? Select all that apply.

1. Client acuity
2. State regulations
3. Availability of staff
4. Accreditation standards
5. Level of competence

7 A director of a radiology department plans to include a positive emission radiological device in the budget; the cost of this equipment is $150,000. To which budget should the director add this piece of equipment?

1. Personnel budget
2. Capital budget
3. Cash budget
4. Operating budget

8 A nurse manager prepares to work on the budget for the next fiscal year. What should the manager do first?

1. Implement the current budget.
2. Develop a draft budget.
3. Plan for the needs of the unit.
4. Evaluate any deficits or excesses from the previous year's budget.

9 A nurse manager has collected data for the budget, developed a plan, and allocated monies to priorities. Which step should the nurse manager take next?

1. Implement the approved budget.
2. Develop a secondary or backup budget if the proposed budget is denied.
3. Plan for the subsequent year's budget.
4. Evaluate the current budget.

10 The nurse manager who is managing fiscal resources would consider which of the following to be a variable cost?

1. Lease
2. Medications
3. Electricity
4. Telephone service

➤ *See pages 196–197 for Answers and Rationales.*

I. RESOURCE MANAGEMENT

A. The nurse leader is responsible for facilitating a climate that provides professional growth to support allocation and use of human resources by:

1. Encouraging critical thinking

2. Providing opportunities for ongoing educational programs

3. Promoting new ideas and projects through staff development and training

B. As a resource manager, the nurse leader must seek to balance human and fiscal resources against escalating healthcare costs; using resources wisely while controlling rising labor costs requires knowledge of:

1. Healthcare finance and funding

2. Access to care

3. Governmental action

4. The aging population

5. Increasing incidence of life-threatening disease

6. Integrated systems of care, which:

    a. Deliver care across the health illness continuum

    b. Provide geographic coverage

    c. Accept risk

II. HEALTHCARE FINANCE

A. Economics focuses on how consumers, business firms, government entities, and other organizations make choices in an environment of scarce resources

B. Healthcare economics: a specialty area of economics that analyzes how different parts of the healthcare system work together to deliver services that meet the needs of clients

C. Demand, in health care, refers to the varying amount of care that a consumer is willing and able to purchase depending on possible prices

D. Supply of healthcare service refers to the ability of providers to deliver healthcare

E. In a provider-driven system the location of services, types of providers, and technology available are controlled by dominant providers such as physicians and hospitals

F. In a market-driven system, the provider's level of education and location and types of services provided are determined by the needs and location of consumers rather than those of providers

G. *Third-party payers* are insurance companies and government agencies that provide insurance coverage; they are financial intermediaries that pay providers for services and collect premiums from enrolled clients

H. A fee-for-service payment system gives providers maximum control of services provided to consumer; preapproval for services is usually not required in this system

I. The *prospective payment system (PPS)* has emerged in response to concerns about access to healthcare and spiraling healthcare costs

1. It is a pay scale to compensate hospitals and other providers for Medicare or other government-funded healthcare services

2. Medicare pays a fixed amount for covered client's procedure or service regardless of actual amount incurred by provider

3. The system is designed to encourage providers to deliver services in a cost-effective manner

III. HEALTHCARE FUNDING

A. ***Managed care*** **is defined as a healthcare system that combines financing and delivery of health services into a single entity; the healthcare system is willing to be held accountable for both clinical and financial outcomes of the enrolled population**

1. Managed-care organizations: entities that arrange for provision of services for a group of clients enrolled in the health plan

2. Managed care has changed the healthcare delivery system:

    a. Total expenditures on healthcare have drastically increased over recent decades, consuming greater and greater portions of the nation's resources; this is primarily the result of hospitalization costs and prescription drug expenses

    b. Managed care is an attempt to control healthcare costs

    c. Managed care has health promotion and prevention, not illness treatment, as the primary goal

3. Types of managed care organizations:

    a. Health Maintenance Organization (HMO): provides healthcare services for a predetermined fixed fee per covered person

    b. Preferred Provider Organization (PPO): contracts with independent healthcare practitioners to provide services for covered persons at a reduced rate

    c. Point-of-Service Organization (POS): covered clients choose to receive services within defined network or may go outside network and pay higher fee

    d. Physician Hospital Organization (PHO): a corporation formed between hospital and physicians for purpose of joint contracting with managed-care organizations

4. Refer back to Chapter 1 for additional information about managed care

B. **Causes of healthcare cost escalation**

1. Inflation: healthcare inflation has escalated at a faster rate than inflation in other segments of economy

2. Demographic changes: there are more elderly people who use a disproportionately high level of healthcare services due to chronic illnesses and the aging process itself

3. An estimated 47 million uninsured population does not seek primary and preventive care; they do not seek care until acuity is high and then they seek care at emergency departments, which is the least cost-effective type of care

4. Medicare and Medicaid: insure the elderly and poor and introduced more consumers into the system, thereby increasing the demand for healthcare services

5. Third-party payment: by health insurance companies, causes price insensitivity, increased demand, and cost escalation

6. New, expensive technologies and drugs: require investment of research and development dollars, which are then passed on to the client

7. Fraud and abuse of payment systems: particularly Medicare and Medicaid upcoding (charging for higher levels of care than given) have helped to account for upwardly spiraling costs

C. Cost-containment efforts and impact on nursing practice

1. Previously when healthcare costs rose, employers looked to the personnel budget for cost savings; they substituted less well-educated caregivers, such as licensed practical/vocational nurses (LPNs/LVNs) or unlicensed assistive personnel (UAPs), for registered nurses and increased nurse-client ratios

2. Managed care has offered opportunities for nurses to function as case managers; nurses are uniquely qualified to fill this role because of their education, holistic view of clients, organizational and communication skills, and information and referral skills

3. Advanced practice nurses have moved into roles as primary caregivers in many settings; this is more cost-effective than physician care and the care provided for routine acute and chronic health problems promotes positive client outcomes

4. Cost containment has also caused stress on nurses

   a. Hospitalized clients are sicker and have shorter lengths of hospital stay than in the past

   b. They are discharged while still requiring skilled nursing care

   c. The home health industry has capitalized upon this trend and more nurses are employed outside hospitals than ever before

D. Impact of managed care on cost containment and healthcare consumers

1. During the 1990s the rapid growth of HMOs and related managed-care organizations raised concerns that quality of care might suffer; care decisions (formerly based on client needs) were increasingly influenced by business interests; managed-care plans set stricter limits than other health insurance plans on types of services covered; this drove the development of care paths

2. In 1996 a serious development became known about managed-care efforts to regulate physicians who advised their clients about treatment options; some plans offered physicians bonuses for limiting services and referrals for clients; such bonuses placed physicians in conflict between best interest of clients and their own economic best interests; these practices evoked concern by organized medical groups, organized nursing groups, consumer groups, and the U.S. Congress

3. Laws were passed to protect clients, but there remains intense interest in decreasing costs, sometimes to the detriment of client care

4. Nurses must speak out when cost control initiatives create a situation in which they cannot provide quality nursing care; economic forces and philosophical shifts experienced today are encouraging nurses to demonstrate their contributions to client outcomes

5. Health report cards are being used to summarize information about physician and hospital performance and cost-effectiveness measures are being used to determine whether the prescribed treatment has accomplished desired outcome at the lowest possible cost

6. Consumer satisfaction studies have been designed for consumers/clients and healthcare buyers

7. In spite of cost containment, healthcare costs continue to rise faster than any other segment of the nation's economy and more Americans than ever (nearly 47 million) are uninsured

IV. TYPES OF BUDGETS

A. Nurse leaders are responsible for fiscal/financial planning; includes knowing how to balance revenues and expenses during a projected period of time for all areas of their budget

B. By using various types of budgets, the nurse leader can formulate a fiscal plan to allocate fiscal resources

    1. Personnel budget: allocates budget expenses related to nursing personnel

        a. Type of expenses include salary, vacation, holidays, education, unemployment, social security, and retirement benefits

        b. When planning for the personnel budget, the nurse leader forecasts the number of staff needed to provide nursing care for a specific timeframe; for example, 24 hours a day, 365 days per year for an acute care hospital

    2. Operating budget:

        a. Budget contains expense items such as medical and nonmedical supplies, small equipment, utilities, and equipment maintenance

        b. Projected revenues are also included in the operating budget

        c. Sources of revenue include payment from private payers, government (Medicare/Medicaid), and other insurance streams; other sources are income from rent, interest, and sale of equipment or property

    3. Cash budget: covers monthly receipts and expenses to department and/or organization; is considered an important component of the organization's operations

    4. Fixed asset or **capital expenditure budget**: a long-range budget (3 to 5 years)

        a. A capital budget includes planned acquisitions of all items or projects that have a useful life of longer than one year and a purchase price greater than a pre-established amount

        b. Many healthcare organizations set an amount of $1,500 to $2,500 to determine which items will be assigned to a capital budget

        c. Items costing less than the amount set to qualify as a capital asset are assigned to a noncapital budget or to the supply budget

        d. Major capital items are considered to be equipment, inventory, furniture, or space renovation/design

        e. This budget is planned for long term, but is prepared annually

        f. It is prioritized and monitored closely; these items are considered to be assets that will depreciate over time

V. BUDGET PROCESS

A. Requires the nurse leader to be responsible for developing and monitoring budget

    1. Budget: a document that reflects the operational goals and objectives of the organization; within the context of the entire organizational operation are individual costs centers (the smallest areas of activity within an organization for which costs accumulatc)

    2. As a unit or department (such as surgical intensive care unit or nursing department), each cost center has an individualized budget that is part of the organization's overall budget

Box 9-1	1. Understand the budgeting process in your organization.
Tools for Budgeting and Managing Resources	2. Determine the number of full-time equivalents necessary to staff the unit.
	3. Compute the salary and nonsalary budget, including salary increases and various additional factors.
	4. Monitor variances over the budget period and identify negative variances, responding promptly as appropriate.
	5. Understand that factors out of your control, such as changes in technology or indirect or direct costs that may be assigned to your budget, affect your budget and its performance.
	6. Encourage staff to monitor resource use, including time and supplies.

Source: Sullivan, E. J. & Decker, P. J. (2005). *Effective leadership and management in nursing* (6th ed.). Upper Saddle River, NJ: Pearson Education, p. 181. Reprinted by permission.

Practice to Pass

Explain the nurse leader's role and responsibility in the budgetary process for his or her assigned unit.

B. Three phases of the budget process:
   1. Planning
      a. Gather information based on organizational or unit goals and objectives
      b. Set priorities
      c. Perform an environmental assessment
      d. Identify financial objectives
   2. Development
      a. Collect and analyze data from previous budgets
      b. Allocate dollar amounts based on organizational/unit priorities
      c. Approve operational and capital budgets
   3. Implementation
      a. Analyze variances and adjust for changes through fiscal year
      b. Negotiate and revise budget as needed
      c. Allocate unit/departmental and cash budgets
      d. Evaluate
      e. Obtain performance reports and analyze efficiency
C. See Box 9-1 for tools that are helpful in budgeting and managing resources

VI. COST CATEGORIES

A. *Fixed costs*
   1. Not affected by volume (typically the number of clients served)
   2. Costs that remain constant
B. *Variable costs*
   1. Affected by changes in volume
   2. An increase in volume of client admissions increases the number of items needed to care for clients—for example, type and number of supplies, medications, and possible staff costs
C. Controllable costs are those costs that a nurse leader can regulate or control
D. Uncontrollable costs are costs that a nurse leader cannot regulate or control—for example, a nurse leader cannot control indirect costs allocated to the cost center, but he or she can control the costs of personnel and supplies

E. ***Direct costs*** are associated with a specific service or product (doctor visit or medication)

F. ***Indirect costs*** cannot be associated with a specific service or product

VII. RESOURCE ALLOCATION

A. Enhances and preserves the quality of client services

B. Productivity represents the ratio of outputs (products and services) to inputs (resources consumed)

    1. Input factors

        a. Staff characteristics (including experience, interpersonal communication styles, time management, and variable or fixed staffing)

        b. Client age and acuity

        c. Extent of treatment setting

        d. Unit layout

        e. Supplies

        f. Management structure

    2. Output factors

        a. Client satisfaction

        b. Medical records

        c. Acuity

C. Productivity must be reviewed over time and requires evaluation of budget, client acuity system, staffing levels, client satisfaction, and continuous quality improvement

    1. Healthcare organizations must demonstrate productivity and measure effectiveness and efficiency of services

    2. Effectiveness measures the ways an organization is achieving its stated objectives; objectives can be measured by:

        a. Evaluation of nursing care provided

        b. Quality improvement data

        c. Performance appraisal

        d. External reviews from Joint Commission on Accreditation of Health Care Organization (JCAHO)

D. Nurse leaders can impact unit productivity by:

    1. Coaching staff on unit goals and client safety

    2. Mentoring and role modeling quality objectives and measures

    3. Providing clear expectations and directions to meet unit productivity measures

E. ***Average daily census*** provides for a key measure of the unit's activity or productivity and provides a measure to project the workload of the unit

    1. Is a measure of the average number of clients cared for in budgeted beds on the unit over a period of time

    2. Formula for calculating average daily census:

$$\frac{\text{Client days for given period of time}}{\text{Number of days in time period}}$$

Example: 600 client days in January $= 600/31 =$ ADC of 19.3

VIII. *STAFFING*

A. Allows for hiring and deployment of human resources to meet the needs of client care; key functions of the nurse leader for coordinating staffing responsibilities include:

1. Follow structure, goals, and standards of the organization
2. Fulfill staffing requirements according to job specifications
3. Ensure that job descriptions fit requirements and role responsibilities of staff member
4. Provide appropriate numbers and mix of nursing staff
5. Establish staffing needs based on daily client acuities, budgeted nursing hours of care, yearly targets, and projected volumes
6. Use personnel budget to balance staffing plan and unit schedule
7. Monitor, evaluate, and modify annual staffing plan

B. The staffing process is driven by factors internal and external to the organization; the nurse leader will use personnel budget allocations to determine the staffing plan and unit schedule

1. Internal factors:
   a. Volume of services required
   b. Complexity and intensity of care
   c. Availability of staff
   d. Skill level and credentials/qualifications of nursing personnel
2. External factors:
   a. State licensing standards: recommendations of minimum number of professional nurses required on a unit at a given time
   b. JCAHO and other regulatory agency standards: recommend that organizations provide an adequate number and mix of staff consistent with their staffing plans
   c. Staff mix: skill level and ratio of individuals providing professional services for client care
3. Nurse leader must consider the unit census and acuity of clients
   a. Census: number of clients admitted to nursing unit for service
   b. Census and severity of client illness: complexity of those services allows the nurse leader to allocate an appropriate skill mix
   c. Effectiveness of staffing models and staffing ratios are evaluated according to 2005 JCAHO Standards using two clinical/service indicators with two human resources indicators selected according to clinical focus of the designated unit (see Box 9-2 for full list of possible clinical/service indicators and human resource indicators)
   d. The American Nurses Association (ANA) *Principles for Safe Staffing* provide guidance and support for nurse leaders to consider when making their unit staffing plans in relation to budget requirements
   e. Studies show a correlation between RN staffing levels and quality client care outcomes, including decreasing length of stay, and fewer postoperative infections and hospital-acquired complications

C. Staffing levels: plans focused on the level of care needed to ensure a safe environment; in the acute care setting, staffing is required for 24 hours/7 days per week coverage

1. Staffing pattern: number of persons in each job classification on duty per shift per day

Box 9-2	Clinical/Service Indicators	Human Resource Indicators
Staffing Effectiveness Indicators	Length of stay	Staff satisfaction
	Client complaints	Staff turnover rate
	Family complaints	Staff vacancy rate
	Injuries to client	Understaffing
	Client falls	Nursing care hours per day
	Adverse drug events	Sick time
	Postoperative infections	On the job staff injuries
	Pneumonia	Use of on call or temporary personnel
	Skin breakdown	
	Urinary infection	
	Shock/cardiac arrest	
	Upper gastrointestinal bleed	

2. Calculate the staffing pattern on the following three components:
   a. Client care requirements and staffing hours per client day
   b. Unit characteristics
   c. For inpatient settings
      1) Number of beds
      2) Average daily census
      3) Occupancy rate
      4) Type and classification of unit
      5) Census fluctuation
      6) Unit architecture
      7) Availability of technology
   d. For outpatient clinic settings
      1) Number of clients
      2) Number of visits per client
      3) Average level and length of visit
      4) Number of exam/treatment rooms
      5) Hours of operation
      6) Availability of technology
3. Characteristics of staff:
   a. Staff expertise and level of competency and experience
   b. Education and preparation of licensed and unlicensed staff
   c. Length of time on assigned unit
   d. Skill mix or licensed and unlicensed staff'
   e. Type of delivery system (primary, team, functional, or client)

D. Client classification systems
   1. Method of grouping clients according to the amount and complexity of nursing care required; client classification systems also use a standard unit of measure for productivity
      a. Several types of systems in market

  b. Determine nursing care hours

  c. Determine full time equivalents (FTEs)

  d. Determine staff mix

  e. Determine distribution of staff

  f. Determine staffing and scheduling

2. Nurse leaders can use a formal client classification system to aid in determining client need based on defined criteria, which can then be used to allocate staff and provide care

3. At the unit level, acuity data is essential in preparing month-end justification for variances in staff utilization

4. At the organization level acuity data can be used to cost out nursing services for a specific client population and global client types

5. Acuity data is also used in preparation of nursing staffing budget for the upcoming fiscal year

6. Client classifications systems: tools for describing client acuity for a designated unit; provide information about:

  a. Status of client acuity; sicker clients obtain higher classifications scores, thus revealing the need for more nursing care

  b. Needed adjustments in unit staffing plan for given time period

  c. Acuity trends over time that can be applied to staffing need projections in the annual budget

7. Types of client classification systems

  a. Prototype evaluation classifies client care on the **diagnostic related group (DRG)** prospective payment system used by Medicare to determine payment rates for hospital services, which are categorized into 495 case types

   1) Descriptive and subjective data

   2) Broad categories for client classification

   3) Uses client categories to predict client need

   4) Advantage: reduction of work for nurse by not classifying clients daily

   5) Disadvantages: no ongoing measure of actual nursing work required by individual clients; no ongoing data to monitor accuracy of pre-assigned nursing care requirements

  b. Factor systems evaluation classifies client care into different interventions for each client using the Nursing Intervention Classification (NIC)

   1) Objective data

   2) Rates client care tasks and activities

   3) Rating results help determine number of direct care hours needed for each client

   4) Uses units of measure that equate to nursing time

   5) Attempts to capture assessment, planning, intervention, and evaluation of client outcomes along with written documentation processes

   6) Most popular type of classification system

   7) Advantages:

    a) Data are readily available for day-to-day operations

    b) Provide information against which one can justify changes in staffing requirements

8) Disadvantages:

    a) Create ongoing workload for nurse in classifying clients every day

    b) Do not capture client needs for psychosocial, environmental, and health management support

    c) Calculate nursing time based on "typical" nurse

E. Standard formula for calculating nursing care hours

    1. After a healthcare organization determines the client classification system, the number of nursing care hours can be determined for each classification

    2. Nursing care hours (NCH) per client (patient) day (PPD) is the number of nursing care hours worked in 24 hours divided by client census:

$$\text{NCH} = \frac{\text{Nursing hours worked in 24 hours}}{\text{Client census}}$$

Example: Client census = 20 as divided below

    a. Number of nursing care hours needed for each acuity level and number of clients is:

        Category 1 = 2.3 hours, 8 clients

        Category 2 = 3.0 hours, 4 clients

        Category 3 = 4.2 hours, 4 clients

        Category 4 = 5.1 hours, 4 clients

    b. Calculate number of nursing care hours per client; multiply each category (acuity level) by the number of clients in each category:

        Category 1 = 2.3 hours × 8 clients = 18.4

        Category 2 = 3.0 hours × 4 clients = 12

        Category 3 = 4.2 hours × 4 clients = 16.8

        Category 4 = 5.1 hours × 4 clients = 20.4

    c. Add all hours from four categories together

        Example: 18.4 + 12 + 16.8 + 20.4 = 67.6

    d. Divide the total number of nursing care hours (67.6) by the number of clients receiving care (20); equals 3.38 hours per client per day

$$\text{Example:} \frac{67.6 \ (\text{nursing care hours})}{20 \ (\text{client census})} = 3.38$$

    3. The nurse leader is responsible for knowing the budgeted hours per client per day; calculating the number of nursing care hours required for any given day allows the nurse leader to determine unit staffing needs and thus helps the nurse leader to avoid understaffing or overstaffing the unit

F. Unit staffing and determining FTEs

    1. Full-time equivalent (FTE): a full-time position that can be equated to 40 hours of work per week for 52 weeks a year, or 2,080 hours per year

        To calculate FTEs, divide the number of hours worked per week by 40 hours:

$$\frac{16 \ \text{hours/week}}{40 \ \text{hours}} = 0.4 \ \text{FTE}$$

An employee working two 12-hour shifts per week:

$$\frac{12 \ \text{hours/shift} \times 2 \ \text{shifts}}{40 \ \text{hours}} = 0.6 \ \text{FTE}$$

2. One FTE equals 80 hours in 2-week pay period
3. To determine number of FTEs required to staff unit for 24 hours a day the nurse leader would require the following information:
   a. Hours of work for staff for 2-week period
   b. Average daily census
   c. Hours of care
   d. Average nursing care hours
4. Formula:

$$\frac{\text{Average nursing care hours} \times \text{days in staffing period} \times \text{average client census}}{\text{Hours of work per FTE in 2 weeks}}$$

G. Benefit time/nonproductive time

1. Once the number of FTEs is determined, the nurse leader can then calculate replacement personnel needed for **benefit paid time** (**nonproductive time**), which is paid time for which there is no work output
2. Calculate hours of replacement time by determining:

Benefit Time	Hours/Shift	Replacement Hours
20 average number of vacation days	× 8 hours	= 160
10 paid holidays	× 8 hours	= 80
4 personal days	× 8 hours	= 32
8 sick days	× 8 hours	= 64
	Total	**336**

3. Determine FTE requirement:

$$\text{Divide replacement time by hours per year:} \frac{336}{2080} = .16$$

H. Determining staffing mix

1. Skill mix: know the type of staff required to provide care (RN, LPN, and UAP)
2. Identify type of care required and who is qualified to provide that care
3. Assess staff competency to fulfill the nursing care needs of clients
4. Be sure to adhere to nurse practice act and other state regulations when making staffing decisions
5. Distribute staff according to when staff is needed for peak hour care: days vs. evenings, or nights, weekends and holidays
6. Use the staffing model to meet client needs during high workload times, maximize the use of nursing personnel and satisfy staff's work needs and requests

I. Staffing models

1. Fixed staffing: specified by a projected workload requirement; uses a standard hourly shift schedule, 8-hour or 12-hour schedule
2. Flex-time: variation in scheduled hours, such as four 10-hour shifts per week, three 12-hour shifts per week, weekends only

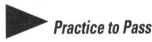

Practice to Pass

Describe how nurse leaders design and determine appropriate skill mix on their assigned units.

3. Rotating/alternating: a varied schedule of one type of shift within single work period and a different shift within another work period (such as an alternating days and evening pattern)

4. Block/cyclic: the same schedule is repeated over a specified period of time

IX. *SCHEDULING*

A. Nurse leaders are responsible for scheduling staff and ensuring that appropriate nursing personnel are on hand to care for clients

B. There are several issues to consider in scheduling staff:

1. Client need:

   a. Measured by the client classification system used by the healthcare organization

   b. Staffing patterns adjust for client acuity and support providing staff when needed

   c. It changes when the types of clients change, resulting in a change in staffing requirements

2. Volume:

   a. Client volume numbers reflect peaks and valleys in census and client acuity

   b. Scheduling adjusts as necessary

3. Experience and capability of staff:

   a. Different degrees of knowledge, experience, and critical thinking skills are required to care for clients

   b. Number of inexperienced staff (adds hours)

   c. Number of experienced staff

   d. Need for staff with special skills

C. Scheduling methods

1. A centralized scheduling method is one that is completed by nursing service or the nursing office for an entire healthcare organization

2. A decentralized method is one that is completed by a nursing division or unit of the healthcare organization

3. Self-scheduling allows nursing staff to develop and create criteria for staffing the unit or division; it requires nursing staff to accept full responsibility for their schedule, including:

   a. Having staff collectively decide and implement monthly work

   b. Agreeing upon a scheduling protocol

   c. Establishing role and responsibilities of scheduling committee members

   d. Establishing general boundaries

   e. Educating unit staff in development of self-scheduling process

   f. Ensuring staff is committed to providing safe staffing on all shifts

D. Factors impacting staffing

1. Shift variations:

   a. 8-, 10-, or 12-hour shifts

   b. Weekend rotation programs

1) Possible disruption of continuity of care

2) Weekend staff should be familiar with clients and recent care events

3) Financial implications

4) Weekend programs are more expensive than traditional staffing patterns

5) Can be used as a recruitment and retention tool

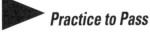

Practice to Pass

Describe the ways nurse leaders can familiarize themselves with learning how to staff and schedule nursing personnel on their units.

2. Number of part-time staff

3. Approved benefit time for preapproved schedule

4. Approved time for continuing education programs, seminars, or orientation

5. Staff vacancies and filled positions

E. See Box 9-3 for a summary of strategies for handling staffing and scheduling

X. NURSING INFORMATICS

A. A growing specialty that combines clinical knowledge and skills with informatics expertise; integrates nursing science, computer science, and information science to manage and communicate data, information, and knowledge in nursing practice

1. Informatics: use of knowledge technology

2. Information technology: use of computer hardware and software to process data

3. Goal: to improve health of populations, communities, families, and individuals by optimizing information management and communication

4. Is a specialty represented by several professional associations, supported by advanced education, and credentialed through certification

5. Primary interest: to expand how data, information, and knowledge are used within nursing practice; **electronic medical record (EMR):** a computer-based client record that features electronic data processes; **electronic medication administration record**: an electronic format of centralized information pertaining to client medication administration

6. Telehealth: telecommunications and information technologies for healthcare to clients at a distance and transmission of information provided for care; involves use of two-way interactive video-conferencing, high-speed phone lines, fiber-optic cable and/or satellite transmission

7. Information competencies: integration of knowledge, skills, and attitudes in performance of various nursing activities that involve data

8. Health management information systems: hardware and software necessary to process data into information for multiple uses; few systems can address every

---

Box 9-3	**1.** Familiarize yourself with the current patient classification or acuity system in use.
Strategies for Handling Staffing and Scheduling	**2.** Determine the nursing care hours needed.
	3. Determine FTEs needed.
	4. Create or modify a schedule that best meets your patients' needs.
	5. Supplement staff as needed.
	6. Consider self-staffing if appropriate.

Source: Sullivan, E. J. & Decker, P. J. (2005). *Effective leadership and management in nursing* (6th ed.). Upper Saddle River, NJ: Pearson Education, p. 239. Reprinted by permission.

Box 9-4	
Tools for Using Healthcare Technology Systems	**1.** Become familiar with the clinical information system used in your facility.
	2. Take advantage of every opportunity to update and upgrade your skills to use technology.
	3. Keep up to date on clinical research in your field; your patients surely are.
	4. Maintain strict adherence to privacy standards and regulations.
	5. Welcome the future of technology.

Source: Sullivan, E. J. & Decker, P. J. (2005). *Effective leadership and management in nursing* (6th ed.). Upper Saddle River, NJ: Pearson Education, pp. 200–201. Reprinted by permission.

component of healthcare, so generally there is an overriding information system, which includes clinical and administrative components

> ***Practice to Pass***
>
> Explain the nurse leader's role and responsibilities regarding nursing informatics and technology.

9. In practice, nurses use computers most commonly for documentation of client care and to access client data; the **computerized patient record (CPR)** is an electronic version of the client record; see Box 9-4 for tips to staff nurses on using healthcare technology systems

10. The diversity of informatics projects and programs has led to tremendous professional career and interdisciplinary opportunities

XI. HEALTH INSURANCE PORTABILITY AND ACCOUNTABILITY ACT (HIPAA)

A. **This act is a federal law that mandates a centralized database and assurance of public confidentiality about each client's healthcare**

1. Enacted by Congress in 1996 to ensure any individual who changed jobs or stopped working did not automatically lose employer-provided health insurance

2. The HIPAA privacy rule ensures that individuals' health information is protected while allowing flow of information needed to provide good care; protected information includes information placed in medical record, conversations between physician and nurse about client, personal information in health insurer's computer system, and billing information

3. The privacy rule applies to covered entities that transmit health information electronically

4. Covered entities are nurses and others employed by hospitals, clinics, and physicians' offices, as well as insurance companies and medical-billing or data-collection companies

B. **Most states have privacy laws; however, the HIPAA privacy rules (2003) mandate healthcare providers are to follow medical privacy laws that are most stringent; in some cases, state law will supersede HIPAA requirements; disclosures related to treatment do not require client authorization**

C. **Exempt from disclosure authorization are certain public records and reports, including births, deaths, and communicable disease incidence and exposure**

D. **Authorization is not required if other federal, state, tribal, or local laws mandate disclosure**

E. **Clients can request reporting of most disclosures but those made to facilities for treatment, billing, or other healthcare operations are excluded**

Table 9-1	Violation	Preventive Measures
Typical HIPAA Violations	1. Faxing or mailing medical records to the wrong hospital department or to someone with no connection to the client	1. Preprogram numbers on fax machine and verify number prior to pressing send button
	2. Incorrect client data	2. Verify client's full name, birth date, and address
	3. Inaccurate address	3. Ensure the address is complete and correct on the envelope
	4. Incomplete name and title	4. Put full name and title with appropriate department on the outside of all interoffice mail

F. Clients are entitled to know about disclosures to state cancer registries, vital statistics agencies, public health agencies, and child welfare authorities even though some of these agencies do not require authorization

G. HIPAA law requires healthcare institutions to record complaints and actions taken to address and prevent violations

H. Inappropriate use or disclosure of client personal health information occurs when given to people who do not need it to do their jobs or should not have it at all (see Table 9-1)

I. Healthcare providers should be careful not to inadvertently disclose client medical information; the following steps must be taken to prevent disclosure of personal health information:

1. Refrain from speaking in public about clients

2. Shred discarded documents rather than placing them in a trash bin

3. Prevent unauthorized access to personal health information by refusing to share computer or voice-mail passwords

4. Do not leave medical records unattended

5. Log off computer when data entry is completed so as not to display a client's personal health information

J. Violation in HIPAA laws may result in civil fines of up to $25,000/year for each requirement or prohibition violated; $50,000 to $100,000 and 1 to 5 years in prison for offenses committed under false pretenses; criminal penalties of up to 10 years in prison and $250,000 in fines for offenses with intent to sell, transfer, or use protected health information for commercial use advantage, personal gain, or malicious harm

▶ *Practice to Pass*

What action would you take if you witnessed confidential client information being released without the client's consent?

Case Study

You have recently accepted a position as the nurse manager of a new 25-bed unit for clients with psychiatric disorders. As part of your role, you are responsible for unit staffing and the allocation of full time equivalencies (FTEs) of the nursing positions on the unit.

1. What process would you use to determine the appropriate number and type of healthcare personnel needed to care for clients on this unit?

2. Explain how you would determine the number, acuity, and type of clients that will be admitted to this unit.

3. On what regulatory requirements and unit requirements would you base the staffing needs?

4. As the newly appointed nurse manager, you are concerned about appropriate staffing levels on your unit. What would you do?

5. Discuss how regulatory agencies such as the Joint Commission on Accreditation of Healthcare Organizations (JCAHO) address the issue of staffing effectiveness in an organization.

For suggested responses, see page 238.

POSTTEST

1 The nurse manager considers that which of the following items represents an output factor of resource allocation?

1. Staff experience
2. Supplies
3. Client age
4. Client satisfaction

2 A nurse overhears a nurse manager request information by telephone about the average daily census. The nurse is aware that the manager is most likely using this information to do which of the following?

1. Determine staff development and training.
2. Project the number of staff needed to work.
3. Calculate the types of client supplies needed.
4. Assist with electronic claims and reimbursement.

3 The nurse manager would include allocations for vacation time and sick time when preparing which type of budget?

1. Personnel budget
2. Operating budget
3. Cash budget
4. Capital expenditure budget

4 Which primary element should a nurse manager on a medical nursing unit use to calculate staffing patterns?

1. Client care requirements
2. Physician rounds
3. Number of outpatient surgeries
4. Vacation time

5 Clients are grouped by which of the following according to the complexity of their condition and the amount of care required by the nursing staff?

1. Third-party payers
2. Provider system
3. Classification systems
4. Staffing model

6 When determining the number of full time equivalents (FTEs) needed for the unit, the nurse manager should start with:

1. The number of hours of work for staff.
2. Client safety factors.
3. The time needed to account for staff breaks.
4. The currently used client classification system.

7 An acute care facility uses a nursing-centered classification system that focuses on the client care activities completed by nurses. A potential applicant for a nurse manager vacancy understands that which type of classification system is being utilized?

1. Managed care system
2. Prospective payment system
3. Nursing intervention classification system
4. Diagnostic related group (DRG)

8 A nurse manager needs to determine the staff mix for the unit. What should the manager do first?

1. Schedule staff to work when the needs are more critical.
2. Consider mandated staff ratios.
3. Identify staff competency to meet the needs of clients.
4. Assess the type of care required by the clients.

9 A nurse manager uses the same nurse staffing schedule over a period of two months and that pattern then repeats. Which staffing model does this represent?

1. Flex-time
2. Fixed staffing
3. Cyclic model
4. Rotating schedule

10 A nurse signs up to work two 10-hour shifts in one week, three 12-hour shifts in another week and two 8-hour shifts the following week. Which type of staffing schedule does this represent?

1. Cyclic schedule
2. Rotating schedule
3. Fixed schedule
4. Flex-time schedule

➤ *See page 197–199 for Answers and Rationales.*

ANSWERS & RATIONALES

Pretest

1 **Answer: 3** Resource management is a great resource for planning and providing educational opportunities, staff development, and training. Information technology may be used for professional growth, but must be done in conjunction with other activities. The other options do not apply.
Cognitive Level: Knowledge **Client Need:** Safe Effective Care Environment: Management of Care **Integrated Process:** Nursing Process: Analysis **Content Area:** Leadership/Management **Strategy:** Choose an option that addresses professional growth, which in this case is option 3. Electronic medical record and information technology do not match the description of professional growth. Resource allocation does not describe professional growth. **References:** Finkelman, A. W. (2006). *Leadership and management in nursing.* Upper Saddle River, NJ: Pearson Education, pp. 450–451; Sullivan, E. J., & Decker, P. (2005). *Effective leadership and management in nursing* (6th ed.). Upper Saddle River, NJ: Pearson Education, pp. 59–60.

2 **Answers: 1, 2, 3** A nurse manager needs knowledge about healthcare financing to manage budgets, government resources for funding and reimbursement, and consumer demographics to identify trends and types of future services that will be needed. Nursing process and use of adaptive equipment (options 4 and 5) are areas in which staff nurses should be knowledgeable.
Cognitive Level: Comprehension **Client Need:** Safe Effective Care Environment: Management of Care **Integrated Process:** Nursing Process: Planning **Content Area:** Leadership/Management **Strategy:** Note that options 4 and 5 do not require the use of human and fiscal responsibility. However, healthcare finance, government resources, and consumer demographics require the use of knowledge in human and fiscal resources. Apply principles of fiscal responsibility to select the correct answer. **References:** Finkelman, A. W. (2006). *Leadership and management in nursing.* Upper Saddle River, NJ: Pearson Education, pp. 450–451; Sullivan, E. J., & Decker, P. (2005). *Effective leadership and management in nursing* (6th ed.). Upper Saddle River, NJ: Pearson Education, pp. 59–60.

3 **Answer: 4** Demand determines the customer's willingness to buy goods and services, but supply is the industry's ability to meet the customer's demand for goods and services. Insurance companies determine the ser-

vices that will be reimbursed and the reimbursement rate. Efficiency is not a term used in relation to supply and demand.
Cognitive Level: Knowledge **Client Need:** Safe Effective Care Environment: Management of Care **Integrated Process:** Nursing Process: Analysis **Content Area:** Leadership/Management **Strategy:** Choose an option that fits the sentence. Demand and supply make sense in each part of the sentence. The other options do not balance with the term *demand* in the question. **Reference:** Finkelman, A. W. (2006). *Leadership and management in nursing.* Upper Saddle River, NJ: Pearson Education, pp. 450–453.

4 **Answer: 2** Cigna is a private insurance company that collects premiums from enrollees for coverage. Third-party payers provide a variety of services, which depend on the type of coverage granted by the company. Medicare and Medicaid are part of the prospective payment system. CMS is the abbreviation for Centers for Medicare and Medicaid Services.
Cognitive Level: Knowledge **Client Need:** NA **Integrated Process:** NA **Content Area:** Leadership/Management **Strategy:** Note that option 1 refers to an organization that umbrellas options 3 and 4 and then also note that options 3 and 4 are not third-party payers. The only plausible choice is option 2. Identify the critical words *third party* in the stem of the question to select the correct option. **References:** Finkelman, A. W. (2006). *Leadership and management in nursing.* Upper Saddle River, NJ: Pearson Education, pp. 435–438; Sullivan, E. J., & Decker, P. (2005). *Effective leadership and management in nursing* (6th ed.). Upper Saddle River, NJ: Pearson Education, pp. 16–18.

5 **Answer: 3** A major goal of the managed care is to hold providers accountable for the treatments and diagnostic tests ordered in an effort to reduce the cost of healthcare spending. Options 1, 2, and 4 represent potential pitfalls in the healthcare system, regardless of structure; however, these are not "expected" results of this system.
Cognitive Level: Comprehension **Client Need:** Safe Effective Care Environment: Management of Care **Integrated Process:** Nursing Process: Analysis **Content Area:** Leadership/Management **Strategy:** Consider that options 1, 2, and 4 are not necessarily based on factual data; however, option 3 is based on requirements of insurance companies, so it is the best choice of all options. Note the critical word *expects* to help you look for an intended consequence. **References:** Finkelman, A. W. (2006). *Leadership and management in nursing.* Upper Saddle

River, NJ: Pearson Education, pp. 433–440; Sullivan, E. J., & Decker, P. (2005). *Effective leadership and management in nursing* (6th ed.). Upper Saddle River, NJ: Pearson Education, p. 18.

6 **Answers: 1, 3, 5** Options 1, 3, and 5 all represent internal factors (with the healthcare organization) that influence staffing. Options 2 and 4 are external factors (outside the organization) that impact staffing. **Cognitive Level:** Comprehension **Client Need:** Safe Effective Care Environment: Management of Care **Integrated Process:** Nursing Process: Analysis **Content Area:** Leadership/Management **Strategy:** Choose options that are internal factors and rule out external factors. Options 2 and 4 are external factors; rule them out. Option 1, 3, and 5 are internal factors. Apply knowledge of productivity and staffing to make the correct selections. **References:** Finkelman, A. W. (2006). *Leadership and management in nursing*. Upper Saddle River, NJ: Pearson Education, pp. 366–370; Sullivan, E. J., & Decker, P. (2005). *Effective leadership and management in nursing* (6th ed.). Upper Saddle River, NJ: Pearson Education, pp. 231–235.

7 **Answer: 2** The capital budget is long term and includes large items with sizable costs, such as a positive emission radiological device. The personnel budget includes expenses related to nursing personnel. Other items included in the personnel budget are vacation, benefits, salary, and holidays. A cash budget covers smaller items. The operating budget includes daily expenses such as medical supplies and equipment maintenance. **Cognitive Level:** Application **Client Need:** NA **Integrated Process:** Nursing Process: Planning **Content Area:** Leadership/Management **Strategy:** Due to the high cost of the equipment, the best option is capital budget. Apply knowledge of budget principles to select the correct answer. **References:** Finkelman, A. W. (2006). *Leadership and management in nursing*. Upper Saddle River, NJ: Pearson Education, p. 455; Sullivan, E. J., & Decker, P. (2005). *Effective leadership and management in nursing* (6th ed.). Upper Saddle River, NJ: Pearson Education, p. 178.

8 **Answer: 3** When preparing the budget, the manager should have some idea of the amount of financial resources that will be needed to cover expenses. The manager should start with the vision, mission, and goals, determine how the nursing unit works within them, then plan for the needs of the unit during the upcoming year. A draft budget would be developed after the planning stage. Implementing and evaluating the current budget are ongoing items that would not be complete before the next year's budget is due. **Cognitive Level:** Application **Client Need:** NA **Integrated Process:** Nursing Process: Planning **Content Area:** Lead-

ership/Management **Strategy:** Think about the nursing process. The first step is establishing goals for the unit. Budget development is the second step. The third step is implementation. Finally, the nurse must evaluate the budget plan. Note that this question addresses the upcoming year's budget to realize that implementation and evaluation of the current budget could not be completed in their entirety before the next budget needs to be submitted for approval. **Reference:** Sullivan, E. J., & Decker, P. (2005). *Effective leadership and management in nursing* (6th ed.). Upper Saddle River, NJ: Pearson Education, pp. 172–175.

9 **Answer: 1** The manager has developed a plan, step one (planning) and has allocated monies to various priorities, step two (development). The next step is implementation. **Cognitive Level:** Application **Client Need:** NA **Integrated Process:** Nursing Process: Implementation **Content Area:** Leadership/Management **Strategy:** Identify the correct stage of the budget process. In this case, monies have been allocated, so it is time to implement the budget plan. Apply knowledge of budget principles to select the correct answer. **References:** Finkelman, A. W. (2006). *Leadership and management in nursing*. Upper Saddle River, NJ: Pearson Education, pp. 455–460; Sullivan, E. J., & Decker, P. (2005). *Effective leadership and management in nursing* (6th ed.). Upper Saddle River, NJ: Pearson Education, pp. 178–181.

10 **Answer: 2** Variable costs include items such as medications and supplies. Fixed costs include items that do not fluctuate such as the lease. Electricity and telephone service constitute indirect costs, which are not associated with a specific item, but are necessary for operation. **Cognitive Level:** Comprehension **Client Need:** NA **Integrated Process:** Nursing Process: Analysis **Content Area:** Leadership/Management **Strategy:** Note the definition of the term variable to mean an item that changes or can fluctuate. Then choose an option that is an example of a variable cost. Options 1, 3, and 4 are not variable costs. Use the process of elimination to make the correct selection. **References:** Finkelman, A. W. (2006). *Leadership and management in nursing*. Upper Saddle River, NJ: Pearson Education, pp. 455–460; Sullivan, E. J., & Decker, P. (2005). *Effective leadership and management in nursing* (6th ed.). Upper Saddle River, NJ: Pearson Education, pp. 178–180.

Posttest

1 **Answer: 4** Output factors include client satisfaction, client outcomes, and medical records. Staff experience (option 1), supplies (option 2), and client age (option 3) are input factors. **Cognitive Level:** Knowledge **Client Need:** NA **Integrated Process:** Nursing Process: Analysis **Content Area:**

Leadership/Management **Strategy:** Specific knowledge of input and output factors is needed to answer the question. Apply knowledge of staffing to make the correct selection. **References:** Finkelman, A. W. (2006). *Leadership and management in nursing.* Upper Saddle River, NJ: Pearson Education, pp. 326–329; Sullivan, E. J., & Decker, P. (2005). *Effective leadership and management in nursing* (6th ed.). Upper Saddle River, NJ: Pearson Education, pp. 183–185.

2 **Answer: 2** Managers use the average daily census to determine the number of nurses and nursing assistants needed on the unit. The census is not used to determine staff development and training (option 1), calculate amount of necessary client supplies (option 3), or assist with electronic claims or reimbursement (option 4). **Cognitive Level:** Application **Client Need:** NA **Integrated Process:** Nursing Process: Planning **Content Area:** Leadership/Management **Strategy:** The average daily census is not needed for staff development, so rule out option 1. The daily census does not impact client supplies and electronic claims; rule out options 3 and 4. Apply knowledge of staffing to make the correct selection. **Reference:** Finkelman, A. W. (2006). *Leadership and management in nursing.* Upper Saddle River, NJ: Pearson Education, pp. 374–377.

3 **Answer: 1** The personnel budget includes expenses related to nursing personnel. Other items included in the personnel budget are vacation, benefits, salary, and holidays. The budget's time frame typically includes a full year with nursing coverage 24 hours per day. A cash budget covers smaller items. The operating budget is focused on daily expenses such as medical supplies and equipment maintenance. The capital budget is planned long-term and includes large items with sizeable costs. **Cognitive Level:** Application **Client Need:** NA **Integrated Process:** Nursing Process: Planning **Content Area:** Leadership/Management **Strategy:** Apply knowledge of budget principles to select the correct answer. Note the correlation between personnel benefits such as vacation and sick time and the word personnel in the correct option. Also note that options 2, 3, and 4 are not typically included in the personnel budget. **References:** Finkelman, A. W. (2006). *Leadership and management in nursing.* Upper Saddle River, NJ: Pearson Education, pp. 455–456; Sullivan, E. J., & Decker, P. (2005). *Effective leadership and management in nursing* (6th ed.). Upper Saddle River, NJ: Pearson Education, pp. 175–177.

4 **Answer: 1** The critical element in calculating staffing patterns is client care requirements. Physician rounds and vacation time do not directly impact staffing patterns. This is a medical nursing unit. Outpatient surgeries are not typically admitted to medical floors, those

clients are discharged home. Should something occur and they need further medical attention, these clients are admitted to the surgical nursing unit. **Cognitive Level:** Application **Client Need:** NA **Integrated Process:** Nursing Process: Evaluation **Content Area:** Leadership/Management **Strategy:** Choose an option that directly impacts staffing patterns. Physician rounds may indirectly impact staffing patterns. Clients who have outpatient surgeries are discharged home. Staffing needs are influenced by vacation time, but staffing needs are most impacted by the types of clients who require care. Apply knowledge of productivity and staffing to make the correct selection. **References:** Finkelman, A. W. (2006). *Leadership and management in nursing.* Upper Saddle River, NJ: Pearson Education, pp. 467–471; Sullivan, E. J., & Decker, P. (2005). *Effective leadership and management in nursing* (6th ed.). Upper Saddle River, NJ: Pearson Education, pp. 231–236.

5 **Answer: 3** There are different types of classification systems; one of the oldest classification systems is the Diagnosis Related Groupings (DRGs), which was created by Medicare to determine reimbursement for healthcare organizations. **Cognitive Level:** Knowledge **Client Need:** NA **Integrated Process:** Nursing Process: Analysis **Content Area:** Leadership/Management **Strategy:** Option 3 is an umbrella of specific types of systems that group clients. Third-party payers or provider systems are not widely used as classification systems. Option 4 is not applicable. Apply knowledge of productivity and staffing to make the correct selection. **References:** Finkelman, A. W. (2006). *Leadership and management in nursing.* Upper Saddle River, NJ: Pearson Education, pp. 374–375; Sullivan, E. J., & Decker, P. (2005). *Effective leadership and management in nursing* (6th ed.). Upper Saddle River, NJ: Pearson Education, pp. 231–234.

6 **Answer: 1** When calculating FTEs, the unit manager should consider the number of FTEs per pay period. The other options, such as client safety, staff breaks, and client classification systems, do not impact the number of FTEs needed to staff for a 24-hour day. **Cognitive Level:** Application **Client Need:** NA **Integrated Process:** Nursing Process: Implementation **Content Area:** Leadership/Management **Strategy:** Select an option that impacts FTEs. Client safety, staff breaks, and classification systems do not influence FTE needs. Apply knowledge of staffing to make the correct selection. **References:** Finkelman, A. W. (2006). *Leadership and management in nursing.* Upper Saddle River, NJ: Pearson Education, pp. 267–268; Sullivan, E. J., & Decker, P. (2005). *Effective leadership and management in nursing* (6th ed.). Upper Saddle River, NJ: Pearson Education, pp. 234–235.

ANSWERS & RATIONALES

7 **Answer: 3** The nursing intervention classification system is devoted to interventions provided by nurses. It measures the time it takes to provide the care nurses give. Managed care and prospective payment systems are used to finance healthcare. A DRG is a label for a medical diagnosis that is used for billing in relation to healthcare services.
Cognitive Level: Application **Client Need:** NA **Integrated Process:** Nursing Process: Evaluation **Content Area:** Leadership/Management **Strategy:** Identify the critical words in the question, *nursing-centered classification system*. Choose an option that closely fits the critical words, *nursing intervention classification*. Eliminate each of the incorrect options after considering that each of them relates in some way to payment for healthcare services. **References:** Finkelman, A. W. (2006). *Leadership and management in nursing.* Upper Saddle River, NJ: Pearson Education, pp. 374–375; Sullivan, E. J., & Decker, P. (2005). *Effective leadership and management in nursing* (6th ed.). Upper Saddle River, NJ: Pearson Education, pp. 231–234.

8 **Answer: 4** From a nursing process approach, the manager should first assess the needs of the clients, which are determined by acuity, then assess the competency of staff. The nurse must now schedule staff according to regulated ratios dictated by the regulating bodies.
Cognitive Level: Application **Client Need:** NA **Integrated Process:** Nursing Process: Assessment **Content Area:** Leadership/Management **Strategy:** Think nursing process and start with assessment. Option 1 is premature. Option 2 is a function of regulating bodies. Option 3 does not apply to the scenario. **References:** Finkelman, A. W. (2006). *Leadership and management in nursing.* Upper Saddle River, NJ: Pearson Education, p. 375; Sullivan, E. J., & Decker, P. (2005). *Effective leadership and management in nursing* (6th ed.). Upper Saddle River, NJ: Pearson Education, pp. 235–236.

9 **Answer: 3** Rationale: The cyclic model is characterized by the same schedule that is repeated over a predetermined length of time. Flex-time (option 1) consists of shifts of varying lengths. Fixed staffing (option 2) utilizes a standard shift schedule, such as 8 hours or 12 hours. A rotating schedule (option 4) utilizes assignment to a single shift during any single week or a longer work period, and the shift assignment changes during another work period (such as a day and night shift rotation).
Cognitive Level: Knowledge **Client Need:** NA **Integrated Process:** Nursing Process: Analysis **Content Area:** Leadership/Management **Strategy:** Identify the critical words in the question, *same schedule over four months*. Choose the option that best describes these words, cyclic model. Options 1, 2, and 4 are staffing models, but they are not defined by the critical words. Apply knowledge of staffing to make the correct selection. **References:** Finkelman, A. W. (2006). *Leadership and management in nursing.* Upper Saddle River, NJ: Pearson Education, pp. 367–370; Sullivan, E. J., & Decker, P. (2005). *Effective leadership and management in nursing* (6th ed.). Upper Saddle River, NJ: Pearson Education, pp. 235–239.

10 **Answer: 4** The flex-time schedule allows for variation in scheduling time. The advantage of the flex schedule is the variation in the hours and days. The disadvantage is the lack of consistency in the days and hours worked. A cyclic schedule (option 1) is a pattern that is utilized over a period of weeks to months and then repeats. A rotating schedule (option 2) assign staff to different shifts during different weeks or pay periods. Such a position might be labeled "days with night rotation." A fixed schedule (option 3) uses a standard length of shift, such as 8-hour or 12-hour.
Cognitive Level: Knowledge **Client Need:** NA **Integrated Process:** Nursing Process: Analysis **Content Area:** Leadership/Management **Strategy:** From the stem, one can surmise there is flexibility in scheduling. Choose an option that includes flexibility in scheduling, flex-time. Cyclic, rotating, and fixed schedules are not characteristic of flex-time. Apply knowledge of staffing to make the correct selection. **References:** Finkelman, A. W. (2006). *Leadership and management in nursing.* Upper Saddle River, NJ: Pearson Education, pp. 366–368; Sullivan, E. J., & Decker, P. (2005). *Effective leadership and management in nursing* (6th ed.). Upper Saddle River, NJ: Pearson Education, pp. 235–239.

References

American Nurses Association. (2005). *Principles for nurse staffing.* Washington, DC: Author.

American Nurses Association. (2001). *Scope and standards of nursing informatics practice.* (Publication No. NIP21 3M 05/02). Washington, DC: Author.

Anderson, F. (2007). Finding HIPAA in your soup. *American Journal of Nursing, 107*(2), 66–71.

Bodeheimer, T., & Grumbach, K. (2005). *Understanding health policy: A clinical approach* (4th ed.). New York: McGraw-Hill.

Clarke, S. P. (2005). The policy implications of staffing-outcomes research. *Journal of Nursing Administration, 35*(1), 17–19.

Finkleman, A. (2006). *Leadership and management in nursing.* Upper Saddle River, NJ: Pearson Education.

ANSWERS & RATIONALES

Page, J. S. (2005). Nurse staffing and outcomes. Lessons learned: Safe scheduling practices for nursing staff. *Voice of Nursing Leadership, 3*(4), 4–5.

Rohloff, R. (2006). Full-time equivalents: What needs to be assessed to meet patient care and create realistic budgets. *Nurse Leader,* 49–54.

Sullivan, E. J., & Decker, P. J. (2005). *Effective leadership and management in nursing* (6th ed.). Upper Saddle River, NJ: Pearson Education.

Yoder-Wise, P. S. (2007). *Leading and managing in nursing* (4th ed.). St. Louis, MO: Mosby.

Nursing Leadership and Challenges in the 21st Century

10

Chapter Outline

Engaged and Empowered Nursing Leadership

Successfully Navigating Change

Critical Thinking: A Tool for the 21st Century Nurse Leader

Evidence-Based Leadership

Culture and Nursing Practice

Spirituality

Death and Dying

Objectives

➤ Identify the theories of change.

➤ Apply the stages of unfreezing, moving, and refreezing to a client situation for managed change.

➤ Describe the roles and characteristics of an effective change agent.

➤ Identify driving and restraining forces of change within a structured setting context.

➤ Define the term *critical thinking*.

➤ Explain the assumptions associated with critical thinking.

➤ Describe the judgments needed in clinical decision making.

➤ Discuss the role of evidenced-based leadership in nursing.

➤ Examine barriers to instituting evidence-based care.

➤ Explore the concepts of death, dying, and spirituality.

➤ Differentiate among spirituality, religion, and faith.

➤ Discuss the influences of spiritual beliefs on healing and health.

NCLEX-RN® Test Prep

Use the CD-ROM enclosed with this book to access additional practice opportunities.

Review at a Glance

change agents persons with formal or informal power whose responsibility it is to initiate, motivate, or champion the change

change process that involves creating something different than what once was; a complex process involving alteration, revision, or re-creation from an established pattern

change process series of continuous efforts applies to managing change

chaos theory theoretical construct of random-appearing, yet deterministic characteristics of complex organizations

culture a specific group of people defined by their behaviors, norms, belief sets, values, and folk laws

culturally competent care care that is sensitive to issues related to culture, race, gender, and sexual preference

cultural diversity the range of cultural differences that represent a set of beliefs or values

cultural sensitivity capacity to understand, feel, and react to the habits, customs, or traditions of other groups or individuals

driving force behaviors that facilitate change by encouraging individuals to move in the desired direction

ethnicity certain group of people whose identifiers include religious beliefs, country of origin, race, language, values, and meaningful traditions

ethnocentrism belief that one's own cultural ways are superior to others

evidence-based practice integrates the best of research evidence with clinical expertise and client values

moving developing new values, behaviors, and attitudes

planned change expected and deliberate change directed to achieve a desired outcome

refreezing instituting new supports, resources, and systems to secure and maintain a change

restraining forces behaviors that impede change by discouraging individuals from making specific changes

unfreezing reducing the forces pressing for the status quo

spirituality integration of beliefs in a higher power, an awareness of life and its meaning, the centering of a person with purpose in life, and meaningful relationships

PRETEST

1 In working to prepare nursing staff for changes that will soon be occurring on the nursing unit, the nurse leader is aware that change is a process that is which of the following?

1. Dynamic and fluid
2. Constant and predictable
3. Unavoidable and easy
4. Difficult and misleading

2 A nurse who wishes to complete a graduate degree in critical care to increase annual income is contemplating which of the following types of change?

1. Personal change
2. Professional change
3. Organizational change
4. Forceful change

3 A chief executive officer (CEO) plans major changes on the medical units. The CEO assigns the nurse leader as the implementer of the changes. The administration represents which of the following types of forces for change?

1. Driving force
2. Restraining force
3. Refreezing force
4. Unfreezing force

4 A nurse manager implements change on the unit. The manager observes the desired behavior in the staff. Which stage of Lewin's change process does the nurse manager observe?

1. Stagnation
2. Unfreezing
3. Moving
4. Refreezing

5 A nursing unit shows little time for orderly change and order comes in the form of rapid and unplanned fluctuations. The nurse leader understands that this unit experiences change that is best described by which change theory?

1. Lewin's change theory
2. Chaos theory
3. Havelock Model of Change
4. Rogers's Innovation-Diffusion process

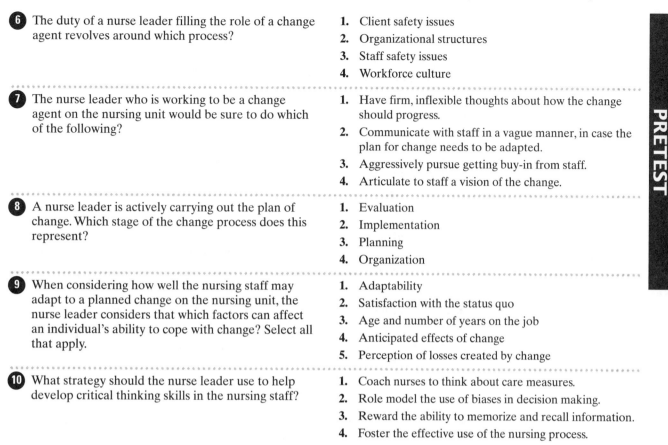

6 The duty of a nurse leader filling the role of a change agent revolves around which process?

1. Client safety issues
2. Organizational structures
3. Staff safety issues
4. Workforce culture

7 The nurse leader who is working to be a change agent on the nursing unit would be sure to do which of the following?

1. Have firm, inflexible thoughts about how the change should progress.
2. Communicate with staff in a vague manner, in case the plan for change needs to be adapted.
3. Aggressively pursue getting buy-in from staff.
4. Articulate to staff a vision of the change.

8 A nurse leader is actively carrying out the plan of change. Which stage of the change process does this represent?

1. Evaluation
2. Implementation
3. Planning
4. Organization

9 When considering how well the nursing staff may adapt to a planned change on the nursing unit, the nurse leader considers that which factors can affect an individual's ability to cope with change? Select all that apply.

1. Adaptability
2. Satisfaction with the status quo
3. Age and number of years on the job
4. Anticipated effects of change
5. Perception of losses created by change

10 What strategy should the nurse leader use to help develop critical thinking skills in the nursing staff?

1. Coach nurses to think about care measures.
2. Role model the use of biases in decision making.
3. Reward the ability to memorize and recall information.
4. Foster the effective use of the nursing process.

➤ *See page 224–226 for Answers and Rationales.*

I. ENGAGED AND EMPOWERED NURSING LEADERSHIP

A. Professional nursing must recruit and sustain a cadre of engaged, spirited, and involved leaders; nurse leaders must be ready to face unprecedented challenges and opportunities in the 21st century, including:

1. Recruiting

2. Retaining

3. Motivating frontline staff

4. Ensuring client safety

B. Engagement

1. Seeks to provide an optimistic culture where staff can feel hopeful and are free to grow and mature in their roles

2. Engaged nurse leaders know, recognize, and celebrate the unique strengths and interests of those around them

3. Engaged nurse leaders match the talents and strengths of their staff with their assigned work

4. Engaged nurse leaders create an atmosphere of attention to work, an ambiance of friendliness, pride in work, and are filled with energy and enthusiasm

C. **Empowerment**: each nurse leader has the opportunity to empower and cultivate transformational behaviors through:

1. Building relations and influence with groups to achieve organizational goals
2. Sustaining influence that is both formal and informal, innate or acquired
3. Guiding and motivating others by clarifying roles and tasks requirements
4. Setting aside self-interests for the interest of the organization
5. Demonstrating a profound and extraordinary effect on followers
6. Supporting risk taking
7. Tolerating failure
8. Delegating decision making to the point of client service

D. **Engaged and empowered nurse leaders use emotional intelligence**

1. Engaged and empowered nurse leaders possess the capabilities and competencies to cope with the chaos and pressures instilled on the organization by external and internal forces
2. These emotional intelligence factors include:

   a. Self-awareness: knowing one's emotions and how they impact others

   b. Self-management: possessing self-control, adaptability, initiative, and optimism being able to show empathy, organizational astuteness, and dedication toward service

   c. Relationship management: building influence, inspiration, and commitment toward development of others; serving as change agents, and managing conflict

   d. Management of difficult team members who do not comply with organizational standards and safety measures

E. **Additional nursing skills and strategies for 21st century leadership**

1. Self-mastery: traits of self-mastery and emotional maturity

   a. Self-respect

   b. Self-incentive

   c. Care for one's own body and soul

   d. Sense of personal accountability

   e. Generate energy in yourself and those around you

   f. Share your passion and noble principles

   g. Connect human to human through your heart

   h. Stand up for what is right

   i. Challenge others to what they don't believe is possible

2. Interpersonal competence: interacting with others in ways that are:

   a. Culturally sensitive

   b. Caring

   c. Respectful

3. Professional skills

   a. Competence

   b. Ability to engage in respectful and honest relationships

   c. Problem solving

   d. Critical thinking

      e. Decision making

      f. Professionalism; lifelong learning

  4. System and organizational skills

      a. Nurse leaders realize that system and organizational skills are essential in managing the complexities of today's workplace

      b. Skills require nurse leaders who have demonstrated competencies in fostering the following:

         1) Creating networks of relationship and board based alliances

         2) Negotiating with diverse groups of individuals

         3) Knowing how to effectively mediate conflict

         4) Using a "system thinking" approach to managing human and fiscal resources

         5) Seeing the "big picture"

II. SUCCESSFULLY NAVIGATING CHANGE

A. Nurse leaders must stand ready and be prepared to lead change by:

  1. Possessing effective diagnostic skills and the ability to adapt their leadership style to the situation and the change

  2. Allowing followers to verbalize their concerns

  3. Providing a thorough rationale for the change

  4. Encouraging human emotions to be expressed

  5. Providing information, often and frequently

  6. Helping followers cope with the change

B. *Change*

  1. Is inevitable within the profession of nursing

  2. Is often influenced by external and internal forces

  3. Is a process that involves creating something different than what once was

  4. Has been associated with the following terms

      a. Constant

      b. Inevitable

      c. Pervasive

      d. Difficult

      e. Challenging

      f. Unpredictable

      g. Intense

      h. Unavoidable

      i. Influenced by individuals, technology, and systems

C. Types of change

  1. Personal change is voluntary change with the goal of self-improvement

  2. Professional change is deliberate change with the goal of improving professional ability/status

  3. Organizational change is mandated change with the goal of improving the organization's efficiency or quality of service/product

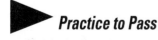

Practice to Pass

Explain the nurse leader's role in implementing change.

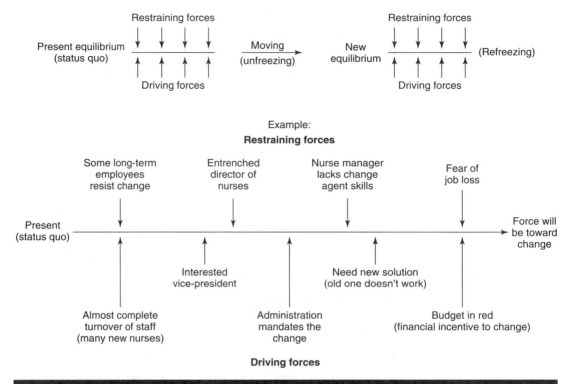

Figure 10-1

Lewin's force-field model of change.

Source: Lewin, K. (1997). *Field theory in social science.* New York: Harper Row. Cited in Sullivan, E. J. & Decker. P. J. (2005). *Effective leadership and management in nursing* (6th ed.). Upper Saddle River, NJ: Pearson Education, p. 219. Reprinted by permission.

D. Theories of change

1. Lewin's Force-Field Model (see Figure 10-1):
   a. Provides a social-psychological view of the change process
   b. Behavior is viewed as a dynamic balance of forces working in opposing directions; forces include:
      1) **Driving forces**—those that facilitate change because they push towards the desired direction
      2) **Restraining forces**—those that impede change because they push in the opposite direction
      3) Change occurs because these forces shift the balance; this is a three-step process:
         - **Unfreezing:** reducing the forces pressing for the status quo
         - **Moving:** developing new values, behaviors, and attitudes
         - **Refreezing:** instituting new supports, resources, and systems to secure and maintain the change
      4) Attention is aimed at increasing driving forces, decreasing restraining forces or both
2. Havelock's Model—a six-step process:
   a. Modified Lewin's model to expand the stages to include 3 substeps under *unfreezing*, and 2 under *moving*, which totals 6 steps after adding *refreezing*
   b. Unfreezing or planning stage:
      1) Building a relationship

      2) Diagnosing the problem

      3) Acquiring resources

   c. Moving stage:

      1) Choosing the solution

      2) Gaining acceptance

   d. Refreezing stage—stabilization and self-renewal

3. Lippit's phases of change:

   a. Builds on Lewin's work and considers human motivation, multiple causation, and habits

   b. Focuses attention on the change agent's actions

   c. Emphasizes key member's involvement throughout the process

   d. Adds importance of communication, rapport, and problem-solving strategies

   e. Incorporates a seven-step process of change:

      1) Diagnose the problem

      2) Assess motivation

      3) Assess change agent's motivation and resources

      4) Select progressive change objects

      5) Choose change agent role

      6) Maintain change

      7) Terminate helping relationships

4. Havelock's change model:

   a. Contains major concepts of role, linkages, and communication

   b. Adds steps to three stages of change, with heightened communication and interpersonal activities

   c. Seven steps in the change process:

      1) Perception of the need

      2) Diagnosis of the problem

      3) Identification of the problem

      4) Devising a plan of action

      5) Gaining acceptance

      6) Stabilizing the plan

      7) Self-renewal

5. Rogers's innovation-diffusion process

   a. Five-stage view of change:

      1) Knowledge

      2) Persuasion

      3) Decision

      4) Implementation

      5) Confirmation

   b. Considers five factors that influence rate of adoption of innovation that may be used as evaluation criteria in the change process

   c. Seven roles for change agent are highlighted in this model; general roles include:

      1) Assessor

      2) Evaluator

        3) Communicator

        4) Translator

        5) Encourager

        6) Mediator

        7) Consultant

   6. Dessler's organizational change process

      a. Is an eight-step process

        1) Create a sense of urgency

        2) Create a guiding coalition and mobilize commitment

        3) Develop and communicate a shared vision

        4) Empower employees to make the change

        5) Generate short-term wins

        6) Consolidate and produce more change

        7) Anchor the new ways of doing things in the organizational culture

        8) Monitor progress and adjust the vision as required

      b. Is consistent with Lewin's theory of change

   7. Emerging theories of change: are more complex and respond to more complex situations than some traditional theories; e.g., **chaos theory**:

      a. Order emerges through fluctuation and chaos

      b. Process is cyclical

      c. There is little time for orderly, linear change

      d. An organization must be able to act with speed, adaptability, and intensity

!   **E. Nurse leaders as *change agents***

   1. Are responsible for implementation of a change project

   2. Manage dynamics of the change process such as:

      a. Organizational structures

      b. Nursing labor force

      c. Cost controls

      d. Quality controls

      e. Client-centered systems

      f. Information systems

      g. Client safety

   3. Characteristics of a change agent:

      a. Elicits trust and respect from executors and recipients of change

      b. Is credible

      c. Is flexible

      d. Maintains and articulates the change vision

      e. Is an exceptional communicator

      f. Is an effective manager of interpersonal relationships

      g. Involves and empowers others in change process

   4. Change agent skill set: the art of combining resources and ideas:

      a. Identify the problems warranting the needed change

      b. Build and sustain relationships and partnerships

    c. Remain flexible

    d. Do not get discouraged when things fail

    e. Understand that change really does take time

    f. Understand the need to be realistic

    g. Model the change at every opportunity

    h. Obtain support from executive leadership

    i. Understand the true benefits of the change

    j. Seek agreement on the need for change

    k. Provide ongoing feedback about the change

F. Human response to change

  1. Change is inevitable for all humans and impacts their personal and professional lives; some individuals are more receptive to change than others

  2. Factors affecting an individual's ability to cope with change include:

    a. Adaptability

    b. Satisfaction with status quo

    c. Anticipated effects of change

    d. Perception of benefits/losses created by change

  3. Environmental or situational factors relative to individuals, families, and groups provide relevant information about resistance to change

  4. Past experience, stress and coping factors, motivational clues, and resources are important data that can assist the nurse leader to understand the emotional impact of change as a human response; potential emotional responses to change:

    a. Equilibrium

    b. Denial

    c. Anger

    d. Bargaining

    e. Chaos

    f. Depression

    g. Resignation

    h. Openness

    i. Readiness

    j. Re-emergence

  5. Resistance as a natural response to change

    a. Nurse leaders must be able to easily recognize the signs of resistance:

      1) Fear of disorder

      2) Adjusting to interruptions in daily routines

      3) Fear of losing one's job

      4) Fear of loss of formal and informal power sources

      5) Fear of loss of resources

    b. Typical responses to change: each person may respond to change differently; however, knowing about the typical responses to change will assist the nurse leader to recognize how others embrace change

      1) Innovators: embrace change

2) Early adopters: are open and receptive to change

3) Early majority: enjoy status quo, but readily adopt change

4) Late majority: are skeptical of change, but will accept it

5) Laggards: prefer the status quo and accept change with reluctance and suspicion

6) Rejecters: oppose and will attempt to sabotage change processes

c. Positive and negative aspects of resistance

1) Positive aspects: change agent must be focused, be ready to clarify information, keep interest high; resistance creates energy and movement

2) Negative aspects: wears down supporters; hard to stay focused among the constant challenges

d. Effective ways to handle resistance: because resistance to change is common in today's healthcare environment, nurse leaders must address it as it arises within their team members:

1) Be sure to communicate—often!

2) Be clear and accurate about tasks and activities

3) Be open and flexible

4) Acknowledge the negative consequences of resistance

5) Acknowledge the positive consequences of change

6) Maintain close contact with those who are most resistant

7) Promote trust, support, and confidence before, during, and after the change

8) Keep the energy moving forward to achieve the change with the fewest disturbances

e. Dealing with resistance and using power as a change agent: the nurse leader can use any of the following strategies depending on their power base:

1) Power-coercive: use authority and threat of job loss to gain compliance with change (power, economic, or political)

2) Normative–re-educative: use social orientation and the need to have satisfactory relationships in the workplace as a method of inducing support for change; focus on the relationship needs of workers (social norms and values)

3) Rational-empirical: use knowledge as power base; assume that once workers understand the organizational need for change or the meaning of the change for them as individuals and the organization as a whole, they will change (knowledge)

G. Low vs. high levels of change

1. **Planned change** is low-level complexity change with these characteristics:

a. Lots of structure

b. Stable

c. Incremental

d. Sequential and directional

2. Planned change is easier to accept because it usually is a choice and has a deliberate process; not a coercive act or accident

3. Planning change examines the situational elements of the organizational structure:

a. People

    b. Resources

    c. Structure

  4. High-level change has these characteristics:

    a. More fluid

    b. More complex

    c. Accomplished in fast-changing environments

H. Change involves use of these nurse leader functions:

  1. Planning

  2. Organizing

  3. Implementing

  4. Evaluating

I. Change as a continual unfolding process:

  1. Successful change initiatives occur because the nurse leaders understand that the **change process** unfolds in three phases:

    a. Present state

    b. Transition state

    c. Desired state

  2. Nurse leaders who are involved in organizational change are required to:

    a. Be knowledgeable about the organization

    b. Understand its restraining and driving forces

    c. Maintain a positive attitude

    d. Be receptive to new ideas and people

    e. Involve other people in the change

    f. Continue to refine skills

    g. Re-evaluate the situation

    h. Preserve stability and morale throughout the process

  3. Box 10-1 suggests strategies for the nurse manager in initiating and managing change

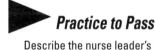

Practice to Pass

Describe the nurse leader's role in implementing change.

Box 10-1	
Strategies for Initiating and Managing Change	**1.** Identify the problem or opportunity.
	2. Collect necessary data and information.
	3. Select and analyze data.
	4. Develop a plan for change, including time frame and resources.
	5. Identify supporters or opposers.
	6. Build a coalition of supporters.
	7. Help people prepare for change.
	8. Prepare to handle resistance.
	9. Provide a feedback mechanism to keep everyone informed of the progress of change.
	10. Evaluate effectiveness of the change and, if successful, stabilize the change.

Source: Sullivan, E. J. & Decker, P. J. (2005). *Effective leadership and management in Nursing* (6th ed.). Upper Saddle River, NJ: Pearson Education, p. 226. Reprinted by permission.

III. CRITICAL THINKING: A TOOL FOR THE 21ST CENTURY NURSE LEADER

A. Critical thinking is a formalized, rational, and organized process for addressing the changes and challenges of nursing practice; as a disciplined process it allows the nurse leader to think, decide, and act in a way that is both systematic and explicit

1. A purposeful, self-regulatory judgment that results in interpretation, analysis, evaluation, and inference as well as explanation of the evidential, conceptual, methodological, or contextual considerations upon which that judgment is based

2. Involves the intellectually disciplined process of actively and skillfully conceptualizing, applying, analyzing, synthesizing, or evaluating information gathered from, or generated by, observation, experience, reflection, reasoning, or communication toward a belief and action

3. The National League of Nursing (NLN) describes critical thinking as a discipline-specific, reflective reasoning process that guides a nurse in generating, implementing, and evaluating approaches for dealing with client care and professional concerns

B. Descriptions of an ideal critical thinker:

1. Habitually inquisitive
2. Well-informed
3. Open-minded and flexible
4. Fair-minded in evaluation
5. Honest in facing personal biases
6. Prudent in making judgments
7. Clear about issues
8. Orderly in complex matters
9. Diligent in seeking relevant information
10. Reasonable in the selection of criteria
11. Focused in inquiry
12. Persistent in seeking results

C. Developing characteristics of a critical thinker:

1. Be open to views that are new and to different viewpoints
2. Be able to express and present ideas in an organized manner
3. Have evidence and logical reasoning to support ideas and views
4. Listen to others but think for oneself

D. Critical thinking and nursing leadership

1. Nurse leaders must recognize that critical thinking is an essential skill for processing client data; two major components of critical thinking:
   a. Cognitive skills are specific to a particular situation
   b. Disposition skills act as motivating factors for development and use of the cognitive skills used in clinical judgment

2. Critical thinking disposition is encouraged by:
   a. Coaching nurses to use megacognition (thinking about thinking)
   b. Asking questions such as:
      1) What is the purpose of my thinking?

2) How well am I articulating the question I am trying to answer?

3) What is my frame of reference?

4) What am I taking for granted/what assumptions am I making?

5) Once I have come to a conclusion, what are the implications?

  c. Using methods such as case study analyses

  d. Clinical journals specifically for critical thinking

3. Critical thinking is applied in each step of the nursing process and requires clinical judgment:

  a. Decide which assessment parameters are important

  b. Decide which, if any, diagnoses of human responses are highly accurate

  c. Decide which of many possible nursing inventions are the most appropriate

  d. Decide which client-behavioral outcomes are most relevant to the clinical situation

  e. Remember that clinical judgment consists of both informed opinions and decisions based on empirical knowledge and experience

  f. Clinical judgment develops gradually, nurse leaders gain a broader knowledge base and clinical experience; extensive direct client contact is the best means of developing clinical judgment

E. Application of critical thinking principles occurs when nurse leaders learn to:

  1. Analyze the nature of the problem or situation

  2. Apply factual information to predict an outcome based on cognitive principles

  3. Analyze the nature of the problem or situation, asking "why" questions (see Figure 10-2)

F. Factors affecting critical thinking

  1. Anxiety

  2. Attitude

  3. Level of preparation

  4. Learning styles

  5. Gender

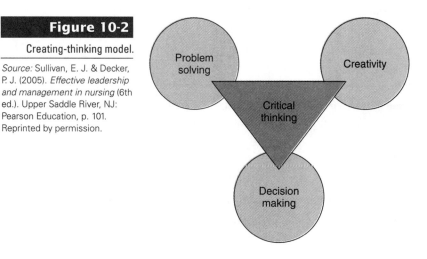

Figure 10-2

Creating-thinking model.

Source: Sullivan, E. J. & Decker, P. J. (2005). *Effective leadership and management in nursing* (6th ed.). Upper Saddle River, NJ: Pearson Education, p. 101. Reprinted by permission.

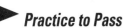

Practice to Pass

In your own words write a definition of critical thinking and how it relates to your use of the nursing process in caring for clients.

G. Becoming an effective thinker: to build capacity as a critical thinker, nurse leaders can use reflective, reflection, and reactive thinking:

   1. Reflective thinking: active, persistent, and careful consideration of any belief or supposed form of knowledge

   2. Reflection thinking: intellectual and affective activities in which individuals engage to explore their experiences to lead to new understandings and appreciations

   3. Reactive thinking: a response to what is and not to what may yet be

H. Critical thinking and evidence-based nursing

   1. Nurse leaders have an obligation to ensure critical thinking is a normal expectation of clinical practice; critical thinking occurs within a particular knowledge base and is paralleled by clinical experience where a nurse leader applies the knowledge base to the situation, using clinical reasoning to make a nursing judgment

   2. Model critical thinking approaches that demonstrate effective thinking, application, and evaluation of nursing practice

   3. Support curiosity, inquisitiveness, and exploration of evidence-based practices toward higher levels of excellence in nursing

IV. EVIDENCED-BASED LEADERSHIP

A. Nurse leaders must promote a positive work environment while promoting client safety based on sound nursing practice and research

   1. Adopt transformational leadership and evidence-based management practices

   2. Maximize workforce capability

   3. Design work structures to reduce errors

   4. Create and sustain a culture of safety

B. Linking to evidence-based nursing practice

   1. Become a consumer of research who uses and applies research in an active manner

   2. Understand the research process

   3. Develop critical evaluation skills needed to judge the merit and relevance of evidence before applying them to practice

   4. Use research to develop policy and clinical standards

   5. Understand how research works and participate in research studies

   6. Identify nursing problems that require investigation

   7. Participate in research studies by collecting and recording relevant data

   8. Promote ethical principles of research and protection of human rights

C. *Evidence-based practice:* integration of individual clinical experience with the best available external evidence from research; precise definition of a client problem

D. Evidence-based practice translates into action:

   1. Nurse leaders must facilitate and promote best practices in nursing care; using evidence-based nursing practice integrates the best of research evidence with clinical expertise and client values

     a. Nursing research links theory, education, and practice

     b. Research studies emphasize clinical issues, problems, and outcomes

     c. Research utilization transfers research finding to nursing practice that is carried out by individual nurses, groups of nurses, and interdisciplinary teams

2. Nurse leaders can find four major sources for evidence-based nursing:

    a. Research

    b. Clinical experience

    c. Client experience

    d. Information from the local context

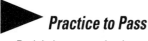
Practice to Pass

Explain how nurse leaders facilitate and promote evidence-based nursing practice.

3. Barriers to evidence-based care:

    a. Time constraints

    b. Limited access to the literature

    c. Lack of training in information seeking and critical appraisal

    d. A professional ideology emphasizing practical rather than intellectual knowledge

    e. A work environment that does not encourage information seeking

4. Each nurse must care enough about own practice to want to make sure it is based on the best possible information

5. Evidence must be relevant for the particular client

6. Clinical expertise should be balanced with the risks and benefits of alternative treatments for each client

7. A client's unique clinical circumstances including co-morbid conditions and preferences should be taken into account

8. A client has his or her preferences for care by choosing alternative treatments, refusing treatment, and by preparing advance directives

E. Evidence-based care information

1. The U.S. Department of Health and Human Services sponsors a national guideline clearinghouse: www.guideline.gov

2. National Institute of Nursing Research: www.nih.gov/ninr

3. International Society for Nursing Research: www.nursingsociety.org

F. Using evidence-based information

1. Understand that external validity deals with the possible problems of generalizability of the investigation's findings to additional populations and to other environmental conditions

2. Understand that reliability refers to the ability of the study measurements to be replicated and achieve the same outcome

3. Ask the following pertinent questions about the evidence:

    a. Are the results valid?

    b. What are the results?

    c. How can the results be applied to client care?

G. Nursing research

1. The Cabinet and Council on Nursing Research of the American Nurses Association propose all nurses share a commitment to the advancement of nursing science by conducting research and using research findings in practice; nurses are required to be accountable for the quality of client care they deliver

2. Characteristics of nursing research:

    a. Focus of nursing research is on a variance that makes a difference in improving client care

> **b.** Research has potential for contributing to theory development and the body of scientific nursing knowledge
>
> **c.** A problem is amenable to nursing research when nurses have access to and control over the phenomenon being studied
>
> **d.** A research nurse has an inquisitive, curious, and questioning mind

3. Nursing research process follows these steps:

   a. Problem area identification

   b. Formulation of a problem statement

   c. Data management

   d. Analysis of results

   e. Dissemination of results

4. Knowing the rights of research participants: comply with these guidelines to uphold the rights of human subjects in research:

   a. Give an explanation of the study

   b. Discuss the procedures to be followed and their purposes

   c. Provide a clear description of any physical and mental discomforts, any invasion of privacy, and any threat to dignity

   d. Describe the methods used to protect anonymity and ensure confidentiality of data

   e. Examine the subject's rights and protections

V. CULTURE AND NURSING PRACTICE

A. *Cultural diversity*

1. An essential aspect of 21st-century nursing practice; derives its conceptual base from nursing, other cross-cultural health disciplines, and the social sciences such as anthropology, sociology, and psychology

2. Nurse leaders have obligation to ensure their nursing workforce is well prepared to engage client, families, and other health providers who have diverse cultural backgrounds with respect and openness

B. *Culture* **is conceptualized broadly to encompass the belief systems of a variety of groups:**

1. Every individual belongs to a culture

2. Each culture has its own behaviors, norms, belief sets, values, and folk laws that are shared, learned, and passed on to generations of social groups

C. Culture consists of patterns of acquired behavior and transmitted symbols, constituting the distinctive achievement of human groups, including their embodiment in artifacts; the essential core of culture consists of historically derived and selected ideas and especially their attached values

D. Culture involves a combination of social, familial, religious, national, and professional characteristics that affect the way we think, act, and interact with others; differences among groups and subgroups produce diversity that can lead from uni-culturalism to appreciation of a multicultural environment and healthcare behaviors

E. Characteristics of culture include that it:

1. Is learned

2. Is unequally shared by its members

3. Is dynamic

    4. Provides diversity

    5. Is reasonable

    6. Is not easily described

    7. Has habituated assumptions

    8. Is ethnocentric

    9. Is relative

    10. Is pervasive

    11. Has common and observable rituals

F. Cultural diversity refers to differences between people based on a shared ideology and valued set of beliefs, norms, customs, and meanings evidenced in a way of life

    1. Diversity includes consideration of socioeconomic class, gender, age, religious belief, sexual preference, and physical disabilities, as well as race and ethnicity

    2. Diversity and equality of opportunity recognize that individuals learn from:

        a. Exposure to and interaction with others who have backgrounds and characteristics different from their own

        b. Recognizing and valuing diversity and equal opportunity also means knowledge, and appreciation

        c. Support of different learning styles

        d. Ways of interaction, and stimulating forms of discourse derived from interaction

        e. Collaboration with persons from diverse backgrounds and experiences

    3. Building culturally diverse and competent organizations

        a. Nurse leaders can value diversity by accepting and respecting differences through the organization

        b. Perform an organizational cultural assessment

        c. Acknowledge the dynamics of cross-cultural interactions such as differences in religious beliefs, values, and cultural experiences

        d. Allow for flexibility within organizational activities to fit cultural norms of staff and client

G. Nursing models

    1. Leininger's framework for transcultural nursing

        a. Highlights the commonalities and differences among worldviews that reflect different aspects of society to diverse health systems

        b. Cultural care is synthesized and culturally constituted to be assistive, supportive, and facilitative caring acts toward self or others, focused on evident or anticipated needs for the client's health or well-being, or to face disabilities, death, or other human conditions

    2. Campinha-Bacote has proposed *The Process of Cultural Competence in the Delivery of Healthcare Services Model* to include five constructs:

        a. Cultural awareness

        b. Cultural knowledge

       c. Cultural skill

        d. Cultural encounters

        e. Cultural desire

H. Characteristics related to culture:

    1. Ethnicity or ethnic identity

2. Minority

3. Race

4. Racism

5. Subculture

6. Stereotype

I. **Ethnic identity is self-conscious about its symbols**

1. **Ethnicity** is a way for people to create a social identity, to define themselves as different from other ethnic groups

2. Ethnic identity is a culturally informed identity

3. Individuals describe themselves as being from a certain group of society that represents ethnic identifiers such as religious beliefs, country of origin, race, language, values, and physical attributes

J. **Nurses need to understand how cultural groups understand life processes:**

1. How cultural groups define health and illness

2. What cultural groups do to maintain wellness

3. What cultural groups believe to be the causes of illness

4. How healers cure and care for members of cultural groups

5. How the cultural background of the nurse influences the way in which care is delivered

K. **Integrating culture into nursing care:**

1. Provide culturally sensitive nursing care

2. Be aware of biocultural variations

a. Growth and development

b. Nutritional tolerance

c. Body odor

d. Skin color

L. **Conducting nursing assessment based on client's perspective:**

1. Use the following techniques as appropriate:

a. Open-ended interviewing

b. Ethnographic interview

c. Key informant technique

2. Be aware of possible language differences between client and nurse

M. **Increasing the effectiveness of client education:** when working with clients from a different culture

1. Observe for patterns of unusual behavior

2. Analyze clusters of similar tales about unfamiliar cultures

3. Use ethnographic interview or key informant technique to gather information

4. Observe client's environment

N. **Nurses as client advocate**

1. Recognizing cultural diversity, integrating cultural knowledge, and acting, when possible, in a culturally appropriate manner enables nurses to be more effective in initiating nursing assessments and to serve as client advocates

2. **Culturally competent care** is sensitive to issues related to culture, race, gender, and sexual preference

3. Nurse leaders must use their knowledge of cultural diversity to develop and implement culturally sensitive nursing care; using cultural nursing theory, models, and research principles, nurse leaders demonstrate competence in identifying healthcare needs of their clients

   a. Nurses bring their personal cultural heritage as well as the cultural and philosophical views of their education into the professional setting

   b. Nurses must understand that nurse-client encounters include the interaction of three cultural systems:

      1) Culture of the nurse

      2) Culture of the client

      3) Culture of the setting

4. Cultural relativism asserts that any culture is different from, not superior to, any other culture

5. **Cultural sensitivity** is an awareness of which issues and concerns are important to one culture and to the culture of others

6. Transcultural reciprocity is the exchange of cultural respect and understanding between nurse and client; both are equal participants, with the nurse shaping care to meet the client's cultural needs

7. **Ethnocentrism** is belief that one's own culture is superior to all others

   a. It is common to all cultural groups; all groups regard their own culture as not only the best but also the correct, moral and only way of life

   b. It is unconscious and is imposed on every aspect of day-to-day interaction and practices including healthcare

   c. It creates problems between nurses and clients of diverse cultural groups

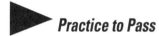

Practice to Pass

Describe ways in which nurse leaders can build a culturally diverse and competent workforce within their healthcare organizations.

VI. SPIRITUALITY

A. **Nurse leaders understand that all humanity confronts the issues of death and dying when confronted with a serious or disabling illness; therefore, the concept of spirituality is important to contemporary nursing practice; spirituality provides an inner resource and value that guides and gives meaning to life**

B. *Spirituality* **is belief in or relationship with a higher power, divine being, or creative force**

   1. Involves the inner part of a person that permeates all aspects of the person

   2. Is manifested through creative expressions, familiar rituals, meaningful work, and religious practices and beliefs

   3. Spiritual needs have been identified as a need for purpose and meaning, need for love and relatedness, a need for forgiveness, and a need for hope

   4. Spiritual beliefs:

      a. Help people cope with life stressors and crisis

      b. Provide a sense of purpose

      c. Develop a sense of inner tranquility that allows people to love and trust others

C. **Religion**

   1. An organized system of worship with central beliefs, rituals, and practices

   2. Has four dimensions:

      a. Theoretical (myths, beliefs, and doctrine)

      b. Practical (rites, prayers, and moral codes)

      c. Sociological (relating to churches, leaders, and functionaries)

      d. Experiential (pertaining to emotions, vision, and various sentiments)

D. Relationship between spirituality, religion, and health

    1. Spiritual and religious beliefs and practices overlap with cultural beliefs about illness causation and methods of caring

    2. Can help people find solace; spiritual needs may increase during crisis situations

    3. Spirituality is an aspect of well-being; clients who do not see themselves as religious may greatly benefit from spiritual support during periods of crisis or illness

    4. To help others, we must help ourselves:

      a. We must accept that illness, suffering, and death are all natural occurrences of the human condition

      b. We must come to terms with our own spirituality

      c. What are our beliefs?

      d. What gives us hope, peace, and spiritual well-being?

E. Nursing assessment for spiritual distress

    1. Spiritual distress is the questioning of life's purpose and its meaning as well as refusing to participate in one's religious practices

    2. Nurse must assess for signs of spiritual distress: note whether a client:

      a. Is withdrawn, sullen, silent, and depressed

      b. Is restless, irritable, and has complaints

      c. Is excitable, garrulous, and wants to talk a lot

      d. Displays by word or other sign undue curiosity and anxiety about self

      e. Takes a turn for the worse, critical, or terminal

      f. Displays conversational interest and curiosity in religious questions

      g. Inquires about a chaplain, chapel, worship, and religious material

      h. Has few or no visitors

      i. Has had or faces particularly traumatic or threatening surgical procedures

F. Spirituality and nursing responsibility

    1. Providing nursing care in an intercultural context:

      a. Culture and religion must be understood and incorporated into the care plan if nursing care is to be effective

      b. Religion affects client's:

        1) Consent to treatments

        2) Schedule of care or room arrangement

        3) Birth or death practices

        4) Food preferences

    2. Nurses need to become aware of and familiar with spiritual resources such as chaplains and clergy in the hospital and community

    3. Gain knowledge about specific tenets of religion:

      a. Christianity is founded on teaching of Jesus Christ (includes Roman Catholicism, Eastern Orthodoxy [Greek, Armenian, Ukrainian, and Syrian], Protestantism)

      b. Judaism

      c. Islam

       d. Hinduism

       e. Buddhism

       f. Atheism

G. Spiritual and cultural nursing assessment

    1. Determine client's concept of God or Deity

    2. Determine client's sources of hope and strength

    3. Determine client's religious practices

    4. Relation between spiritual beliefs and health

    5. Ask questions to avoid cultural stereotypes

    6. Learn the client's views about health

    7. Learn about accepted ways to show respect

    8. Understand relationships

    9. Consider privacy needs

H. Nursing assessments build cultural awareness: effective nursing assessment leads to a cultural encounter between the nurse and the client:

    1. Refines or modifies existing knowledge about a specific cultural group

    2. Encourages self-analysis of one's own prejudices and biases

    3. Builds cultural skill and generates accurate nursing diagnoses

    4. Includes intercultural collaboration of other members of the healthcare team, such as dietitians, social workers, hospital chaplains, or pastoral counselors

VII. DEATH AND DYING

A. Grief is a bereavement state of desolation that occurs as the result of a loss, especially the death of a significant other

B. Mourning is a social response to the death of a significant other; including behavioral responses that may be culturally based and culturally prescribed

C. Signs and symptoms of grief:

    1. Dejected physical appearance

    2. Slowed motor function

    3. Weeping

    4. Anger and emotional blunting

    5. Sleep disturbance

    6. Appetite disturbance with weight loss or gain

    7. Inability to express joy

    8. Inability to speak of the deceased without intense emotion

D. Personal grieving is influenced by:

    1. Meaning of the loss to the individual

    2. Circumstances of the loss

    3. Religious beliefs and cultural practices

    4. Personal resources and stressors

    5. Sociocultural resources and stressors

> **!** ▷ **E. Dysfunctional grieving:**
> 1. Extends beyond three years and is more pronounced
> 2. Falls outside the range of normal response to grief
> 3. Manifests by exaggerated grief, prolonged grief, or absence of grief
> 4. Expends excessive energy and leaves no energy for normal activities

> **!** ▷ **F. Dimensions of hospice care:**
> 1. Hospice care focuses on quality vs. quantity of life
> 2. Empowers clients and families to retain control over their lives as much as possible
> 3. Clients may be kept in a hospital/facility or home
> 4. Provides for comfort care in pain and nausea control, as well as other comfort measures
> 5. Assists the clients and their families to prepare for death

▶ **Practice to Pass**

Explain the factors that might influence an individual's grieving.

POSTTEST

Case Study

You are the nurse manager on a 15-bed infectious disease unit that has a variety of clients from diverse cultures and ethnicities who are primarily diagnosed with acquired immunodeficiency syndrome (AIDS). Your responsibility is to support the staff in identifying information about the culture and ethnicity of their assigned clients in an effort to enhance provision of culturally competent nursing care.

1. What type of information does the staff need to be able to deliver care effectively to these clients?

2. What are some of the challenges inherent in delivering care to this client population?

3. What are potential barriers to caring for these clients by healthcare workers?

4. How can you stress to your assigned staff the importance of valuing cultural and ethnic differences and the need for sensitive awareness of others?

5. What are potential positive outcomes for caring for a variety of clients from diverse cultures and ethnicities?

See page 238 for suggested responses.

POSTTEST

1 A nurse responds to change by being open and receptive to the new process. The nurse leader implementing the change recognizes that this nurse is a(n):

1. Innovator.
2. Early adopter.
3. Laggard.
4. Early majority.

2 A nurse reports in a staff meeting about being unaware of the status of a planned changed on the nursing unit. Which strategy should the nurse leader use to resolve this problem?

1. Communicate with staff more frequently.
2. Acknowledge negative consequences to resisting the change.
3. Maintain close contact with resisters to facilitate buy-in to the change.
4. Remain open and flexible to hearing the staff's concerns about the change.

3 A nurse leader provides orientation to an upcoming change in wound care procedures. The leader builds relationships and supports the staff in implementing the new procedures. Which type of approach is the leader using to manage resistance to change?

1. Rational-empirical
2. Power-coercive
3. Normative–re-educative
4. Country club

4 The nurse leader of a nursing unit would like to pilot a new automated medication dispensing system on the nursing unit. Which of the following roles does the nurse leader need to focus on to facilitate this option?

1. Communication liaison
2. Care manager
3. Unit manager
4. Change agent

5 Which elements of the organizational structure should the nurse leader consider when planning change on the nursing unit? Select all that apply.

1. People
2. Resources
3. Structure
4. Materials management
5. Rate of admissions

6 A nurse leader determines the effectiveness of the plan of change and modifies the plan. Which step in the change process does this represent?

1. Evaluation
2. Implementation
3. Planning
4. Organization

7 The nurse leader who is contemplating change would recall that the first step in the change process is to:

1. Identify the problem in need of change.
2. Fractionize the problem for clarification.
3. Provide ongoing rationale about the change.
4. Build relationships and partnerships.

8 Which of the following should be done by the nurse leader who is involved in change on the nursing unit? Select all that apply.

1. Use coercive power to maintain change.
2. Be knowledgeable about the organization.
3. Use a limited number of people in the change.
4. Show receptiveness to new ideas and people.
5. Demonstrate an understanding of restraining forces.

9 A nurse stays well informed on issues involving client care; the nurse is aware of personal biases and asks many questions. The nurse leader interprets that this nurse exhibits which of the following?

1. Cultural sensitivity
2. Leadership
3. Critical thinking skills
4. Research ability

10 A nurse leader observes behavior and hears words that indicate anger and bitterness in a certified nursing assistant (CNA) who opposed the use of a new computerized documentation system. The nurse manager recognizes that the CNA's expression of anger:

1. Also represents the feelings of other staff members about the new system.
2. Is a likely coping mechanism in response to the change.
3. Is the unfreezing of current behavior and the CNA will make the adjustment.
4. Is aggressive behavior that should not be tolerated.

➤ *See pages 226–228 for Answers and Rationales.*

POSTTEST

ANSWERS & RATIONALES

Pretest

1 **Answer: 1** The characteristics of change include that it is constant, dynamic, inevitable, challenging, unpredictable, intense, and unavoidable, and that change may have positive or negative consequences. Change is not easy or predictable. **Cognitive Level:** Knowledge **Client Need:** Safe Effective Care Environment: Management of Care **Integrated Process:** Nursing Process: Analysis **Content Area:** Leadership/Management **Strategy:** The wording of the question tells you that the correct answer is a true statement or option. Choose the option that logically fits the sentence. Focus on characteristics of change. Option 2 is incorrect because change is not always predictable. Options 3 and 4 are false statements. Change is dynamic and fluid; a true statement. **References:** Finkelman, A. W. (2006). *Leadership and management in nursing.* Upper Saddle River, NJ: Pearson Education, pp. 40–41; Sullivan, E. J., & Decker, P. (2005). *Effective leadership and management in nursing* (6th ed.). Upper Saddle River, NJ: Pearson Education, pp. 217–218.

2 **Answer: 1** This nurse is furthering educational advancement to increase annual income. The benefits of this change reap personal advantages. If the rationale was one of professional growth to provide better care to clients and facilitate positive client outcomes, then the answer would be professional change (option 2). Organizational change (option 3) is reflective of improving the overall efficiency or quality of the service provided by the organization. The term forceful (option 4) is not a term used to categorize a type of change. **Cognitive Level:** Comprehension **Client Need:** Safe Effective Care Environment: Management of Care **Integrated Process:** Nursing Process: Planning **Content Area:** Leadership/Management **Strategy:** Identify the critical words in the stem, *educational advancement and increased income.* Begin by eliminating options 3 and 4, which are not applicable. Because the impetus to return to college for an advanced degree is one of personal gain, the correct answer is option 1. This is a professional change, but the nurse's desire to change stems from a personal goal. Use knowledge of the change process to select the correct answer. **References:** Finkelman, A. W. (2006). *Leadership and management in nursing.* Upper Saddle River, NJ: Pearson Education, pp. 43–48; Sullivan, E. J., & Decker, P. (2005). *Effective leadership and management in nursing* (6th ed.). Upper Saddle River, NJ: Pearson Education, pp. 221–223.

3 **Answer: 1** Driving forces are those who support the change and provide resources to make the change possible. In this case, the plan for change is derived from the CEO, which reinforces the CEO's role as a driving force. Restraining forces prohibit change and fight to prevent any change. Refreezing and unfreezing are not forces that affect change; they are steps in the change process that affect the desired behavior. **Cognitive Level:** Comprehension **Client Need:** Safe Effective Care Environment: Management of Care **Integrated Process:** Nursing Process: Analysis **Content Area:** Leadership/Management **Strategy:** Eliminate option 2 first as incorrect because the CEO does not function in an inhibitory capacity. Next, note that options 3 and 4 are steps in the change process to directly impact behavioral responses to change; rule these options out. The CEO functions in supportive and administrative roles, which makes option 1 correct. **References:** Finkelman, A. W. (2006). *Leadership and management in nursing.* Upper Saddle River, NJ: Pearson Education, pp. 42–43; Sullivan, E. J., & Decker, P. (2005). *Effective leadership and management in nursing* (6th ed.). Upper Saddle River, NJ: Pearson Education, pp. 217–218.

4 **Answer: 3** The staff member demonstrates the desired behavior as a direct result of the change. This action shows the manager the staff has accepted the change and has modified behavior, which is the indicator of effective change. In the refreezing phase of Lewin's change process (option 4), new resources are implemented to maintain the change. Unfreezing (option 2) is characterized by reducing the restraining forces and gathering driving forces. Stagnation (option 1) is not a phase in Lewin's change process. **Cognitive Level:** Comprehension **Client Need:** Safe Effective Care Environment: Management of Care **Integrated Process:** Nursing Process: Evaluation **Content Area:** Leadership/Management **Strategy:** Identify critical words in the question or stem to select the right answer. First, note that stagnation is not a step in Lewin's change process; rule it out. Option 2 is not described in the stem, so that is eliminated next. The stem does not provide data to support option 4, making this option incorrect. Desired behavior is an indication of change; this is the moving stage. **References:** Finkelman, A. W. (2006). *Leadership and management in nursing.* Upper Saddle River, NJ: Pearson Education, pp. 42–43; Sullivan, E. J., & Decker, P. (2005). *Effective leadership and management in nursing* (6th ed.). Upper Saddle River, NJ: Pearson Education, pp. 217–218.

5 **Answer: 2** Chaos theory is characterized by order that emerges from rapid and unplanned fluctuations. Change is not orderly, but linear. Lewin's theory is orderly and process driven along with Havelock's and Rogers's theories on change. **Cognitive Level:** Comprehension **Client Need:** Safe Effective Care Environment: Management of Care **Integrated Process:** Nursing Process: Analysis **Content Area:** Leadership/Management **Strategy:** The stem does not support data for Lewin's change theory, so eliminate option 1 first. Options 3 and 4 are not supported by the data provided in the stem, so they are also eliminated. The stem indicates rapid fluctuations and lack of order, both indicating chaos. **References:** Finkelman, A. W. (2006). *Leadership and management in nursing.* Upper Saddle River, NJ: Pearson Education, pp. 11–12; Sullivan, E. J., & Decker, P. (2005). *Effective leadership and management in nursing* (6th ed.). Upper Saddle River, NJ: Pearson Education, pp. 15–16.

6 **Answer: 2** Organizational structures are the likely places where change will occur and incorporates client safety and staff safety issues. Workforce culture can influence the staff's readiness to change. **Cognitive Level:** Knowledge **Client Need:** Safe Effective Care Environment: Management of Care **Integrated Process:** Nursing Process: Analysis **Content Area:** Leadership/Management **Strategy:** Identify critical words in the question or stem to select the right answer. Note that options 1 and 3 fall under the more global category of organizational structures to eliminate them as possible answers. Recall that workforce culture is a characteristic of a group that can influence the process of change. **References:** Finkelman, A. W. (2006). *Leadership and management in nursing.* Upper Saddle River, NJ: Pearson Education, pp. 48–50; Sullivan, E. J., & Decker, P. (2005). *Effective leadership and management in nursing* (6th ed.). Upper Saddle River, NJ: Pearson Education, pp. 225–226.

7 **Answer: 4** The change agent must be able to communicate the vision as it relates to change. The nurse leader should remain flexible to the change process (option 1). Communications need to be clear rather than vague (option 2). Aggression (option 3) is not a characteristic that facilitates change. **Cognitive Level:** Comprehension **Client Need:** Safe Effective Care Environment: Management of Care **Integrated Process:** Communication and Documentation **Content Area:** Leadership/Management **Strategy:** Choose an option that describes the characteristics of a change agent. Look for true statements. Options 1, 3, and 4 are false statements; rule them out. Use knowledge of the change process to select the correct answer. **References:**

Finkelman, A. W. (2006). *Leadership and management in nursing.* Upper Saddle River, NJ: Pearson Education, pp. 50–52; Sullivan, E. J., & Decker, P. (2005). *Effective leadership and management in nursing* (6th ed.). Upper Saddle River, NJ: Pearson Education, p. 217.

8 **Answer: 2** The implementation phase is characterized by the actual carrying out of the plan. In the evaluation step of the change process, the nurse determines the effectiveness of the current plan and makes necessary changes. The planning phase provides a detailed step-by-step blueprint of actions that must be implemented to make the change possible. In the organization phase, the resources are aligned to meet the needs of the change event. **Cognitive Level:** Knowledge **Client Need:** Safe Effective Care Environment: Management of Care **Integrated Process:** Nursing Process: Analysis **Content Area:** Leadership/Management **Strategy:** The critical words in the stem are *actively carrying out.* In other words, implementing the change. The stem does not provide evidence to support the other options. Use knowledge of the change process to select the correct answer. **References:** Finkelman, A. W. (2006). *Leadership and management in nursing.* Upper Saddle River, NJ: Pearson Education, p. 65; Sullivan, E. J., & Decker, P. (2005). *Effective leadership and management in nursing* (6th ed.). Upper Saddle River, NJ: Pearson Education, pp. 220–222.

9 **Answers: 1, 2, 4, 5** Adaptability, satisfaction with the status quo, anticipated effects of the change, and the perception of losses that will be created by the change can all affect an individual's ability to cope with change. Typically, age and number of years on the job do not impact or influence one's ability to cope with the effects of change. **Cognitive Level:** Knowledge **Client Need:** Safe Effective Care Environment: Management of Care **Integrated Process:** Nursing Process: Analysis **Content Area:** Leadership/Management **Strategy:** Choose options that are true statements. Rule out false statements. Consider that age and number of years on the job have no impact on an individual's ability to cope with change to rule this single option out. **References:** Finkelman, A. W. (2006). *Leadership and management in nursing.* Upper Saddle River, NJ: Pearson Education, pp. 45–49; Sullivan, E. J., & Decker, P. (2005). *Effective leadership and management in nursing* (6th ed.). Upper Saddle River, NJ: Pearson Education, pp. 223–225.

10 **Answer: 4** The nursing process is a guide that assists in developing critical thinking skills. Critical thinking skills may also be developed by the formation of specific questions, use of case study analyses and reading clinical journals focused on critical thinking. Nurses should be coached to think about their thought processes in relation to frame of reference, assumptions, and cues. Memorization of information (option 3) does not foster the development of critical thinking skills. Nurses must identify biases and prevent their biases from influencing their thoughts (option 2). Thinking about care measures (option 1) does not imply that critical thinking is also involved, which has an analytic component. **Cognitive Level:** Application **Client Need:** Safe Effective Care Environment: Management of Care **Integrated Process:** Nursing Process: Implementation **Content Area:** Leadership/Management **Strategy:** Consider that ordinary thinking about care measures will not develop critical thinking to eliminate option 1. Note that critical thinkers should be aware of their biases when making decisions to eliminate option 2. Recall that memorization (option 3) is not a critical thinking method, but the nursing process is. Identify the critical words *critical thinking* in the question and *effective use* in the correct option to help you choose option 4. **References:** Finkelman, A. W. (2006). *Leadership and management in nursing*. Upper Saddle River, NJ: Pearson Education, p. 56; Sullivan, E. J., & Decker, P. (2005). *Effective leadership and management in nursing* (6th ed.). Upper Saddle River, NJ: Pearson Education, pp. 101–102.

Posttest

1 **Answer: 2** The early adopter is open and receptive to change. The innovator (option 1) embraces change, and the laggard (option 3) prefers not to change, but will do so with reluctance. The early majority (option 4) prefer the current systems, but succumb to change readily. **Cognitive Level:** Comprehension **Client Need:** Safe Effective Care Environment: Management of Care **Integrated Process:** Nursing Process: Assessment **Content Area:** Leadership/Management **Strategy:** Choose an option that fits closely with the description in the stem. Rule out laggard; it clearly stands out. The stem does not provide data to support options 1 and 4. The early adopter fits the description provided in the stem. Apply knowledge of responses to change and the process of elimination to make the correct selection. **References:** Finkelman, A. W. (2006). *Leadership and management in nursing*. Upper Saddle River, NJ: Pearson Education, pp. 43–46, 51; Sullivan, E. J., & Decker, P. (2005). *Effective leadership and management in nursing* (6th ed.). Upper Saddle River, NJ: Pearson Education, pp. 222–223.

2 **Answer: 1** The problem in this scenario is a lack of communication. The staff nurse does not know the progress or the status of the change. The leader should use clear, concise communication to convey the status of the change with the staff. The other options do not address communication.

Cognitive Level: Application **Client Need:** Safe Effective Care Environment: Management of Care **Integrated Process:** Communication and Documentation **Content Area:** Leadership/Management **Strategy:** Choose an option containing a true statement. The problem identified in the stem is one of communication. Option 1 provides a solution to improve communication. Options 2 and 3 do not address the issue. Option 4 is true, but it does not solve the problem. Use knowledge of the change process to select the correct answer. **References:** Finkelman, A. W. (2006). *Leadership and management in nursing*. Upper Saddle River, NJ: Pearson Education, pp. 50–53; Sullivan, E. J., & Decker, P. (2005). *Effective leadership and management in nursing* (6th ed.). Upper Saddle River, NJ: Pearson Education, pp. 220–223.

3 **Answer: 3** The normative–re-educative approach focuses on building relationships, using orientation to educate staff and social orientation in the workplace. Power-coercive strategies (option 2) use punitive measures, fear, and authority to achieve compliance with change. The rational-empirical approach (option 1) uses knowledge and empowerment to gain compliance from staff. The country club approach (option 4) is social in nature. **Cognitive Level:** Comprehension **Client Need:** Safe Effective Care Environment: Management of Care **Integrated Process:** Nursing Process: Implementation **Content Area:** Leadership/Management **Strategy:** First rule out option 4 because it is inapplicable. Next option 2 can be ruled out based on the force of power suggested by the term power-coercive. The stem does not provide data to support option 1 (rational-empirical) so that is eliminated as the third incorrect option. Option 3 best describes the leader. Identify critical words in the question or stem to select the right answer. **Reference:** Finkelman, A. W. (2006). *Leadership and management in nursing*. Upper Saddle River, NJ: Pearson Education, pp. 222–223.

4 **Answer: 4** The change agent uses the change process, which includes planning, organizing, implementing, and evaluating. The unit manager role encompasses all aspects of the day-to-day operations of the unit. Communication liaison and care manager are not applicable to the situation described.

Cognitive Level: Comprehension **Client Need:** Safe Effective Care Environment: Management of Care **Integrated Process:** Nursing Process: Planning **Content Area:** Leadership/Management **Strategy:** Note that the question is addressing an intention to make a change on the nursing unit. Therefore, choose the option that focuses on the change process. The care manager and staff nurse may use the change process; however, in doing so they function in the role of a change agent. The more specific answer is option 4. Use knowledge of the change process to select the correct answer. **References:** Finkelman, A. W.

(2006). *Leadership and management in nursing.* Upper Saddle River, NJ: Pearson Education, pp. 50–52; Sullivan, E. J., & Decker, P. (2005). *Effective leadership and management in nursing* (6th ed.). Upper Saddle River, NJ: Pearson Education, p. 217.

5 Answers: 1, 2, 3 Planned change should consider situational elements of the organization such as people, resources, and structure. Materials management falls under the umbrella of resources, and rate of admissions is not applicable because it is too specific and may or may not relate to any specific change that is planned. **Cognitive Level:** Application **Client Need:** Safe Effective Care Environment: Management of Care **Integrated Process:** Nursing Process: Planning **Content Area:** Leadership/Management **Strategy:** Select options that are important in change, people, resources, and structure. Rule out options that are directly impacted by organizational change such as materials management and rate of admissions. Apply knowledge of the change theories to select the correct answer. **References:** Finkelman, A. W. (2006). *Leadership and management in nursing.* Upper Saddle River, NJ: Pearson Education, pp. 57–65; Sullivan, E. J., & Decker, P. (2005). *Effective leadership and management in nursing* (6th ed.). Upper Saddle River, NJ: Pearson Education, pp. 223–226.

6 Answer: 1 In the evaluation step of the change process, the nurse determines the effectiveness of the current plan and makes necessary changes. The implementation phase is characterized by the actual carrying out of the plan. The planning phase provides a detailed step-by-step blueprint of what must be done to make the change possible. In the organization phase, the resources are aligned to meet the needs of the change event. **Cognitive Level:** Comprehension **Client Need:** Safe Effective Care Environment: Management of Care **Integrated Process:** Nursing Process: Analysis **Content Area:** Leadership/Management **Strategy:** Think about the nursing process. The leader now evaluates the effectiveness of the plan. The stem does not provide data to support the other options. Use knowledge of the change process to select the correct answer. **References:** Finkelman, A. W. (2006). *Leadership and management in nursing.* Upper Saddle River, NJ: Pearson Education, pp. 65–67; Sullivan, E. J., & Decker, P. (2005). *Effective leadership and management in nursing* (6th ed.). Upper Saddle River, NJ: Pearson Education, p. 222.

7 Answer: 1 The first step in the change process is to constantly be aware of those processes and/or procedures in need of change. Change agents should look at the whole picture when dealing with change. Rationale should be given once the process starts along with alliance building.

Cognitive Level: Knowledge **Client Need:** Safe Effective Care Environment: Management of Care **Integrated Process:** Nursing Process: Planning **Content Area:** Leadership/Management **Strategy:** Use knowledge of the change process to select the correct answer. Think nursing process: assess first. Identifying the areas in need of change stems from continual assessment. Option 2 is an incorrect statement; rule it out. Options 3 and 4 are important, but are not first steps in the change process. **References:** Finkelman, A. W. (2006). *Leadership and management in nursing.* Upper Saddle River, NJ: Pearson Education, pp. 57–58; Sullivan, E. J., & Decker, P. (2005). *Effective leadership and management in nursing* (6th ed.). Upper Saddle River, NJ: Pearson Education, p. 221.

8 Answers: 2, 4, 5 Change is only effective if all who must carry out the change are involved. Coercive power may be used, but is often ineffective in maintaining change. Nurse leaders must be knowledgeable about the organization, show receptiveness to new ideas and people, and understand restraining and driving forces.

Cognitive Level: Knowledge **Client Need:** Safe Effective Care Environment: Management of Care **Integrated Process:** Nursing Process: Implementation **Content Area:** Leadership/Management **Strategy:** Choose options that are stated in true terms. Option 1 is incorrect because coercive power may not be very effective in maintaining change. Option 3 is an incorrect statement. Leaders should involve many individuals in the change process. Apply knowledge of the change theories to select the correct answer. **References:** Finkelman, A. W. (2006). *Leadership and management in nursing.* Upper Saddle River, NJ: Pearson Education, pp. 49–52; Sullivan, E. J., & Decker, P. (2005). *Effective leadership and management in nursing* (6th ed.). Upper Saddle River, NJ: Pearson Education, pp. 225–226.

9 Answer: 3 Critical thinkers are inquisitive, well-informed, and aware of personal biases that may influence decisions. They also possess an open mind that is objective. The characteristics in this question do not address cultural sensitivity, leadership, or research. **Cognitive Level:** Application **Client Need:** Safe Effective Care Environment: Management of Care **Integrated Process:** Nursing Process: Evaluation **Content Area:** Leadership/Management **Strategy:** The information in the stem of the question does not support options 1 or 2. Researchers are well-informed, but may not be aware of personal biases. Critical thinkers are aware of biases and stay informed on client care issues. Identify critical words in the question or stem to select the right answer. **References:** Finkelman, A. W. (2006). *Leadership and management in nursing.* Upper Saddle River, NJ: Pearson Education, p. 56; Sullivan, E. J., & Decker, P. (2005). *Effective leadership and management in nursing*

(6th ed.). Upper Saddle River, NJ: Pearson Education, pp. 101–102.

10 Answer: 2 Each individual responds to change differently. Anger is a coping mechanism that occurs in employees who may resist change. These coping mechanisms are influenced by previous experience with change. While anger is aggressive, it should be recognized as a coping response. Unfreezing does not apply to this scenario. The feelings of one staff member cannot be generalized to all members of the staff. **Cognitive Level:** Comprehension **Client Need:** Safe Effective Care Environment: Management of Care **Integrated Process:** Nursing Process: Assessment **Content Area:**

Leadership/Management **Strategy:** Rule out any false statements; option 1 falls in this category. The stem does not provide data to support option 3. Option 4 is a true statement, but the nurse should understand the meaning of the behavior as option two suggests. Apply knowledge of responses to change and the process of elimination to make the correct selection. **References:** Finkelman, A. W. (2006). *Leadership and management in nursing.* Upper Saddle River, NJ: Pearson Education, pp. 56–59; Sullivan, E. J., & Decker, P. (2005). *Effective leadership and management in nursing* (6th ed.). Upper Saddle River, NJ: Pearson Education, pp. 222–223.

References

American Association of Critical Care Nurses. *AACN's Healthy Work Environment Initiative.* Retrieved August 7, 2007, from www.aacn/pubpolcy.nsf/vwdoc/worken?opendocument.

Baker, A. M., Sullivan, D. T., & Emery, M. J. (2006). *Leadership competencies for clinical managers: The renaissance of transformational leadership.* Sudbury, MA: Jones and Bartlett Publishers.

Campinha-Bacote, J. (2003). *The process of cultural competence in the delivery of healthcare services: A culturally competent model of care* (4th ed.). Cincinnati, OH: Transcultural C.A.R.E. Associates.

Campinha-Bacote, J. (2002). The process of cultural competence in a delivery of healthcare services: A model of care. *Journal of Transcultural Nursing, 13*(3), 181–184.

D'Avanzo, C. E., & Geissler, E. M. (2003). *Pocket guide to cultural health assessment* (3rd ed.). St. Louis: Mosby.

De Groot, H. A. (2005). Evidenced-based leadership: Nursing's new mandate. *Nurse Leader, 3*(2), 37–41.

Dessler, G. (2004). *Management: Principles and practices for tomorrow's leaders.* Upper Saddle River, NJ: Pearson Education.

Flesner, M. K., Scott-Cawiezell, J., & Rantz, M. (2005). Preparation of nurse leaders in the 21st century workplace. *Nurse Leader, 3*(4), 37–40.

Geoffee, R., & Jones, G. (2005). Managing authenticity. *Harvard Business Review, 83*(12), 85–94.

Hancock, C. (2004). Unity with diversity: ICN framework of competence. *Journal of Advanced Nursing, 47*(2), 119.

Havelock, R. (1973). *The change agent's guide to innovation in education.* Englewood Cliffs, NJ: Educational Technology Publications.

Jones, M. E., Carson, C., & Bond, M. L. (2004). Cultural attitudes, knowledge, and skills of a health workforce. *Journal of Transcultural Nursing, 13*(3), 189–192.

Jourard, S. M. (1971). *The transparent self.* New York: Litton Educational.

Leininger, M. (2002). Essential transcultural nursing care concepts, principles, examples, and policy statements. Cited in M. Leininger, & M. R. McFarland. (2002). *Transcultural nursing: Concepts, theories, research, and practice* (3rd ed.). New York: McGraw-Hill Medical Publishing Division.

Mazanec, P., & Tyler, M. K. (2003). Cultural considerations in end-of-life care. *American Journal of Nursing, 103*(3), 50–59.

Websites

A-Z of Jewish and Israel related resources: www.ort.org:80/anjy/a-z

Cyber Muslim Information Collective: www.uoknor.edu/cybermuslim

CyberZen: http://indy.net/~bdmoore.cyberzen.html

Distinctive Churches: www.best.com/~nodakid/church.html

Global Hindu electronic network: http://rbhatnagar.csm.us.edu:8080/hindu-universe.html

Library of God: http://convex.uky.edu80/~rtcrit00/atemple.html

Transcultural C.A.R.E. Associates: www.transculturalcare.net.

Yahoo Religion Subdirectory: www.yahoo.com/society-and-culture/religion

Appendix

➤ *Practice to Pass Suggested Answers*

Chapter 1

Page 10: *Answer*—Mentoring of the new graduate by experienced professional nurses can be a key component in producing beneficial outcomes for both the mentor and mentee. Key components of leadership that are beneficial to the new nurse leader would include someone who:

- Is trustworthy and will act as a counselor or guide
- Encourages questions and questioning
- Will assist in overcoming professional barriers
- Will help the mentee focus on the future
- Will offer constructive feedback
- Acts in a nonthreatening manner
- Views the mentee's weaknesses as opportunities and provides a safe haven for exploration, risk taking, and failure.

Additionally, consider asking yourself the following questions prior to choosing your mentor: Is the mentor competent or valued because of his or her position? Is the mentor on the way up or down or out of the organization? Is the mentor respected in his or her field? Can the mentor teach and motivate me? Do our communication styles match? The right mentor can foster self-confidence and instill important professional values. When choosing a mentor, remember to select someone who can be trusted to act as your coach or teacher.

Page 11: *Answer*—A response to a staff nurse who delegated to an unlicensed assistive personnel (UAP) an assigned task for which the UAP is not prepared and is beyond the scope of practice would require that the nurse leader speak directly to the staff nurse in private. The nurse leader should be prepared to offer guidance or direction in what the leader witnessed the UAP doing. The nurse leader must be sure to explain what was done and why it is beyond the UAP's scope of practice. It is vital that the communication between the nurse leader and the staff nurse is clear and direct. Timely follow-up must be done promptly to ensure future execution of delegated activities and orders follow the scope of technical knowledge of the UAP. Finally, the nurse leader should strive to maintain a positive working relationship with the staff nurse.

Page 12: *Answer*—Empowering new nurse leaders with the self-confidence they need to be leaders is critical to future leadership. The knowledge and skills needed to enhance self-confidence and ability to lead include being able to recognize and feel personal strength and using power to keep clients safe as well as to transform work environments. Empowered nurses have freedom and autonomy to practice professional nursing through collaboration, connectedness, and sharing information and power openly and freely. They encourage the development of community over individualism and equitable partnerships with other healthcare providers. Nurse leaders who empower frontline nurses to be engaged in decisions that affect their work life and client care provide for ways for nursing to have a clear and profound voice in clinical practice.

Page 12: *Answer*—Hospitals must continue to reduce tragic errors and prevent near misses by describing the result of successful and unsuccessful healthcare encounters in specific and measurable ways, describing client's behavior and reactions to interventions and treatments, using standard data systems or tools for quality and performance measures and formulating ethical and legal standards of practice. In this case, the hospital leadership needs to explore the process of blood transfusion from the time of initial type and cross match through blood administration, with a focus on ensuring that the right type of blood is administered to the right client. It also means actively involving all affected departments in the process of investigation and also in a problem-solving process to identify and revise policies and problematic systems.

Page 15: *Answer*—Important measures used to manage violent behaviors in the workplace include ensuring there are adequate resources dedicated to support nursing staff in the acquisition of new knowledge and skills to maintain clinical competence. Nurses must be involved in identifying staffing levels and methods to improve safety, such as providing (in this case) additional support staff to assist in meeting patient requests.

Chapter 2

Page 27: *Answer*—Three important terms that best describe leadership potential and leadership style include passionately leading and influencing others to perform to the best of their ability toward goal achievement, compassionately advocating and changing the behavior of another, and building consensus around the vision of getting others to want to do what one deems valuable for client care and safety.

Page 28: *Answer*—An effective follower understands and uses a follower style that supports the goals and objectives of the leader. This involves knowing and deciding how to achieve the organization's vision from the perspective of the leader. It also means that the leader assists the follower's efforts to realize the vision by providing coaching, feedback, and role modeling; recognizing and rewarding success; and learning not to blame others when things go wrong.

Page 30: *Answer*—The nurse leader must ensure that staff understand that patients come first. However, the nurse leader can ask the staff their preference for meal time and breaks. This response demonstrates to the staff that patient needs are the priority but staff needs are not ignored.

Page 33: *Answer*—The difference between the terms leadership and management is leadership is the ability to influence others toward goal achievement. The leader creates a vision and supports the abilities of others to get the job done. These abilities include a combination of courage, decisiveness, assertiveness, and innovation. Leaders involve followers in the decision-making process. Leaders have the total organization as a focus with the knowledge to consider a broad range of consequences of any decisions they make.

Managers accomplish the goal through others by using the management process: planning, directing, controlling and the problem-solving process to accomplish goals. Managers will use human, financial, and information resources to implement the organization's goals.

Page 38: *Answer*—The nurse leader may understand similarities between the management process and the problem-solving process as both starting with the ability to identify a problem through data collection. Then, once the nurse leader has the data collected, the next step includes determining possible solutions to the problem and determining consequences of each possible solution. Both the management process and the problem-solving process use implementation and evaluation to determine the effectiveness of the results.

Chapter 3

Page 51: *Answer*—Personal morality includes one's personal values and applies only to situations involving the self. Professional values and ethics are universal and represent a standard of conduct that is upheld by all professionals during client interventions and situations.

Page 53: *Answer*—Principles of healthcare ethics are defined as autonomy through maintaining independence and self-direction, beneficence by doing or promoting good, and non-maleficence, by avoiding harm to a client. Justice relates to the principle of fairness, meaning that nurses treat all clients equally and fairly. Ethical rules that guide healthcare decision making include veracity, fidelity, privacy, and confidentiality.

Page 55: *Answer*—An ethical dilemma results when there are conflicting choices to be made and it is difficult to determine which is best because either one will not solve all of the problems. The first step is to begin by identifying the feelings of all those involved in the situation. Next, describe the known facts. Identify the alternative choices. Focus on outcomes that provide for consistency in the goals for the client. Seek to clarify who is accountable for each aspect of the client's care plan. Ensure that the plan is carried out and verify that all those involved in the plan have completed their responsibilities. If the ethical dilemma cannot be resolved, it can always be referred to the organization's ethics committee for recommendations and resolution.

Page 57: *Answer*—Nurse leaders must be familiar with the Code of Ethics for Nurses because it provides a decision-making framework for solving ethical problems and offers ways to resolve them. Additionally, the nurse leader can role model ethical principles and ensure that frontline staff adhere to ethical conduct in the practice setting as well as create an ethically principled environment that seeks to uphold the standards of conduct set by the code.

Chapter 4

Page 70: *Answer*—The best way nurses can reduce potential liability and protect their license is to know the scope of nursing practice contained in their state nurse practice act. This includes the definition of the practice of nursing, requirements for licensure (initial and renewal), actions or conditions that can result in the loss or limitations of a license, actions that the nurse can take independently, and actions that require a physician's order before completion. In the U.S., most nurse practice acts are similar in content and hold professional nurses legally responsible for licensure requirements and regulations of practice as defined by the home state in which they practice.

Page 74: *Answer*—First, explore the client's concerns and explain the benefits of the infusion to prevent dehydration. If the client continues to refuse, document your teaching and the client's comments in the medical record. Notify the nursing supervisor and the surgeon, and document these communications as well. Complete an incident report as required by agency policy. Finally, realize that your obligations are to the client at this time and you must follow her wishes if she refuses medical treatment. As the nurse responsible for this client, you must be aware that by hanging the next infusion without consent you may face allegations of assault and battery or violation of the client's bill of rights.

Page 76: *Answer*—You must promptly report this incident. This is a deviation from the routine operation within a healthcare organization. Verbal abuse to clients is a violation of their right to safety. You must be familiar with the policy and procedure for reporting, investigating, and taking corrective action when incidents occur. This is a serious incident and must be reported immediately. Your supervisor should be contacted by telephone and informed about the incident, and a written report must be completed within 24 hours.

Page 78: *Answer*—Nurses may be called upon as expert witnesses in a client case from within their own hospital. Therefore, it requires that as employees of the hospital, nurses should be aware of their rights and obligations in regards to legal action before giving a deposition and/or testimony. First and foremost, the nurse should be sure to carry their own individual malpractice insurance. The hospital is not responsible for malpractice for individual staff members but may cover an employee as a part of an organizational policy. The nurse should confer with the hospital attorney and become familiar with and comply with any policies related to this type of activity.

Chapter 5

Page 91: *Answer*—The essential skills required by the nurse leader in order to effectively delegate include knowing that delegation transfers to a competent individual the authority to perform a selected nursing task in a selected situation. Because the nurse leader is usually unable to perform all assigned activities, he or she must delegate some of these to unlicensed assistive personnel. Therefore, the nurse leader must ensure that the task being delegated is within the delegate's scope of practice and that the person has the competency to perform the task. It is very important that during the delegation process, the nurse leader gives clear, concise, correct and complete directions for the delegated task and provides appropriate feedback.

Page 93: *Answer*—Standards of care are expected at all levels of performance; they act as guidelines in providing nursing care and are useful in malpractice situations and in cases where a nurse's license is at stake because of failure to perform within the standard of care. The nurse leader needs to document the reason when nursing staff deviate from the standard of practice because a breach of standards of care or performing tasks outside their scope of practice may lead to nursing personnel being found negligent.

Page 96: *Answer*—The nurse leader is accountable for the care given to clients even if that care has been delegated to a staff nurse or unlicensed assistive personnel (UAP) because the nurse leader is legally liable for their actions and is answerable for the overall nursing care for designated clients. This means the nurse leader makes sure that team members understand their jobs, accept their responsibility, and commit to deliver the desired results. Liability is the responsibility for one's own actions and those that the nurse leader supervises

during the delegation process. The nurse leader is responsible for knowing all tasks that are within the scope of practice within the state's nurse practice act, the scope of practice of the assigned nursing staff members, and the competency of the nursing staff assigned to the task.

Page 97: *Answer*—Continuity of nursing care is an essential component of the delegation process because not all relevant information about a client is included in the medical record. Some information may be outdated or incorrect; other information is intentionally omitted or was never recorded. The nurse and/or UAPs may have an ongoing relationship with a client and may be able to recognize significant changes or client reports, in part because of having a referent period (the client has his or her own control).

Page 99: *Answer*—When a client is fully dependent, the nurse is accountable for the overall management of nursing care. The responsibility for client care has been transferred to licensed professional nurses within a healthcare system. Clients may or may not be competent or capable of participating in self-care. When assistive personnel are used, they are authorized to perform care through the delegation process.

Chapter 6

Page 116: *Answer*—The DMAIC methodology includes the following: define (project, goals, and customers/clients both internally and externally), measure (processes to determine performance), analyze (determine root cause(s) of defect), improve (eliminate defect), and control (future process and performance). Using the DMAIC methodology, your answer should define the problem, list measures to increase performance, analyze the causes, think of solutions to improve the problem, and recommend ways to evaluate improved processes and performance in the future. Think about whom you could share these recommendations with.

Page 117: *Answer*—Your answer should include the following elements. Teamwork supports and sustains unit-based quality improvement processes by promoting open communication between nurses and other health professionals, encouraging nurses to act as a team, and ensuring other health professionals are included in unit-based quality improvement activities.

Page 119: *Answer*—Apply the Plan-Do-Study-Act (PDSA) cycle assist in data collection process of quality improvement by asking two key questions: What is the change the nurse leader is trying to accomplish? How will this change be assessed to determine if an improvement occurred? Then determine how best to decrease the delay for surgical beds by using tools for data collection (such as data sheets and check sheets) and data analysis (such as bar and pie charts and the Pareto diagrams).

Page 124: *Answer*—Your answer should include a description of your own witnessed error. The error is reported to the nursing supervisor and the Risk Management Department on an incident form or as a report. Incident forms are not kept with the client record but rather filed separately. To avoid a recurrence of this error, the nurse leader can do a root-cause analysis. This is a retrospective review of the error to identify the sequence leading to the error and the root causes. A root-cause analysis can lead to specific risk-reduction strategies. In some circumstances, the risk-reduction plan is reported to JCAHO.

Chapter 7

Page 136: *Answer*—A nurse leader can go about building a high performance team by setting the stage and expectations for team building, including:

- Providing a clear mission statement that has firm direction and motivates the team toward high performance.
- Creating identifiable goals.
- Mastering the fundamentals—clear roles, competency in skills, constant training, and development of standards of performance.
- Developing clear lines of communication.
- Fostering trust and intimacy.
- Paying attention to team building effectiveness and continuous improvement.
- Promoting mutual support and balance of task and social responsibility.
- Selecting team members for skill and for skill potential.
- Creating a vision and keeping the team on track towards implementing and achieving the visions.
- Finding solutions and creating results.

Page 140: *Answer*—For collaboration to be truly effective, the following essential factors must be present: communication, competence, accountability, trust, administrative support, and equity. Additionally, for collaboration to occur there must be an openness and trust among interested parties. There must be an emphasis on reward for quality work, not simply for quantity and speed of task accomplishment. The organization has the responsibility to ensure resources are sufficiently available to support collaborative activities so that positive attributes of professional interaction can emerge.

Page 143: *Answer*—When you encounter a team member, another health professional, or a client whose nonverbal behavior fails to match his or her verbal messages, translate your message into verbal or nonverbal symbols that will communicate the intended meaning to the receiver. Decide the appropriate degree of intensity of the message. Know that words mean different things to different people. Encode in the simplest terms; if terms are complex, the message should be expressed in several ways or broken down into simple bits (sound bites). Ensure the language used reflects the values, culture, and personality of the receiver.

Page 149: *Answer*—The conflict process involves antecedent conditions (incompatible goals, structural conflicts, competition for resources, values and beliefs, perceived or felt conflict, overt or manifest behavior; outcomes suppression or

resolution, and resolution aftermath). Effective tools for managing conflict include:

- Knowing how to manage conflict among team members.
- Recognizing generational perceptions and how they impact group dynamics.
- Understanding when to use disciplinary action.
- Helping team members to resolve conflict when it occurs.
- Knowing what conflict strategy to select for the situation.

Page 150: *Answer*—Negotiation is a key response in which both parties are willing to give and take on the issues. The nurse leader can use any of the following strategies to successfully negotiate conflict: clarify the common purpose, keep the discussion relevant, get agreement on terminology, avoid abstract principals, use facts, look for potential tradeoffs, use active listening, avoid debating tactics, use persuasion, and look for solutions that satisfy real interests.

Chapter 8

Page 161: *Answer*—Answers to the first question will vary. The common competencies needed by all RNs include managing the nursing process, fulfilling daily job performance, maintaining safety, attending continuing education programs, adhering to policies and procedures, creating a workflow environment free of incidents, errors, and accidents, and being honest, trustworthy, and professional.

Page 163: *Answer*—All nurses are client advocates regardless of their title or position. Nurses are expected to act as client advocates in providing information that is useful to clients and supports their care decisions. Advocacy promotes and protects clients' human and legal rights, ensures clients' needs are addressed and fulfilled, protects and prevents clients from injury, and educates clients and families about the healthcare delivery system.

Page 164: *Answer*—The reason why performance appraisal is considered an important process in guiding and directing nursing staff in their professional development and performance is because it assists staff to improve performance, maintains high standards of care, provides a safe and supportive work environment, and attains work satisfaction for self and others.

Page 168: *Answer*—The nurse leader can help nursing staff to improve their performance over time through day-to-day coaching. Here, the nurse leader states targeted performance in behavioral terms, ties an identified problem to consequences, avoids jumping to conclusions, asks the employee for his or her suggestions and discusses how to solve the problem.

Page 169: *Answer*—Nurse leaders can solve the issue of absenteeism on the nursing unit by increasing the desire and motivation to attend work. The nurse leader can ensure the job itself remains interesting, challenging, and fulfilling by asking the staff about their personal and professional goals and desires. Additionally, the nurse leader can endorse organizational policies and procedures to reward those who come to work. The nursing staff must be educated and informed about "what does it mean to be absent?" They must understand how their job expectations and job responsibilities can be matched, thus encouraging and promoting enhanced advancement opportunities.

Chapter 9

Page 184: *Answer*—Nurse leaders are responsible for fiscal/financial planning. This includes knowing how to balance revenues and expenses during a projected period of time for all human and fiscal responsibilities. By using various types of budgets, the nurse leader can formulate a fiscal plan to allocate fiscal resources. The budget process requires the nurse leader to be responsible for developing and monitoring the budget.

Three phases to the budget process:

1. Planning: gather information based on organizational or unit goals and objectives; set priorities; perform an environmental assessment; identify financial objectives
2. Development: collect and analyze data from previous budgets; allocate dollar amounts based on organizational/unit priorities; approve operational and capital budgets
3. Implementation: analyze variances and adjust for changes through the fiscal year; negotiate and revise budget as needed; allocate unit/departmental and cash budgets; evaluate; obtain performance reports and analyze efficiency

Page 190: *Answer*—Nurse leaders design and determine appropriate skill mix on their assigned units by knowing the type of staff that is required to provide the care (RN, LPN, and UAPs); identifying the type of care that is required and who is qualified to provide that care; assessing the staff competency to fulfill the care needs of clients, adhering to the nurse practice act and other state regulations when making staffing decisions; and distributing staff according to when staff is needed for peak hour care: days vs. evenings, weekends and holidays.

Page 192: *Answer*—Nurse leaders can familiarize themselves with learning how to staff and schedule nursing personnel on their units by understanding client need through a client classification system used by the health organization, using staffing patterns adjusted for client acuity and providing staff when needed. To properly plan for the staffing and schedule needs of the unit, the nurse leader must understand the level of experience and capability of staff, including those different degrees of knowledge, experience, and critical thinking skills that are required to care for different clients. Additionally, the nurse leader may decide to use a variety of scheduling methods, including centralized scheduling, decentralized scheduling, and self-scheduling.

Page 193: *Answer*—The nurse leader's role and responsibilities in nursing informatics includes knowing how to integrate nursing science, computer science, and information science to manage and communicate data, information, and knowledge in nursing practice. The key for the nurse leader is to use nursing informatics to improve the health of populations, communities, families, and individuals by optimizing information management and communication through an electronic medical record (computer-based client record) that features electronic data processes.

Page 194: *Answer*—If client information is inappropriately disclosed without the client's consent, HIPAA law requires that the healthcare organization record the violation or complaint and take actions necessary to address the violation. You would need to report this to a nursing supervisor for further action.

Chapter 10

Page 205: *Answer*—The nurse leader's role in implementing change revolves around the ability to move an idea to action or gather the necessary resources to change the behaviors of others to adapt the change. This implementation requires a high level of energy of the nurse leader, who must believe passionately in the change to raise the level of enthusiasm, energy, and commitment in others. The nurse leader must also demonstrate astute interpersonal skills to effectively communicate the change, manage the change, and respond quickly to problems or concerns as they develop during the implementation process. Because no change is ever implemented seamlessly from beginning to end, the nurse leader must be ready to adjust or be flexible in the change design. The change may not unfold as planned and also may experience complications. If the nurse leader remains open and flexible during implementation, the change will occur but maybe not as intended. This requires that the nurse leader be confident when challenged, knowledgeable about the structure and format of the change in order to re-design if necessary, be able to respond to all levels and kinds of resistance, and be realistic about the implementation timeframe. To demonstrate sound and effective skills in implementing change the nurse leader must remain confident and positive throughout the process.

Page 211: *Answer*—The nurse leader must allow staff to have an opportunity to express their feelings and emotions to the change. The nurse leader should give as much information as needed about the change and provide staff with ample opportunity within limits of the situation to have input into the change process. The nurse leader needs to be aware that the consequences of change will impact self as well as staff, and actively communicate information about the change, offer ways to participate in the change, and support staff as they move through the change process.

Page 214: *Answer*—Your answer should be similar to the following: Critical thinking involves the intellectually disciplined process of actively and skillfully conceptualizing, applying, analyzing, synthesizing, or evaluating information gathered from, or generated by observation, experience, reflection, reasoning, or communication toward a belief and action. It requires clinical judgment consisting of both informed opinions and decisions based on empirical knowledge and experience.

Clinical judgment develops gradually as nurse leaders gain a broader knowledge base and clinical experience. Extensive direct client contact is the best means of developing clinical judgment.

Page 215: *Answer*—Nurse leaders can facilitate and promote best practices in nursing care by using evidence-based nursing practice that integrates the best of research evidence with clinical expertise and client values. This includes nursing research that links theory, education, and practice; research studies emphasizing clinical issues, problems, and outcomes; and research utilization transferring research findings to nursing practice.

Page 219: *Answer*—The nurse leader can build a culturally diverse and competent workforce by accepting and respecting differences throughout the organization; performing an organizational cultural assessment; acknowledging the dynamics of cross-cultural interactions such as differences in religious beliefs, values, and cultural experiences and allow for flexibility within organizational activities to fit cultural norms of staff and clients.

Page 222: *Answer*—Factors that influence an individual's grieving might include the meaning of the loss and the circumstances of the loss. Often, a person's religious beliefs and cultural practices, as well as his or her own personal resources and stressors, will impact the loss. The meaning of loss might include the personal importance of the loss to the individual as well as the object and the age at which this loss occurs. The circumstances of the loss may differ depending on whether the loss is unexpected and violent or expected and natural. The way an individual responds to the circumstance of loss may vary from severe to matter of fact.

➤ *Case Study Suggested Answers*

Chapter 1

1. As the costs of medical care have increased and as medical technology has advanced, society has been forced to confront how to allocate limited healthcare resources responsibly. Managed care has highlighted cost efficacy in decision making about coverage and benefits. It has forced health plans and purchasers not to underwrite approaches to care that are individually desired but not justifiable on the basis of clinical or theoretical scientific grounds. Managed care seeks to cover treatments that are relatively cost-effective compared with other therapies for the same condition or other therapies. Health plans must explain to purchasers and clients the reasoning behind coverage, exclusion, and cost determinations, both for individuals and for general policy decisions. Managed care has attempted to control health care cost by sharing information with purchasers and the public so they can understand the advantages and disadvantages

when contracting for particular benefits at reasonable premiums.

2. Managed care has health promotion as a primary goal by providing an entry point, delivering core medical and preventive care, and helping clients coordinate and integrate care. If manage care works well, each of these dimensions can be instrumental in improving health outcomes and cost performance. Managed care has called for design of a care system that includes an emphasis on promoting health and engaging consumers in their own care. Access to effective primary care through a managed care system offers health consumers opportunities to live healthy, productive lives.

3. a. Health Maintenance Organization (HMO) is a prepayment system established through federal legislation to reorganize healthcare services to reduce the rate of healthcare cost increases and control utilization of services.

   b. Preferred Provider Organization (PPO) contracts with established medical care providers referred to as preferred providers and provides incentives to participants for selecting preferred providers. Participants gain greater flexibility in provider and hospital selection.

   c. Point-of-Service Organization (POS) combines the selection choice of PPO with the lower cost of an HMO and requires participants to choose a primary care provider from within a healthcare network.

   d. Physician Hospital Organization (PHO) is a separate legal entity formed by one or more physicians and one or more hospitals whose objective is to negotiate contracts with payer organizations. The PHO provides financial, marketing, and administrative services to its members.

4. The impact of managed care on cost containment and healthcare consumers centers around restructuring healthcare services to enhance cost containment, maintain quality, and facilitate management of care needs of the health consumer. Managed care has required healthcare providers to submit written justification and seek prior approval for diagnostic tests and interventions or to extend client's length of stay (LOS).

5. Case managers by definition have various roles and responsibilities. They provide a type of care to clients that utilizes specific tools to coordinate case management services, as well as a mechanism to monitor the quality and cost of services at both the individual and client population level. The nurse case manager serves as a client advocate and liaison between the client and all providers of the client's health care services. The nurse case manager bridges that gap to assure that the client has all the information needed to make well-informed health care decisions. Additionally, the nurse case manager provides linkages to other resources and services to assure the client has all their needs cared for. Additionally, the nurse case manager helps the client understand and cope with the medical, insurance, and emotional issues confronting them.

Chapter 2

1. The most appropriate leadership style to manage this crisis is autocratic leadership. This style is authoritarian and directive in nature and is what is needed to manage a crisis situation, when rapid decision-making is required and the goals are clear.
2. Leadership development is important for nurses even if they are not in a formal management position because all nurses must possess the necessary knowledge, skills, and attitudes to work with others in all types of situations, especially emergency situations. This includes having thoughtful and convincing ideas, expert knowledge, and strong interpersonal skills.
3. The core elements of the management process that would be used today by the nurses or nurse managers include the functions planning, organizing, leading, and controlling. Functions known as the management process include:
   1. Planning and setting direction: setting goals and deciding a course of action through an inductive process; gathering data and looking for patterns; building relationships and linkages to help explain things; and creating visions and strategies for what the organization will look like in the future.
   2. Organizing and aligning people: identifying work to be accomplished and goals to be achieved; hiring the right person for the right work; creating interdependence by getting people to move in the same direction; delegating authority by talking to anyone who can help implement the vision and strategies; and coordinating the work of others.
   3. Leading and getting others to believe in the organization's mission and vision: influencing others to accomplish workload responsibilities; keeping the message clear; communicating with integrity and trustworthiness; molding culture and maintaining morale; and insisting on consistency between words and deeds.
   4. Controlling: setting standards for accomplishing the organization's goals and activities; determining the means to measure performance and making sure that quality lapses are spotted immediately; evaluating performance; and providing feedback.
4. The essential leadership characteristics that would be critical for this nurse leader to demonstrate during this emergency include critical thinking; the composite of knowledge, attitudes, and skills; ability to assess the situation by asking open-ended questions about facts and assumptions that underlie it and using personal judgment and problem-solving ability in deciding how to deal with it; using a systematic process to solve a problem; purposeful and goal-directed decision making using a systematic process to choose among options; team building by supporting efforts and work of a number of people associated together by specific tasks or activities and delegation; achieving performance of care outcomes for which an individual is accountable and responsible by

sharing activities with others who have appropriate authority to accomplish work.
5. The nurse leader would use legitimate power, which is granted to an individual who occupies a specific position within the organization. The leader would also use expert power, which involves recognition of the leader's knowledge, experience, and expertise; and charismatic power (the ability to inspire and attract others) in this emergency situation.

Chapter 3

1. The values that influence your decision about the appropriate action to take include nonmaleficence: obligation to do no harm. In this situation, the client was given an accidental medication overdose, and the client was unintentionally harmed during this course of healthcare treatment. The second value is veracity: truthfulness or power of perceiving and conveying truth. Nurses must tell the truth and must not intentionally deceive or mislead. The client's parents have a right to full and accurate information about the health status and treatment of their child and, therefore, must be informed about what occurred.
2. The ethical dilemma that occurred in this situation was one that involved an incompetent nursing action compounded by the unethical behavior of the staff nurse.
3. The problem in this situation involved the safety, dignity, and treatment of a client. The staff nurse did not maintain professional competency by administrating the wrong dose, did not take responsibility for own actions, and was not accountable to the parents for these actions by being untruthful. According to the ANA Code of Ethics for Nurses, clients, families, groups, and/or communities are their first obligation. The nurse leader must seek to ensure that provisions of code are integrated into nursing care.
4. The ethical decision-making a process to use in resolving this issue would include:
   1. Clarifying the ethical dilemma/identifying the problem and investigating why the staff nurse lied to the client's parent about the child's condition.
   2. Gathering additional data: assessing the client's wellbeing and asking the staff nurse to explain the steps in medication preparation and administration to the client.
   3. Identifying potential options and ethical principles; reviewing the values of nonmaleficence and veracity with the staff nurse.
   4. Assisting others in decision making: assisting the staff nurse to understand the ethical decision making process to enhance own personal morality and organizational commitment; affirm the ability to contribute to quality client care outcomes and improve overall organizational success.
   5. Selecting the appropriate course of action to address the ethical dilemma: ensure the staff nurse fully understands how to use a decision-making framework for

solving ethical problems. This will enhance the staff nurse's ability to adhere to ethical conduct in the practice settings as well as uphold the standards of conduct set by the ANA code of ethics.

6. Evaluating results or choice of action. The nurse leader has responsibility to create an ethical climate in the workplace that allows staff nurse to experience congruence between caring for clients, fulfilling organizational mission, and having a supportive work environment. Therefore, the staff nurse would be counseled by the nurse leader and an incident report would be completed.

5. Remind the staff to follow organizational policy for medication administration, encourage staff to seek assistance from another peer if a dosage question emerges, and remind assigned staff they have an obligation to uphold the standards of conduct set by the ANA code of ethics.

Chapter 4

1. The law that the staff nurse's behavior violated is a criminal law. This law consists of conduct considered offensive to the public or society as whole. The nurse committed a crime known as a felony (a major offense) by the diversion of narcotics to self rather than to the client.

2. The nurse manager of this 22-bed surgical unit has an obligation to immediately report this incident to the manager's supervisor. The staff nurse must be spoken to and asked to explain the behavior of signing out narcotics ordered for assigned clients and keeping the narcotics for personal use. The staff nurse's explanation must be documented in a confidential report. The report will include the date(s), time, witnesses, *observed* behavior and action, and adverse consequences to client or staff. The nurse manager may be required to report the incident to the state board of nursing if the nurse practice act calls for such incidents to be reported.

3. The purpose of nursing licensure is for each state to license professionals and institutions under its constitutional power to protect the health and welfare of its citizens. The type of credential provided by state statutes authorizes qualified individuals to perform designated skills and services. Violation of law, such as in the case of this felony, could result in prosecution unless state statute allows for the Board of Nursing to intervene, such as with an impaired nurse program.

Chapter 5

1. The steps in the delegation process include the following:
   - Determine and identify the task and level of responsibility of each task.
   - Evaluate delegate's fit with the assigned task.
   - Decide what level of supervision is needed and describe expectations.
   - Reach agreement on performance and outcome.
   - Provide continuous feedback, monitor performance, and adjust accordingly.

2. Responsibility requires an individual to perform the activity at an acceptable level and to be both reliable and dependable in accomplishing the assigned task or activity. Accountability occurs when a professional nurse leader becomes legally liable for the actions of others and is answerable for overall nursing care for designated clients. Authority is the right to instruct others to carry out orders and to use power to expect compliance. It is derived from the person's rank or position within organization.

3. The nurse manager used overdelegation in this situation. This occurred because the nurse manager became overwhelmed by the situation and lost control by delegating too much authority and responsibility to the unit clerk.

4. The supervision was not appropriate given the assigned task by the nurse manager. It is not within the scope of the unit clerk's responsibility to cover and perform the staffing requirements of the unit, including finding replacements for sick calls because of a sudden influx of clients in active labor.

5. The nurse manager did not delegate appropriately to the unit clerk's abilities. It was inappropriate for the nurse manager to ask the unit clerk to assume the assignment of staffing for the unit based on the unit census and level of client acuity. This is the responsibility of the nurse manager. Each nurse manager must determine the ability of staff to take on the assigned request, and balance requests after prioritizing needs of unit staff and clients.

Chapter 6

1. The first action would be to assess the client status and reaction to IV Demerol, notify the client and physician and then assess and determine why the medication error occurred with the assigned day nurse.

2. A reportable incident is an unusual event, such as injury to a client. A report is completed to document the exact details of the occurrence while they are fresh in the minds of those who witnessed the event. A medical-legal incident is an adverse event in which an injury is caused by medical management. This medical mismanagement may represent a form of negligence or malpractice. The result is a violation of a professional standard of care in which a client is injured. A medication error is any preventable event that may cause or lead to inappropriate medication use or client harm while the medication is in the control of the healthcare professional, client, or consumer.

3. The client's chart should reflect the actual care provided to the client. This includes following the nursing process as it relates to the medication error and the actions taken to report the incident to the client's physician. Nursing documentation clearly describes an assessment of the client's health status, nursing interventions carried out, and the impact of these interventions on client outcomes.

No mention should be made in the client's chart that an incident report was completed since incident reports are administrative risk management tools. Incident reports are used for quality management not punitive purposes. Incident reports completed in hospitals are protected from disclosure in legal proceedings. Therefore, they are retained separately from the client record and no reference to an incident report is made in the client record to protect the incident report from subpoena.

4. The nurse manager's role in risk management includes the following:
   - Identify and report unusual occurrences
   - Identify all potential risks
   - Reduce fear of punishment for acknowledging, reporting, or discussing error
   - Monitor threats to client safety on ongoing basis
   - Recognize staff efforts provider error reflects organizational or system failure
5. An incident report is required for this incident because the client received twice the dose of the ordered medication, and it was given by the wrong (and most dangerous) route. The documentation of a deviation from the routine procedure—in this case, a medication error for wrong dose and wrong route—requires the completion and documentation of an incident report.

Chapter 7

1. The responses that would best indicate the staff nurse is a holistic communicator might include:

   "The night staff informed me that you might not have had sufficient sleep last night. It appears that you are upset about undergoing an additional surgery. Would you like to discuss your frustrations and concerns with me?"

   "Tell me how much you understand about why you need additional surgery."

2. The communication facilitators that would be useful for the nurse to use when communicating with this client include attending to active listening, responding with verbal and nonverbal acknowledgment of the client's messages, and clarifying issues and concerns the client may have to help the messages become clearer or help the client to confront her concerns with additional surgery by working jointly to resolve the problem or conflict.
3. The communication barriers that may be present when the nurse is communicating with this client include social and psychological barriers. The nurse should avoid judgments, emotions, and social values that the client may have regarding her need for additional surgery. This includes knowing that communication cannot be separated from personality and social implications because whatever emotions this client has at this time affects the communication process. Additionally, the nurse will have to realize that there may

be semantic barriers (interpretation of meanings) present as well. This means that the nurse must remember to encode and decode accurately, remembering that difficulties may arise in the verbal and listening processes.
4. The client might already be experiencing an alteration in her body image. Undergoing an additional surgery may be cause for undue anxiety, frustration, and anger for her. The client may believe that her physician may not have performed the surgery correctly the first time.
5. "I have some time right now if you would like to discuss with me your frustrations and concerns about having this abdominal surgical procedure to remove this infected tissue."

Chapter 8

1. The first step that you should take in confronting the staff nurse about a policy violation is to determine whether the staff member is aware of current policy/procedure on hand hygiene between clients. Then inform the staff member by describing that his or her action/behavior has violated the policy. The nurse leader should solicit the staff member's reason for the action/behavior. Then provide appropriate progressive discipline. This action should allow for consistent and ongoing evaluation of the staff member's performance on hand hygiene.
2. Explain that if the procedure for hand hygiene is not followed, the client is at risk for hospital-acquired infection. Restate the policy and ensure the staff member knows proper procedure. It may help to share with the staff member current quality improvement data related to infection rates on the unit over time.
3. The most important guideline in disciplining this employee is for the nurse leader to investigate the incident carefully prior to any disciplinary action. The purpose of discipline is to teach or reinforce skills (hand hygiene in this case) and encourage the staff member to improve performance or behave appropriately in the future.
4. The reason for encouraging the correct behavior is to ensure that staff members carry out their delegated duties and assignments competently. By outlining correct behavior, the nurse manager deals with the performance issue immediately rather than waiting for infection rates to rise. By stating targeted performance in behavioral terms, the nurse manager is able to connect this problem to consequences, ask the staff member for his or her suggestions, and discuss how to solve the problem.
5. The nurse leader must provide appropriate and immediate feedback to the nurse who is noncompliant with the hand hygiene policy. This feedback can consist of the day-to-day coaching approach, which includes:
   - Stating targeted performance in behavioral terms
   - Connecting the problem to consequences
   - Avoiding jumping to conclusions
   - Asking the staff member for his or her suggestions and discussing how to solve the problem

- Documenting required behavioral steps as indicated
- Arranging for a follow-up meeting to evaluate performance and progress towards the agreed-upon target

Should the staff member fail to meet the job expectations, the nurse leader is obligated to discipline the staff member. The steps in progressive discipline include:

- Counseling
- A reprimand, either verbally or in writing
- Suspension
- Agreed-upon terms to return to work
- Termination if necessary

Chapter 9

1. The staffing process would be used to determine the appropriate number and type of healthcare personnel needed to care for clients on this unit by using the personnel budget allocations for the unit schedule. This includes knowing about the internal and external factors affecting need. Internal factors include volume of services required, complexity and intensity of care, availability of staff, and skill level and credentials/qualifications of nursing personnel. External factors include state licensing standards, staff mix, acuity of clients, census, and census in relation to severity of client illness.

2. The patient classification system can be used to determine the number, acuity, and type of clients that would be admitted to this unit. A patient classification system groups clients according to the amount and complexity of nursing care requirements. These classifications systems allow for determining nursing care hours, FTEs, staff mix, and distribution of staff.

3. The regulatory requirement of JCAHO and other regulatory agency standards such as the American Nurses Association (ANA) Principles for Safe Staffing provide guidance and support when staffing the unit. Studies show correlation between RN staffing levels and quality client care outcomes, including length of stay, postoperative infections, and hospital-acquired complications and recommend that organizations provide adequate number and mix of staff consistent to their staffing plan.

4. As a newly appointed nurse manager concerned about appropriate staffing levels on the unit, a staffing plan can be used to justify the level of care needed to ensure safe environment required for 24 hours/7 days week coverage. The staffing level would require determining the number of persons in each job classification on duty per shift per day, calculating staffing pattern on the following three components: client care requirements and staffing hours/client day, number of beds, average daily census, occupancy rate and type, and client classification of the unit. By using a staffing level plan, a determination can then be made if the appropriate level of staffing is available on the unit.

5. JCAHO addresses the issue of staffing in an organization by using Standard HR.1.30: Introduction to Staffing Effectiveness to define the number, competency, and skill mix of staff in relation to the provision of needed care and treatment. Effective staffing has been linked to positive [client] outcomes and improved quality and safety of care. This standard is designed to help healthcare organizations determine and continuously improve the effectiveness of nurse staffing (including registered nurses, licensed practical nurses, and nursing assistants or aides) through an objective, evidence-based approach.

Chapter 10

1. The type of information that the staff needs to be able to deliver care effectively to these clients is understanding that diversity includes consideration of socioeconomic class, gender, age, religious belief, sexual preference, and physical disabilities, as well as race and ethnicity. The staff needs to understand how cultural groups understand life processes, including how culture defines health and illness, what cultural groups do to maintain wellness, what cultural groups believe to be the causes of illness, and how healers cure and care for members of cultural groups.

2. One challenge inherent in delivering care to this client population is learning how best to integrate culturally competent care that is sensitive to issues related to culture, race, gender, and sexual preference while being sensitive to such issues as drug abuse, nutritional tolerance, and body odor.

3. One potential barrier to caring for these clients by healthcare workers is fear of contracting (AIDS) from the clients' body fluids or a contaminated needle.

4. The importance of valuing cultural and ethnic differences and need for sensitive awareness of others is reflected in providing nursing care that is culturally competent and focused on being supportive toward the anticipated needs for the clients' health or well-being and assisting clients in facing their disabilities, death, or other human conditions.

5. One potential positive outcome for caring for a variety of clients from diverse cultures and ethnicities is learning how cultural and ethnic diversity enables nurses to be more effective in initiating nursing assessments and serving as client advocates. Using cultural nursing theory, models, and research principles, nurses demonstrate competency in identifying healthcare needs of their clients. Additionally, nurses begin to recognize how their personal cultural heritage as well as their cultural and philosophical views are integrated in caring for others from diverse cultures and ethnicities.

Index

Page numbers followed by b indicate box; those followed by f indicate figure; those followed by t indicate table.